Hepatocellular Carcinoma: Moving into the 21st Century

Editor

CATHERINE FRENETTE

CLINICS IN LIVER DISEASE

www.liver.theclinics.com

Consulting Editor
NORMAN GITLIN

November 2020 • Volume 24 • Number 4

ELSEVIER

1600 John F. Kennedy Boulevard ● Suite 1800 ● Philadelphia, Pennsylvania, 19103-2899

http://www.theclinics.com

CLINICS IN LIVER DISEASE Volume 24, Number 4
November 2020 ISSN 1089-3261, ISBN-13: 978-0-323-71140-1

Editor: Kerry Holland
Developmental Editor: Donald Mumford

Clinics in Liver Disease (ISSN 1089-3261) is published quarterly by Elsevier Inc., 360 Park Avenue South, New York, NY 10010-1710. Months of issue are February, May, August, and November. Business and Editorial Offices: 1600 John F. Kennedy Blvd., Ste. 1800, Philadelphia, PA 19103-2899. Customer Service Office: 3251 Riverport Lane, Maryland Heights, MO 63043. Periodicals postage paid at New York, NY and additional mailing offices. Subscription prices are $313.00 per year (U.S. individuals), $100.00 per year (U.S. student/resident), $572.00 per year (U.S. institutions), $409.00 per year (international individuals), $200.00 per year (international student/resident), $709.00 per year (international instituitions), $343.00 per year (Canadian individuals), $100.00 per year (Canadian student/resident), and $709.00 per year (Canadian institutions). Foreign air speed delivery is included in all *Clinics* subscription prices. All prices are subject to change without notice. **POSTMASTER:** Send address changes to *Clinics in Liver Disease*, Elsevier Health Sciences Division, Subscription Customer Service, 3251 Riverport Lane, Maryland Heights, MO 63043. **Customer Service: Telephone: 1-800-654-2452 (U.S. and Canada); 314-447-8871 (outside U.S. and Canada). Fax: 314-447-8029. E-mail: journalscustomer service-usa@elsevier.com (for print support); journalsonlinesupport-usa@elsevier.com (for online support).**

Reprints. For copies of 100 or more of articles in this publication, please contact the Commercial Reprints Department, Elsevier Inc., 360 Park Avenue South, New York, NY 10010-1710. Tel.: 212-633-3874; Fax: 212-633-3820; E-mail: reprints@elsevier.com.

Clinics in Liver Disease is covered in *MEDLINE/PubMed (Index Medicus)*, Science Citation Index Expanded, Journal Citation Reports/Science Edition, and Current Contents/Clinical Medicine.

Contributors

CONSULTING EDITOR

NORMAN GITLIN, MD, FRCP (LONDON), FRCPE (EDINBURGH), FAASLD, FACP, FACG
Head of Hepatology, Southern California Liver Centers, San Clemente, California, USA

EDITOR

CATHERINE FRENETTE, MD, FAST, AGAF, FAASLD
Medical Director of Liver Transplantation, Scripps Center for Organ Transplantation, Director, Liver and Hepatocellular Cancer Program, Scripps MD Anderson Cancer Center, Scripps Green Hospital, La Jolla, California, USA

AUTHORS

FARID ABUSHAMAT, MD
Division of Gastroenterology and Hepatology, University of California, San Diego, San Diego, California, USA

SAMANTHA A. ARMSTRONG, MD
Department of Medicine, Division of Hematology and Oncology, Lombardi Comprehensive Cancer Center, MedStar Georgetown University Hospital, Washington, DC, USA

FATIMA BEDIER, BS
Department of Surgery, University of California, Los Angeles, Pfleger Liver Institute, Los Angeles, California, USA

JORDI BRUIX, MD, PhD
Barcelona Clinic Liver Cancer (BCLC) Group, Liver Unit, Hospital Clinic Barcelona, IDIBAPS, University of Barcelona, Centro de Investigación Biomédica en Red de Enfermedades Hepáticas y Digestivas (CIBERehd), Barcelona, Spain

ALLYCE CAINES, MD
Transplant Hepatologist, Henry Ford Hospital, Detroit, Michigan, USA

ANDREW T. CHAN, MD, MPH
Professor of Medicine, Division of Gastroenterology, Department of Medicine, Harvard Medical School, Clinical and Translational Epidemiology Unit, Massachusetts General Hospital, Channing Division of Network Medicine, Department of Medicine, Brigham and Women's Hospital, Broad Institute, Department of Immunology and Infectious Diseases, Harvard T.H. Chan School of Public Health, Boston, Massachusetts, USA

CHIEN PETER CHEN, MD, PhD
Radiation Oncologist, Department of Radiation Oncology, Scripps Radiation Therapy Center, San Diego, California, USA

VINCENT L. CHEN, MD, MS
Division of Gastroenterology and Hepatology, Department of Internal Medicine, University of Michigan, Ann Arbor, Michigan, USA

GUILHERME MOURA CUNHA, MD
Liver Imaging Group, Department of Radiology, University of California, San Diego, San Diego, California, USA

LEONARDO G. DA FONSECA, MD
Clinical Oncology, Instituto do Cancer do Estado de Sao Paulo, University of São Paulo, São Paulo, São Paulo, Brazil

KATHRYN J. FOWLER, MD
Liver Imaging Group, Department of Radiology, University of California, San Diego, San Diego, California, USA

ELLEN W. GREEN, MD, PhD
Department of Medicine, Resident, Internal Medicine Residency, Oregon Health & Science University, Portland, Oregon, USA

AIWU RUTH HE, MD, PhD
Associate Professor, Department of Medicine, Division of Hematology and Oncology, Lombardi Comprehensive Cancer Center, MedStar Georgetown University Hospital, Washington, DC, USA

JULIE K. HEIMBACH, MD
Professor of Surgery, Mayo Clinic College of Medicine, Rochester, Minnesota, USA

YOSHIKUNI KAWAGUCHI, MD, PhD
Research Fellow, Department of Surgical Oncology, The University of Texas MD Anderson Cancer Center, Houston, Texas, USA; Assistant Professor, Hepato-Biliary-Pancreatic Surgery Division, Department of Surgery, Graduate School of Medicine, The University of Tokyo, Tokyo, Japan

YUKO KONO, MD, PhD
Division of Gastroenterology and Hepatology, University of California, San Diego, San Diego, California, USA

LAURA KULIK, MD
Professor of Medicine, Department of Internal Medicine, Northwestern Memorial Hospital, Chicago, Illinois, USA

DEKEY LHEWA, MD
Assistant Professor, Department of Medicine, Division of Gastroenterology and Hepatology, Oregon Health & Science University, Portland, Oregon, USA

HEATHER A. LILLEMOE, MD
Research Fellow, Department of Surgical Oncology, The University of Texas MD Anderson Cancer Center, Houston, Texas, USA

JORGE A. MARRERO, MD, MS
Professor of Medicine, Medical Director Liver Transplant, UT Southwestern Medical Center, Dallas, Texas, USA

NEIL MEHTA, MD
Associate Professor, Department of Medicine, Division of Gastroenterology and Hepatology, University of California, San Francisco, San Francisco, California, USA

WILLSCOTT E. NAUGLER, MD
Medical Director of Liver Transplantation and Multidisciplinary Liver Tumor Group, Professor, Department of Medicine, Division of Gastroenterology and Hepatology, Oregon Health & Science University, Portland, Oregon, USA

ANJANA A. PILLAI, MD
Associate Professor of Medicine, Department of Internal Medicine, University of Chicago Medicine, Chicago, Illinois, USA

MEERA RAMANATHAN, MD
Assistant Professor of Medicine, Department of Internal Medicine, Northwestern Memorial Hospital, Chicago, Illinois, USA

MARIA REIG, MD, PhD
Barcelona Clinic Liver Cancer (BCLC) Group, Liver Unit, Hospital Clinic Barcelona, IDIBAPS, University of Barcelona, Centro de Investigación Biomédica en Red de Enfermedades Hepáticas y Digestivas (CIBERehd), Barcelona, Spain

SAMMY SAAB, MD MPH, AGAF, FAASLD
Departments of Medicine, Surgery, and Nursing, University of California, Los Angeles, Pfleger Liver Institute, Los Angeles, California, USA

REENA SALGIA, MD
Transplant Hepatologist, Medical Director, Liver Cancer Clinic, Program Director, Gastroenterology/Transplant Hepatology Fellowship, Associate Professor of Medicine, Wayne State University, School of Medicine, Henry Ford Hospital, Detroit, Michigan, USA

RANYA SELIM, MD
Transplant Hepatology Fellow, Henry Ford Hospital, Detroit, Michigan, USA

PRATIMA SHARMA, MD, MS
Associate Professor, Division of Gastroenterology and Hepatology, Department of Internal Medicine, University of Michigan, Ann Arbor, Michigan, USA

TRACEY G. SIMON, MD, MPH
Instructor, Division of Gastroenterology, Department of Medicine, Harvard Medical School, Clinical and Translational Epidemiology Unit, Massachusetts General Hospital, Boston, Massachusetts, USA

CLAUDE B. SIRLIN, MD
Liver Imaging Group, Department of Radiology, University of California, San Diego, San Diego, California, USA

JEAN-NICOLAS VAUTHEY, MD, FACS
Professor, Department of Surgical Oncology, The University of Texas MD Anderson Cancer Center, Houston, Texas, USA

MONIKA VYAS, MBBS
Department of Pathology, Beth Israel Deaconess Medical Center, Harvard Medical School, Boston, Massachusetts, USA

ADAM C. WINTERS, MD
UCLA Vatche & Tamar Manoukian Division of Digestive Diseases, Department of Medicine, University of California, Los Angeles, Pfleger Liver Institute, Los Angeles, California, USA

LAVANYA YOHANATHAN, MD
Mayo Clinic College of Medicine, Rochester, Minnesota, USA

XUCHEN ZHANG, MD, PhD
Department of Pathology, Yale School of Medicine, New Haven, Connecticut, USA

KALI ZHOU, MD, MAS
Assistant Professor, Department of Medicine, Division of Gastrointestinal and Liver Diseases, University of Southern California, Los Angeles, California, USA

Contents

Preface: Advances in Hepatocellular Carcinoma   **xiii**

Catherine Frenette

The Changing Global Epidemiology of Hepatocellular Carcinoma   **535**

Allyce Caines, Ranya Selim, and Reena Salgia

Hepatocellular carcinoma is among the leading causes of morbidity and mortality. Owing to the current epidemic of metabolic syndrome, the population affected by nonalcoholic fatty liver disease/nonalcoholic steatohepatitis continues to increase and now comprises a significant portion with those with hepatocellular carcinoma. The World Health Organization goal of obtaining universal hepatitis B virus vaccination has led to a global effort to improve vaccination, prevent mother-to-child transmission, and implement linkage to care to avoid the development of hepatocellular carcinoma. In contrast with the decreased burden of chronic hepatitis C virus, there has been an increase in new-onset acute hepatitis C virus.

Lifestyle and Environmental Approaches for the Primary Prevention of Hepatocellular Carcinoma   **549**

Tracey G. Simon and Andrew T. Chan

Patients with chronic liver disease are at increased risk of developing hepatocellular carcinoma (HCC). Most patients diagnosed with HCC have limited treatment options and a poor overall prognosis, with a 5-year survival less than 15%. Preventing the development of HCC represents the most important strategy. However, current guidelines lack specific recommendations for primary prevention. Lifestyle factors may be central in the pathogenesis of HCC, and primary prevention strategies focused on lifestyle modification could represent an important approach to the prevention of HCC. Both experimental and epidemiologic studies have identified promising chemopreventive agents for the primary prevention of HCC.

Role of Biomarkers and Biopsy in Hepatocellular Carcinoma   **577**

Vincent L. Chen and Pratima Sharma

Hepatocellular carcinoma (HCC) is increasing in prevalence and is the third leading cause of cancer-related death worldwide. Unlike other malignancies, HCC can be diagnosed with dynamic imaging with very high accuracy, and tissue diagnosis is not needed for cancer therapy. There is a unique role of established as well as developing biomarkers in diagnosis, prognosis, and management of HCC. Sequencing HCC tumors has yielded substantial insights into HCC tumor biology and has raised the possibility of precision oncology in which therapy decisions are guided by cancer genetics. However, it is not ready for prime time yet.

Hepatocellular Carcinoma: Role of Pathology in the Era of Precision Medicine   591

Monika Vyas and Xuchen Zhang

Hepatocellular carcinoma (HCC) is a morphologically heterogeneous tumor with variable architectural growth patterns and several distinct histologic subtypes. Large-scale attempts have been made over the past decade to identify targetable genomic alterations in HCC; however, its translation into clinical personalized care remains a challenge to precision oncology. The role of pathology is no longer limited to confirmation of diagnosis when radiologic features are atypical. Pathology is now in a position to predict the underlying molecular alteration, prognosis, and behavior of HCC. This review outlines various aspects of histopathologic diagnosis and role of pathology in cutting-edge diagnostics of HCC.

Surveillance for Hepatocellular Carcinoma   611

Jorge A. Marrero

Patients with cirrhosis of the liver have a very high risk for developing hepatocellular carcinoma (HCC). Therefore, this group of patients should undergo surveillance to improve mortality. Better tools for stratifying the risk of HCC among patients with cirrhosis are needed. The best strategy for surveillance is the combination of alpha-fetoprotein and ultrasound of the liver every 6 months. This strategy shows a sensitivity of approximately 65% and a specificity of 90%, and importantly, has been shown to improve mortality in these patients. Balancing benefits and harms should be performed when deciding to proceed with surveillance.

Imaging Diagnosis of Hepatocellular Carcinoma: The Liver Imaging Reporting and Data System, Why and How?   623

Guilherme Moura Cunha, Kathryn J. Fowler, Farid Abushamat, Claude B. Sirlin, and Yuko Kono

The Liver Imaging Reporting and Data System (LI-RADS) provides standardized lexicon, technique, interpretation, and reporting of liver imaging in patients at risk for hepatocellular carcinoma (HCC). When applied to at-risk populations, LI-RADS achieves higher than 95% positive predictive value for the noninvasive diagnosis of HCC on computed tomography (CT), MRI and contrast-enhanced ultrasound (CEUS). This article focuses on similarities and differences between the CT/MRI diagnostic algorithm (CT/MRI LI-RADS) and the CEUS diagnostic algorithm (CEUS LI-RADS) to inform health care professionals for efficient and appropriate clinical decisions through the management of patients at risk.

Surgical Resection: Old Dog, Any New Tricks?   637

Yoshikuni Kawaguchi, Heather A. Lillemoe, and Jean-Nicolas Vauthey

Patients with hepatocellular carcinoma (HCC) have many treatment options. For patients with surgical indication, consideration of future liver remnant and the surgical complexity of the procedure is essential. A new 3-level complexity classification categorizing 11 liver resection procedures predicts surgical complexity and postoperative morbidity better than reported classifications. Preoperative portal vein embolization can mitigate the risk of hepatic insufficiency. For small HCCs, both liver resection and ablation are effective. New medical treatment options are promising and perioperative use of these drugs may further improve outcomes for patients undergoing liver resection and lead to changes in current treatment guidelines.

The Impact of Allocation Changes on Patients with Hepatocellular Carcinoma   657

Lavanya Yohanathan and Julie K. Heimbach

Since the establishment of the Milan criteria, liver transplantation (LT) has been identified as an optimal therapy for selected patients with early stage, unresectable hepatocellular carcinoma (HCC) complicating cirrhosis, although a major limitation is the critical shortage of available deceased donor liver allografts. This review focuses on the evolution of liver allocation for HCC in the United States and what the most recent revisions to the allocation system mean for patients with HCC.

Downstaging to Liver Transplant: Success Involves Choosing the Right Patient   665

Kali Zhou and Neil Mehta

Hepatocellular carcinoma is a rising indication for liver transplantation in the United States. Downstaging, defined as the reduction of tumor burden using local-regional therapy into Milan criteria, opens an avenue to access cure through transplant for patients who traditionally would not qualify. Approaching the selection of downstaging candidates through an assessment of hepatic function, staying within a modest expansion of tumor burden, and incorporation of serologic/imaging markers for tumor biology provide the best chance for successful downstaging. Following well-defined downstaging protocols with built-in failure criteria ensures excellent post-transplant outcomes.

Locoregional Therapies for Hepatocellular Carcinoma: What Has Changed in the Past Ten Years?   681

Anjana A. Pillai, Meera Ramanathan, and Laura Kulik

The evolution of locoregional therapies in the last decade has been refined with improved patient selection and a development of a more personalized approach. In doing so, there has been associated improved outcomes and less toxicity. With the rapidly changing landscape of systemic therapy, the role of locoregional therapies alone or in combination for downstaging and curative intent will continue to evolve.

Role of External Beam Radiotherapy in Hepatocellular Carcinoma   701

Chien Peter Chen

External beam radiotherapy (EBRT) has improved efficacy and safety with advancements in technology and techniques. EBRT plays an important role in management of hepatocellular carcinoma (HCC). In resectable cases, EBRT serves as a bridge to transplantation or improves local control through adjuvant radiotherapy. In unresectable patients, EBRT offers high local control rates. In metastatic settings, EBRT provides effective palliation. This review presents an overview of radiotherapy treatment modalities used for HCC, current treatment guidelines for the role of EBRT in

HCC, clinical outcomes between various EBRT approaches and other lo-coregional treatments for HCC, and the future role of EBRT for HCC.

Tyrosine Kinase Inhibitors and Hepatocellular Carcinoma   719

Leonardo G. da Fonseca, Maria Reig, and Jordi Bruix

> Sorafenib was the first tyrosine kinase inhibitor (TKI) that showed success in extending survival in patients with advanced hepatocellular carcinoma (HCC). In recent years, additional TKIs have been shown to improve survival and expanded the armamentarium for treating this malignancy. The current landscape includes other classes of drugs, such as immune checkpoint inhibitors and monoclonal antibodies. The challenge is now placed on how to best select, combine, and sequence drugs with the goal of improving efficacy and minimizing toxicities to deliver better outcomes for HCC patients.

Immuno-oncology for Hepatocellular Carcinoma: The Present and the Future   739

Samantha A. Armstrong and Aiwu Ruth He

> Hepatocellular carcinoma is a highly prevalent and lethal cancer that many therapeutics are being tested for this disease. It has the potential to be a highly immune-responsive tumor given its inflammatory origins. The first immunotherapies were anti-programmed death-1 monotherapies, which improved response rates and survival. Novel immunotherapy combinations and immunotherapy show promise in frontline treatment. The novel antibody therapy combination of atezolizumab and bevacizumab may be practice changing. Although these landmark studies seem to offer new treatment options, the role of immunotherapy in the liver transplant setting is uncertain until the safety of this approach is defined.

Management of Side Effects of Systemic Therapies for Hepatocellular Carcinoma: Guide for the Hepatologist   755

Adam C. Winters, Fatima Bedier, and Sammy Saab

> Historically, systemic treatment of advanced hepatocellular carcinoma was limited to the tyrosine kinase inhibitor sorafenib. With the recent approval of several new agents the armamentarium of treatment options available to providers and patients has expanded. Although these promising advances offer hope for patients with advanced hepatocellular carcinoma, they also present new and challenging adverse effects that threaten to limit their efficacy. Immunotherapy with checkpoint inhibitors introduce immune-related adverse events, which may affect a wide array of organ systems. With prompt recognition, however, common side effects of systemic therapies for hepatocellular carcinoma are predictable, manageable, and many improve with appropriate intervention.

Multidisciplinary Team Management of Hepatocellular Carcinoma Is Standard of Care   771

Dekey Lhewa, Ellen W. Green, and Willscott E. Naugler

> Hepatocellular carcinoma (HCC) is a leading cause of cancer mortality, but unlike other leading causes of cancer death, HCC is increasing in mortality

and burden of management. Management of HCC is unique because it usually arises in a diseased liver, which itself may be a driver of mortality. Multidisciplinary teams (MDTs) for the management of complex diseases are becoming more common, but are especially needed in the management of patients with HCC. Liver cancer MDTs are used in most centers providing comprehensive care for patients with HCC, and should be considered the standard of care for these patients.

CLINICS IN LIVER DISEASE

FORTHCOMING ISSUES

February 2021
Liver Transplantation
David Goldberg, *Editor*

May 2021
Complications of Cirrhosis
Andres Cardenas and Thomas Reiberger,
Editors

November 2021
**Challenging Issues in the Management of
Chronic Hepatitis B Virus**
Mitchell L. Shiffman, *Editor*

RECENT ISSUES

August 2020
Consultations in Liver Disease
Steven L. Flamm, *Editor*

May 2020
Hepatic Encephalopathy
Vinod K. Rustgi, *Editor*

February 2020
Drug Hepatotoxicity
Pierre M. Gholam, *Editor*

SERIES OF RELATED INTEREST

Gastroenterology Clinics of North America
www.gastro.theclinics.com
Gastrointestinal Endoscopy Clinics of North America
www.giendo.theclinics.com

THE CLINICS ARE AVAILABLE ONLINE!
Access your subscription at:
www.theclinics.com

Preface

Advances in Hepatocellular Carcinoma

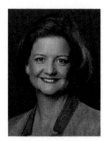

Catherine Frenette, MD, FAST, AGAF, FAASLD
Editor

Hepatocellular carcinoma (HCC) has been increasing in incidence and prevalence for more than 30 years. As hepatologists have become more adept at treating underlying liver disease and cirrhosis, patients with cirrhosis are living longer, and with longer duration of cirrhosis comes an increased risk of HCC development. Cirrhosis is the underlying disease in most patients with HCC, although around 10% of HCC occurs without cirrhosis, often in the setting of chronic hepatitis B infection. Unfortunately, even with improving treatments for viral hepatitis, cirrhosis has continued to increase worldwide, due to the epidemic of nonalcoholic fatty liver disease and increasing alcoholic liver disease. Screening and surveillance have long been shown to improve survival, and despite clear guidelines from the American Association for the Study of Liver Disease, the European Association for the Study of the Liver, and the Asian Pacific Association for the Study of the Liver, rates of compliance with screening and surveillance for patients at risk for HCC remain low. Because of the low rates of screening and surveillance, many patients with HCC continue to present in an advanced stage that precludes curative therapy.

For more than a decade, treatment options for HCC have been limited to surgical (resection and transplant) and locoregional (ablation, chemoembolization, and radioembolization), with limited systemic therapy options. Sorafenib was approved in 2007 and was the sole systemic therapy that has been shown to improve survival in HCC. The previous issue of *Clinics in Liver Disease* dedicated to HCC was published in May 2015. Since that time, significant advances in the field of HCC have been made. I have had the honor of being a guest editor for this issue of *Clinics in Liver Disease*, and our talented and knowledgeable authors have outdone themselves with excellent articles. Dr Salgia outlines how the epidemiology of HCC has changed in recent years. Drs Chan and Simon discuss strategies for prevention of development of malignancy in patients at risk. Dr Sharma discusses new information on biomarkers for screening and

Clin Liver Dis 24 (2020) xiii–xiv
https://doi.org/10.1016/j.cld.2020.08.014
1089-3261/20/© 2020 Published by Elsevier Inc.

diagnosis, as well as the increasing utility of biopsy. Dr Zhang does a magnificent job of discussing the role of pathology in the era of precision medicine, which is significantly progressing in the treatment of all cancers. Dr Marrero discusses strategies to improve our screening and surveillance, while Drs Kono and Sirlin, who were the creators of the LIRADS radiographic diagnostic criteria for HCC, discuss how to appropriately diagnose HCC with imaging. Dr Vauthey is one of the grandfathers of liver resection, and he and Dr Kawagushi wrote an excellent article on resection strategies. Dr Heimbach is a surgeon who has been instrumental in liver transplant for HCC and appropriate allocation changes for liver transplantation and discusses new allocation changes that have altered how our HCC patients will obtain liver grafts for transplantation. Dr Mehta has had multiple publications about downstaging HCC to within transplant criteria, and his data have contributed to the major changes in liver transplantation for HCC, with patients now being eligible for transplant who previously would not have been able to receive a liver graft. Dr Kulik and her team in Chicago discuss locoregional and transarterial strategies for local HCC treatment. Dr Chen is a dear friend and colleague and wrote about his experience and new data for use of external beam radiotherapy for HCC treatment. I can't emphasize enough how much I respect and admire Jordi Bruix, and he and his colleagues were kind enough to discuss the new tyrosine kinase inhibitor therapies. Dr He is a well-respected oncologist in the field of HCC, and she discusses the present and future uses of immunotherapy and immunooncology for HCC treatment. Dr Saab is one of my favorite people to work with and wrote a guide for the hepatologist on management of side effects of systemic therapies for HCC. Dr Naugler and colleagues round out this issue with an article explaining and demonstrating how in this complicated disease state that a multidisciplinary tumor board remains as critical as ever in treatment of HCC.

I hope you enjoy this issue of *Clinics in Liver Disease*. I would like to thank Dr Norman Gitlin for the invitation, and Norm, I hope you are enjoying Southern California. I would also like to thank Kerry Holland and Donald Mumford for their patience, perseverance, and professionalism with helping to bring this issue to fruition. Thank you to our readers for reading this issue, and I hope you are enjoying it with a large cup of coffee!

Catherine Frenette, MD, FAST, AGAF, FAASLD
Scripps Center for Organ Transplantation
Liver and Hepatocellular Cancer Program
Scripps MD Anderson Cancer Center
Scripps Green Hospital
10666 North Torrey Pines Road N200
La Jolla, CA 92037, USA

E-mail address:
Frenette.Catherine@scrippshealth.org

The Changing Global Epidemiology of Hepatocellular Carcinoma

Allyce Caines, MD*, Ranya Selim, MD, Reena Salgia, MD

KEYWORDS

- Hepatocellular carcinoma • Epidemiology • NASH • Opioid crisis • Hepatitis B
- Hepatitis C

KEY POINTS

- Hepatocellular carcinoma is the fifth and ninth most commonly diagnosed cancer in men and women, respectively, and the fourth leading cause of cancer mortality worldwide.
- In developing countries hepatocellular carcinoma is largely attributed to underlying hepatitis B virus infection, with more than 70% of hepatocellular carcinoma cases attributable to hepatitis B virus.
- Until recently, cirrhosis secondary to hepatitis C virus was the most common underlying etiology of hepatocellular carcinoma, accounting for 60% of hepatocellular carcinoma cases.
- More recently, the landscape of HCV and in turn hepatocellular carcinoma is changing owing to direct acting antiviral therapy and the opioid epidemic.
- More recent data show that nonalcoholic steatohepatitis is playing a greater role in hepatocellular carcinoma cases.

INTRODUCTION

Hepatocellular carcinoma (HCC) has been increasing in incidence over the last several decades. Previously limited to Eastern Asia, HCC has become increasingly prevalent in the northern and western hemispheres, particularly Western Europe and the United States.[1] Today, it is the fifth and ninth most commonly diagnosed cancer in men and women, respectively, and the fourth leading cause of cancer mortality worldwide.[2] There is a greater than 2-fold predilection toward males compared with females, especially between the ages of 55 and 64.[3] The annual incidence in the United States has increased from 1.4 in 100,000 cases per year in 1976 to 1980 to 6.2 in 100,000 cases per year in 2011.[1] Worldwide, the incidence was 10.1 in 100,000 in 2017, with an incidence of 24.2 per 100,000 in parts of Africa and 35.5 per 100,000 in Eastern Asia.[4] According to the Centers for Disease Control and Prevention, the age-adjusted death

Henry Ford Hospital, 2799 West Grand Boulevard, Suite K7, Detroit, MI 48202, USA
* Corresponding author.
E-mail addresses: acaines1@hfhs.org; allyce.caines@gmail.com

Clin Liver Dis 24 (2020) 535–547
https://doi.org/10.1016/j.cld.2020.06.001
1089-3261/20/© 2020 Elsevier Inc. All rights reserved.

rate owing to HCC has been increasing by 3% per year. It is estimated that over the next 2 decades, the global burden of HCC will increase to more than 22 million cases.[1]

In developing countries such as those in Asia and Africa where vaccination capabilities can remain limited in remote areas, HCC is largely attributed to underlying hepatitis B virus (HBV) infection, with more than 70% of HCC cases attributable to HBV.[5] Until recently, in Europe and the United States, hepatitis C virus (HCV) cirrhosis was the most common underlying etiology of HCC, accounting for 60% of HCC cases.[6] More recent data show that nonalcoholic steatohepatitis (NASH) is playing a greater role in HCC cases, with a 9% increase in HCC cases attributed to NASH between 2004 and 2009.[7] The contribution of alcohol to the HCC burden is also significant at about 30%, with significant variability between different countries.[8] Aflatoxin exposure is responsible for up to 40% of HCC cases in Africa, with a comparatively negligible contribution in Europe and North America.[9] This worldwide heterogeneity of etiologic epidemiology is driven by several factors, including the availability of vaccination, the prevalence of the metabolic syndrome, and the prevalence of injection drug use. In this article, we discuss the evolving global epidemiology of HCC and the elements driving it.

CHRONIC HEPATITIS B
The Epidemiology of Chronic Hepatitis B

Despite the availability of effective vaccines since 1982 and effective antiviral therapy, HBV remains a prevalent global health problem.[10] Two billion people have serologic evidence of past or ongoing HBV infection and an estimated 257 million people or 3.5% of the world's population are chronically infected with HBV.[11] It is well-known that HBV is associated with significant morbidity and mortality. The lifetime risk of cirrhosis, liver failure, and HCC in patients with HBV is reported to be between 15% and 40%.[12] HBV is the leading cause of incident cases of liver cancer and deaths in the world (33%), followed by alcohol (30%), HCV (21%), and other causes (16%) **(Fig. 1)**.[13] Hepatitis B surface antigen (HBsAg) seroprevalence varies geographically.

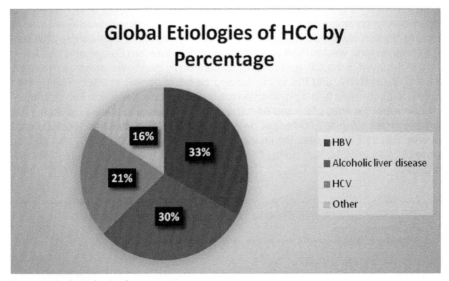

Fig. 1. Global etiologies by percentage.

According to the 2017 World Health Organization (WHO) Global Hepatitis Report, the number of HBsAg-positive individuals was highest in the Western Pacific (115 million, prevalence estimate 6.2%; 95% uncertainty interval, 5.1%–7.6%) and Africa (60 million prevalence estimate 6.1%; 95% uncertainty interval, 4.6%–8.5%), which together accounted for 68% of the global burden.[11] In May of 2016, the WHO adopted a global hepatitis strategy with the goal of eliminating viral hepatitis as a public health threat by 2030. This goal includes a target to decrease new cases of chronic HBV by 90%, decrease mortality owing to HBV and HCV by 65%, and to treat 80% of eligible persons with chronic HBV and HCV infections.[14] Reaching these targets will ultimately decrease the incidence of HCC and its associated mortality.

Hepatitis B Virus as a Risk Factor for Hepatocellular Carcinoma

Among HBV-infected individuals, independent risk factors for HCC include HBeAg seropositivity, high viral load, and genotype C infection.[13] Human immunodeficiency virus/HBV coinfection has a further impact because human immunodeficiency virus promotes a more aggressive natural history of hepatitis B, with often a younger age of disease onset with a more advanced fibrosis stage at diagnosis. The annual incidence of HCC correlates with the geographic HBsAg seroprevalence with the highest incidence found in sub-Saharan Africa and South East Asia.[10] In Africa and East Africa, the population attributable fraction of HCC caused by HBV is reported to be approximately 60%, compared with lower rates in the western hemisphere.[15] In sub-Saharan Africa HBV-related HCC is the most common malignancy among men in 12 countries and the most common cause of premature death. In the same region, HCC is the second most prevalent cancer in men and the third for women. HCC in Africa tends to occur in the late 30s and early 40s, at least a decade earlier than in Western countries.[16] An analysis of the African population chronically infected with hepatitis B has elucidated genotype A, particularly subgenotype A1, to be associated with more aggressive liver disease, and more rapid progression to HCC.[17] Although cirrhosis is the most common risk factor for HCC in the setting of chronic HBV, HCC can also develop independent of cirrhosis in HBV infection. High levels of HBV replication and chronicity of inflammation are known to independently increase the risk for HCC. Although infrequent, inactive HBV carriers or those with occult HBV infection can develop HCC in the absence of cirrhosis. A direct carcinogenic role of viral factors, HBV genotype, integration of viral DNA into the host genome, and direct effects of viral proteins are likely to contribute to the occurrence.[18]

The Impact of Hepatitis B Vaccination on the Global Epidemiology of Hepatocellular Carcinoma

The WHO recommended incorporation of HBV vaccination into the Expanded Program of immunization in 1991 as the most effective way to decrease the global burden of HBV. Universal vaccination has globally decreased HBsAg prevalence in children less than 5 years of age from 4.7% in the prevaccination era to 1.3% in 2015. However, the prevalence of HBsAg in the WHO Africa continent remains high at 3%.[11] The WHO Western Pacific region has decreased their HBsAg prevalence in children less than 5 years of age to 0.9%. By 2013, universal HBV vaccination had prevented 14.2 million cases of chronic HBV infection among children aged 0 to 5 years worldwide and more than 1.3 million deaths.[10] Universal HBV vaccination has also led to a significant decrease in HBV in Taiwan, where universal vaccination (introduced in 1984), together with a catchup vaccination program and improved maternal screening has led to a decrease in the prevalence of HBsAg positivity in children aged less than 15 years from 9.8% in 1984% to 0.3% in 2009.[19,20] In turn, this process has led to a decrease in HCC incidence per 10^5 person-years from 0.92 in unvaccinated to 0.23 in vaccinated cohorts.[21] In many East Asian countries, the implementation of infant HBV immunization programs is expected to decrease HBV-related HCC in the future to a similar degree demonstrated in Taiwan.[21] Universal HBV vaccination, vaccine catchup programs, and mass screening since 1981 have also eliminated acute symptomatic HBV infection and early-onset HCC as a public health threat among Alaskan Native children.[10]

There are several countries that have yet to implement universal HBV vaccination and many individuals are still infected with HBV (approximately 257 million in 2015), mostly in Asia and sub-Saharan Africa, where the prevalence of HBsAg remains high.[22] In Africa, HBV vaccine coverage is only 77%.[23] A major limitation is the access to immunization and HBV treatment specifically in sub-Saharan Africa. The WHO Global Policy Report on the Prevention and Control of Viral Hepatitis reported that only 16.7% of WHO-AFRO countries have publicly funded HBV treatment available.[24,25] Despite the WHO recommendation for use of birth dose vaccine for prevention of chronic HBV infection, as of 2019 only 10 of the 47 African nations have implemented this recommendation. Although an effective HBV vaccine has been available since 1982, there remains a wide range of vaccination rates and challenges associated with global HBV vaccination. It is imperative to recognize and address potential challenges associated with achieving the elimination of HBV, while also realizing that HBV and its associated complications are entirely vaccine preventable.[10] To achieve higher global vaccination rates, every country will need to assess the burden of HBV within its population and have knowledge of seroprevalence and potential high-risk groups. Prevention of mother-to-child transmission (MTCT) also plays a key role in the elimination of HBV.

Mother-to-Child Transmission of Hepatitis B Virus

In the absence of effective MTCT prophylaxis, HBV endemicity and chronicity is established in early childhood, with HBsAg seroprevalence studies showing no difference between children aged 5 to 9 years and adults.[26] The risk of chronic HBV is strongly correlated with the age of acquisition of infection: 90% after neonatal infection (in children born to HBeAg-positive or highly viremic mothers), 20% to 50% with childhood infection (<5 years of age), and less than 5% for adults more than 20 years.[10] HBV MTCT prevention strategies include antenatal HBsAg screening, third trimester antiviral therapy for women with high infectivity risk (HBeAg positive and/or HBV DNA >200,000 IU/mL), hepatitis B birth-dose (HepB-BD) vaccination, administration of hepatitis B immunoglobulin to the newborn, and full HBV vaccine coverage.[27–29] In 2009, the WHO recommended HepB-BD vaccination with a monovalent HBV vaccine administered within 24 hours of delivery for all countries.[14] However, globally in 2014, only 96 of 194 countries (49%) reported offering HepB-BD as part of their national immunization programs and fewer than 38% of babies born worldwide received HepB-BD within 24 hours after birth.[10] Coverage of the HepB-BD vaccine in 2015 was only 38% worldwide and 10% in sub-Saharan Africa. The identification of HBsAg-positive pregnant women also provides the opportunity to identify potentially HBV-infected partners, siblings, and children and thereby link them to care, breaking the ongoing cycles of infection.

Hepatitis Delta Virus and Hepatocellular Carcinoma

Hepatitis delta virus (HDV) is a negative-sense RNA satellite virus of HBV that requires HBsAg for formation of new virions.[30] HDV coexists with HBV and is related to the most severe form of liver failure attributable to chronic viral hepatitis.[31] Accurate data on HDV prevalence in many countries is lacking, leading to a global underestimation of disease burden.[31] The WHO estimates that there are at least 20 million people infected with HDV worldwide, which represents 5% of HBV carriers.[32] Key features of HDV remain unknown. Coinfection of HBV with HDV has been shown to increase the risk of HCC by 2-fold and the risk of cirrhosis 3-fold.[30] It has been suggested that HDV accelerates the disease course compared with HBV monoinfection; however, the potential mechanisms underlying HDV-specific oncogenesis are poorly understood. Apart from enhancing fibrosis and inflammation, there is no evidence to suggest a direct oncogenic mechanism of HDV. Well-designed prospective studies are needed to further evaluate the oncogenic capacity of HBV/HDV co-infection.[31]

NONALCOHOLIC FATTY LIVER DISEASE
The Epidemiology of Nonalcoholic Fatty Liver Disease

First described in the 1980s as an "unnamed disease," nonalcoholic fatty liver disease (NAFLD) has now become the most common etiology of chronic liver disease in the United States, and is increasingly being recognized throughout the world as a frequent cause of liver disease in the setting of globally increasing rates of the metabolic syndrome.[33] NAFLD is an entity that encompasses a wide range of manifestations from steatosis to NASH, with or without cirrhosis. It has been linked with multiple risk factors including metabolic syndrome, insulin resistance, altered gut flora and persistent inflammation. Notably, NAFLD is more common in the elderly, in whom it manifests with more advanced fibrosis staging at diagnosis and with additional associated comorbidities, such as glucose intolerance and cardiovascular disease, as compared with younger patients. One possible underlying mechanism is aging of the liver, resulting in impairment of metabolism and detoxification by hepatocytes, leading to liver injury and inflammation and the generation of pro-oncogenic substances.[34]

The worldwide incidence of NAFLD ranges from 6% to 35% per year,[35] with a prevalence estimated at 9% to 37%.[36] The global disease burden of NAFLD is currently estimated at 1 billion cases, with the highest prevalence existing in Asia, closely followed by the United States. In the United States, the NAFLD burden has doubled over the past 2 decades to a current burden of 80 to 100 million cases, approximately 30% of the population, and has become the most rapidly growing etiology of cirrhosis.[37] It is possible that the increasing prevalence may also in part relate to the advent of newer, more sensitive, noninvasive diagnostic modalities such as ultrasound examination, computed tomography scans, MRI, and elastography. NASH affects about 5% to 7% of the general population, with 3% to 15% of patients with NASH eventually progressing onto cirrhosis. Studies have shown that the risk of developing HCC in this patient population can be as high as 38% over 5 to 10 years.[38] With the enhanced prevention and eradication of HBV and HCV respectively, NAFLD is predicted to supersede viral etiologies in its contribution to the HCC burden, particularly in developed countries around the world.

Progression of Nonalcoholic Fatty Liver Disease to Hepatocellular Carcinoma

Undoubtedly, the pathway of progression from NAFLD to NASH and similarly from NASH to HCC is complex with a pathophysiology that remains incompletely understood. Notable risk factors include genomic instability, obesity, and diabetes. Mechanisms related to these factors stimulate changes in signaling pathways leading to the evolution of dysplastic cells into malignant cells. A 2-hit hypothesis has been proposed, which suggests the initial risk is insulin resistance, which enhances lipolysis and increases serum free fatty acids. High levels of free fatty acids result in delivering triglycerides from the liver to peripheral organs, inducing excess lipid synthesis and accumulation of lipids in the liver, or steatosis. The second hit—oxidative stress—is caused by an accumulation of triglycerides and, in turn, induces lipid peroxidation, proinflammatory factor release, and mitochondrial injury.[39] This cascade of events culminates with hepatocellular damage, inflammation, and fibrosis described as NASH. More recently, a parallel hit hypothesis has been suggested.[40] According to this theory, multiple concurrent processes are involved in the development of NASH, including genetic mutations, lipid metabolism disorders, oxidative stress, mitochondrial disorders, variable immune responses, and abnormal gut flora. Per this theory, inflammation is the first step in the cascade leading to fibrosis rather than steatosis. It is felt that much of the disruption in signaling pathways leading to NASH simultaneously lead to HCC. Important molecules orchestrating coordination between these signaling pathways lead to activation of pro-oncogenic processes and suppression of antioncogenic processes.[41] Regardless of the pathophysiology causing NASH to develop, it is the culmination of cirrhotic architectural changes that is felt to be the common denominator in NASH-related HCC. Several clinical trials are ongoing at this time investigating the various pathways involved to determine treatment targets that may reduce progression to NASH and HCC.[41]

Importantly, there is increasing evidence implicating noncirrhotic NAFLD in HCC development. Several studies have showed that in many patients with HCC of unknown etiology, that only risk factor for liver disease was the presence of metabolic syndrome, thus raising suspicion for underlying NAFLD.[42] Many of those with HCC did have histologically confirmed steatosis in the absence of fibrosis or steatohepatitis. This finding suggests that steatosis alone may be implicated in the development of HCC.[43] Notably, obesity has been identified as an independent risk factor for HCC, with an odds ratio of 2.6 (95% confidence interval [CI], 1.4–4.4).[44] The pathogenesis of nonfibrotic NAFLD leading to HCC is yet to be confirmed at this time, although a few potential mechanisms related to the metabolic syndrome have been suggested: increased release of proinflammatory and pro-oncogenic cytokines, decreased expression of anti-inflammatory hormones, lipotoxicity interfering with cell signaling pathways, and hyperinsulinemia resulting in the activation of proliferative cell signaling cascades.[45]

CHRONIC HEPATITIS C
The Epidemiology of Chronic Hepatitis C

HCV has been shown to be responsible for 10% to 25% of HCC cases worldwide.[46,47] The risk of developing HCV-related HCC is 1.2% to 1.7% per year for patients with chronic hepatitis and 1.4% to 2.5% per year for those with cirrhosis.[48] HCV endemicity is low in northern Europe and North America; intermediate in South America, Eastern Europe, Oceania, and in some Mediterranean countries; and high in some Eastern Asian countries and Western Africa.[49] One of the highest areas of viremic prevalence is Egypt, with a prevalence of 6.3%, equivalent to 5.6 million HCV-infected individuals.[50] Although prior studies among HCV-infected patients reported similar risk factors, for example, HCV genotype, the strongest determinants of HCC risk in these patients are currently the presence (vs absence) of cirrhosis and attaining a sustained virologic response (SVR).[13] Unfortunately, unlike hepatitis B infection, a vaccine for HCV does not exist, making prevention strategies more limited.

Hepatitis C Virus as a Risk Factor for Hepatocellular Carcinoma

Attaining an SVR after HCV treatment is associated with a decreased risk of cirrhosis and its complications including HCC. Before the development of direct-acting antivirals (DAA), HCV therapy consisted primarily of interferon (IFN)-based treatment. Depending on the HCV genotype and the IFN regimen with or without ribavirin, approximately 30% to 50% of patients treated with IFN achieved an SVR compared with more than 95% of patients achieving an SVR with DAA therapy.[51] Despite the challenges with IFN therapy, studies have consistently demonstrated that, among HCV-infected patients, the risk of developing HCC significantly declined from 6.2% to 1.5% with IFN-based SVR[52] and a similar reduction is observed for SVR from DAA agents[53]

Early reports raised concern and controversy about an apparent unexpected increase in the number of HCC cases developing after DAA therapy for HCV, as well as higher than expected rates of recurrence after surgical resection in patients receiving DAA treatment.[54] It was hypothesized that DAAs may adversely impact immune surveillance, resulting in higher HCC risk. Despite the results of these studies, subsequent data have emerged comparing HCC risk in DAA-cured patients with the risk in patients achieving SVR with IFN-based regimens. In a study by Li and colleagues[55] among all treated persons, risk of HCC was similar in the DAA-treated and the IFN-treated cohorts (hazard ratio [HR], 1.07; 95% CI, 0.55–2.08) after adjusting for differences in patient populations, including higher proportions of cirrhosis and portal hypertension among DAA treated patients than those treated with IFN. Among persons with cirrhosis who achieved an SVR, neither HCC incidence nor HCC-free survival was significantly different in the DAA cohort compared with the IFN-treated cohort (21.2 per 1000 person-years vs 22.8 per 1000 person-years; $P = .78$). Collectively, recent data have shown that successful HCV eradication confers a benefit of decreased HCC incidence in DAA-treated patients.

There continues to be debate regarding the risk and aggressiveness of HCC recurrence after DAA therapy in patients with a history of HCC. However, a retrospective cohort study of patients with HCV-related HCC with complete response to resection, local ablation, transarterial chemoembolization, radioembolization, or radiation therapy found that DAA therapy was not associated with HCC recurrence (HR, 0.90; 95% CI, 0.70–1.16) or early HCC recurrence (HR, 0.96; 95% CI, 0.70–1.34).[56] DAA therapy has also been associated with a significant reduction in risk of death as demonstrated by Singal and colleagues,[56] who, in an analysis of nearly 800 patients with HCV-related HCC, found that DAA therapy was associated with a significant decrease in the risk of death (HR, 0.54; 95% CI, 0.33–0.90). The association differed by SVR to DAA therapy, where risk of death was lower in patients with SVR to DAA therapy (HR, 0.29; 95% CI, 0.18–0.47) but not in patients without an SVR (HR, 1.13; 95% CI, 0.55–2.33).

DAA therapy, in addition to curing HCV, has shown benefit in terms of regression of liver fibrosis. However, despite HCV clearance, patients with bridging fibrosis or cirrhosis are still at risk of developing HCC. HCC may occur in patients with bridging fibrosis (METAVIR F3) owing to sampling variation in liver specimens, inaccurate evaluation by noninvasive tests, or the transition to cirrhosis after the F3 stage.[57,58] All international guidelines endorse indefinite HCC surveillance after achieving an SVR in patients with cirrhosis diagnosed before the implementation of antiviral treatment and the development of an SVR.[59–61] The necessity for periodic surveillance of patients with pretherapeutic bridging fibrosis (METAVIR F3) is more controversial. Recent dedicated analyses suggest that this strategy may not be cost effective in F3 patients owing to the lower HCC incidence observed after achieving an SVR than in patients with pretherapeutic documented cirrhosis.[62] Although the regression of cirrhosis is possible, the proportion of patients who will experience such an improvement is not known. Many patients may experience progression, particularly those with comorbidities. Recent large-scale longitudinal studies of noninvasive evaluations (eg, FIB-4 and APRI) suggest that even in cases of regression of these parameters, the risk of HCC remains high enough to justify surveillance[63]

The Impact of the Opioid Crisis on the Incidence of Acute Hepatitis C

It is worth mentioning that the population at risk for HCV has changed over the past several years. This has been reflected in the US Preventive Services Task Force recent changes in HCV screening recommendations. Previously it was felt that the recommendation to screen all adults born between 1945 and 1965 would capture the majority of the at-risk populations. More recently, there has been a sharp increase in the incidence of acute HCV infection. This increase can be almost entirely attributable to the epidemic of opioid use, which has created a crisis in communities across the United States. Over the last 2 decades, a nearly 4-fold increase in opioid sales has occurred from 1999 to 2008.[64,65] Along with an increase in prescription opioid use and addiction, there has also been an acute increase in heroin use. Given these changes in 2019 the US Preventive Services Task Force released a draft recommendation summary to screen for HCV infection in adults ages 18 to 79 years of age.

The rapid increase in injection drug use has resulted in an abrupt increase in HCV transmission among populations at risk. After a remarkable decrease in acute HCV infection over the decade before, the number of acute HCV cases in the United States has nearly tripled between 2011 and 2015.[66] Injection drug use continues to be the principle factor for HCV exposure. It is estimated that up to 1 in 3 persons who inject drugs will develop HCV infection within the first year of injecting drugs.[66] Given the benefits associated with virologic cure, the current AASLD/IDSA HCV guidance document strongly recommends antiviral treatment for all adults with acute or chronic HCV infection (except those with a short life expectancy that cannot be remediated).[67] This includes all persons with ongoing substance use (alcohol or drugs), because several studies have demonstrated that treatment-committed individuals in this disproportionately affected population achieve SVR rates with DAA therapy comparable with those without known, current substance use.[67,68] Although it is unlikely that the opioid crisis is contributing to the current epidemiology of HCC, this factor deserves attention and a focus on antiviral treatment of this generally young population, with the hopes of preventing long-term complications of cirrhosis and HCC.

Alcoholic Liver Disease

Alcohol consumption has been linked to the development of many malignancies including HCC, with a 2.07 relative risk of development of HCC for alcohol abusers compared with nondrinkers. However, alcoholic liver disease in the absence of fibrosis or with very mild fibrosis has not been shown to be associated with an increased HCC risk.[69] Although alcohol accounts for a significant proportion of primary HCC burden in cirrhosis, there is significant geographic variation. Alcohol is a risk factor for HCC development in 6% to 14% of patients in the Middle East and North Africa compared with 50% to 60% in Eastern Europe.[8] The pathophysiology is believed to be related to the effect of alcohol in the disruption of liver architecture and function, with the eventual development of steatosis, steatohepatitis, and cirrhosis. A number of processes have been reported to contribute to carcinogenesis, including the formation of acetaldehyde and reactive oxygen species, increased production of cytochrome P450, and impairment DNA repair.[70]

SUMMARY

HCC has been steadily increasing in incidence and is among the leading causes of morbidity and mortality in the United States and the world. Previously limited to developing countries, it is now impacting the northern and western hemispheres. With the burden of HCC expected to increase in the coming years, prevention of HCC through the modification of risk factors will be imperative. Owing to the current epidemic of metabolic syndrome, the population affected by NAFLD and NASH continues to increase and now comprises a significant portion with HCC.

The majority of efforts to prevent the progression from NASH to cirrhosis and HCC at this time focus on improving the metabolic syndrome and obesity, with an emphasis on dietary and lifestyle changes. As clinical trials for targeted pharmacologic therapy for the treatment of NASH are underway, there is promise that the future will bring medical therapies aimed to prevent fibrosis and decrease the risk for HCC development. The WHO goal of obtaining universal HBV vaccination by 2016 has led to a global effort to improve vaccination efforts, prevent MTCT and implement linkage to care to avoid the development of HCC in addition to cirrhosis.

Finally, the use of highly effective DAA therapies to reduce the burden of chronic HCV has decreased but not eliminated the risk of subsequent HCC development. Ongoing HCC risk factor identification and global attention to the prevention and treatment of chronic liver diseases will be critical to slowing the incidence of HCC.

REFERENCES

1. Ghouri YA, Mian I, Rowe JH. Review of hepatocellular carcinoma: epidemiology, etiology, and carcinogenesis. J Carcinog 2017;16:1.

2. Ferlay J, Soerjomataram I, Dikshit R, et al. Cancer incidence and mortality worldwide: sources, methods and major patterns in GLOBOCAN 2012. Int J Cancer 2015;136(5):E359–86.

3. Kulik L, El-Serag HB. Epidemiology and management of hepatocellular carcinoma. Gastroenterology 2019;156(2):477–91.e1.

4. Arabsalmani M, Mirzaei M, Ghoncheh M, et al. Incidence and mortality of liver cancer and their relationship with the human development index in the world. Biomed Res Ther 2016;3(9):41.

5. Beasley RP. Hepatitis B virus. The major etiology of hepatocellular carcinoma. Cancer 1988;61(10):1942–56.

6. Knudsen ES, Gopal P, Singal AG. The changing landscape of hepatocellular carcinoma: etiology, genetics, and therapy. Am J Pathol 2014;184(3):574–83.

7. Younossi ZM, Otgonsuren M, Henry L, et al. Association of nonalcoholic fatty liver disease (NAFLD) with hepatocellular carcinoma (HCC) in the United States from 2004 to 2009. Hepatology 2015;62(6):1723–30.

8. Ganne-Carrié N, Nahon P. Hepatocellular carcinoma in the setting of alcohol-related liver disease. J Hepatol 2019;70(2):284–93.

9. Liu Y, Wu F. Global burden of aflatoxin-induced hepatocellular carcinoma: a risk assessment. Environ Health Perspect 2010;118(6):818–24.

10. Spearman CW. Towards the elimination of hepatitis B and hepatocellular carcinoma. South Afr Med J 2018;108(8b):13–6.

11. World Health Organization. Global hepatitis report. 2017. Available at: www.who.int/hepatitis/publications/global-hepatitis-report2017/en/. Accessed January 14, 2020.

12. Lozano R, Naghavi M, Foreman K, et al. Global and regional mortality from 235 causes of death for 20 age groups in 1990 and 2010: a systematic analysis for the Global Burden of Disease Study 2010. Lancet 2012;380(9859):2095–128.

13. Singal AG, Lampertico P, Nahon P. Epidemiology and surveillance for hepatocellular carcinoma: new trends. J Hepatol 2020;72(2):250–61.

14. World Health Organization. WHO global health sector strategy on viral hepatitis 2016-2021: towards ending viral hepatitis. Available at: https://apps.who.int/iris/bitstream/handle/10665/246177/WHO-HIV-2016.06-eng.pdf;jsessionid=E7A33F51BE84C5ED2CDB0BE4CA0D6972?sequence=1. Accessed 14 January 2020.

15. Akinyemiju T, Abera S, Ahmed M, et al. The burden of primary liver cancer and underlying etiologies from 1990 to 2015 at the global, regional, and national level: results from the global burden of disease study 2015. JAMA Oncol 2017;3(12):1683–91.

16. Yang JD, Roberts LR. Epidemiology and management of hepatocellular carcinoma. Infect Dis Clin 2010;24(4):899–919.

17. Kramvis A. Genotypes and genetic variability of hepatitis B virus. Intervirology 2014;57(3–4):141–50.

18. Ringelhan M, Heikenwalder M, Protzer U. Direct effects of hepatitis B virus-encoded proteins and chronic infection in liver cancer development. Dig Dis 2013;31(1):138–51.

19. Chen H-L, Chang M-H, Ni Y-H, et al. Seroepidemiology of hepatitis B virus infection in children: ten years of mass vaccination in Taiwan. JAMA 1996;276(11):906–8.

20. Hsu H-M, Chen D-S, Chuang C-H, et al. Efficacy of a mass hepatitis B vaccination program in Taiwan: studies on 3464 infants of hepatitis B surface antigen—carrier mothers. JAMA 1988;260(15):2231–5.

21. Chang M-H, You S-L, Chen C-J, et al. Long-term effects of hepatitis B immunization of infants in preventing liver cancer. Gastroenterology 2016;151(3):472–80.e1.

22. Yuen MF, Chen DS, Dusheiko GM, et al. Hepatitis B virus infection. Nat Rev Dis Primers 2018;4:18035.

23. Tamandjou CR, Maponga TG, Chotun N, et al. Is hepatitis B birth dose vaccine needed in Africa? Pan Afr Med J 2017;27(Suppl 3):18.

24. Cooke GS, Andrieux-Meyer I, Applegate TL, et al. Accelerating the elimination of viral hepatitis: a Lancet Gastroenterology & Hepatology Commission. Lancet Gastroenterol Hepatol 2019;4(2):135–84.

25. Yang J, Mohamed E, Aziz A, et al. Africa Network for Gastrointestinal and Liver Diseases. Characteristics, management, and outcomes of patients with hepatocellular carcinoma in Africa: a multicountry observational study from the Africa liver cancer consortium. Lancet Gastroenterol Hepatol 2017;2(02):103–11.

26. Maynard JE. Hepatitis B: global importance and need for control. Vaccine 1990;8(Suppl):S18–20 [discussion: S21–3].

27. Zhang H, Pan CQ, Pang Q, et al. Telbivudine or lamivudine use in late pregnancy safely reduces perinatal transmission of hepatitis B virus in real-life practice. Hepatology 2014;60(2):468–76.

28. del Canho R, Grosheide PM, Schalm SW, et al. Failure of neonatal hepatitis B vaccination: the role of HBV-DNA levels in hepatitis B carrier mothers and HLA antigens in neonates. J Hepatol 1994;20(4):483–6.

29. Pan CQ, Duan Z, Dai E, et al. Tenofovir to prevent hepatitis B transmission in mothers with high viral load. N Engl J Med 2016;374(24):2324–34.

30. Tu T, Bühler S, Bartenschlager R. Chronic viral hepatitis and its association with liver cancer. Biol Chem 2017;398(8):817–37.
31. Puigvehí M, Moctezuma-Velázquez C, Villanueva A, et al. The oncogenic role of hepatitis delta virus in hepatocellular carcinoma. JHEP Rep 2019;1(2):120–30.
32. WHO. Global hepatitis report 2017. Geneva (Switzerland): World Health Organization; 2017.
33. Kanwal F, Kramer JR, Mapakshi S, et al. Risk of hepatocellular cancer in patients with non-alcoholic fatty liver disease. Gastroenterology 2018;155(6):1828–37.e2.
34. Frith J, Day CP, Henderson E, et al. Non-alcoholic fatty liver disease in older people. Gerontology 2009;55(6):607–13.
35. Dhamija E, Paul SB, Kedia S. Non-alcoholic fatty liver disease associated with hepatocellular carcinoma: an increasing concern. Indian J Med Res 2019;149(1):9–17.
36. Starley BQ, Calcagno CJ, Harrison SA. Nonalcoholic fatty liver disease and hepatocellular carcinoma: a weighty connection. Hepatology 2010;51(5):1820–32.
37. Perumpail BJ, Khan MA, Yoo ER, et al. Clinical epidemiology and disease burden of nonalcoholic fatty liver disease. World J Gastroenterol 2017;23(47):8263–76.
38. White DL, Kanwal F, El-Serag HB. Association between nonalcoholic fatty liver disease and risk for hepatocellular cancer, based on systematic review. Clin Gastroenterol Hepatol 2012;10(12):1342–59.e2.
39. Day CP, James OF. Steatohepatitis: a tale of two "hits"? Gastroenterology 1998;114(4):842–5.
40. Tilg H, Moschen AR. Evolution of inflammation in nonalcoholic fatty liver disease: the multiple parallel hits hypothesis. Hepatology 2010;52(5):1836–46.
41. Caligiuri A, Gentilini A, Marra F. Molecular pathogenesis of NASH. Int J Mol Sci 2016;17(9):1575.
42. Paradis V, Zalinski S, Chelbi E, et al. Hepatocellular carcinomas in patients with metabolic syndrome often develop without significant liver fibrosis: a pathological analysis. Hepatology 2009;49(3):851–9.
43. Guzman G, Brunt EM, Petrovic LM, et al. Does nonalcoholic fatty liver disease predispose patients to hepatocellular carcinoma in the absence of cirrhosis? Arch Pathol Lab Med 2008;132(11):1761–6.
44. Hassan MM, Abdel-Wahab R, Kaseb A, et al. Obesity early in adulthood increases risk but does not affect outcomes of hepatocellular carcinoma. Gastroenterology 2015;149(1):119–29.
45. Baffy G, Brunt EM, Caldwell SH. Hepatocellular carcinoma in non-alcoholic fatty liver disease: an emerging menace. J Hepatol 2012;56(6):1384–91.
46. Donato F, Tagger A, Gelatti U, et al. Alcohol and hepatocellular carcinoma: the effect of lifetime intake and hepatitis virus infections in men and women. Am J Epidemiol 2002;155(4):323–31.
47. El-Serag HB, Rudolph KL. Hepatocellular carcinoma: epidemiology and molecular carcinogenesis. Gastroenterology 2007;132(7):2557–76.
48. Mahale P, Torres HA, Kramer JR, et al. Hepatitis C virus infection and the risk of cancer among elderly US adults: a registry-based case-control study. Cancer 2017;123(7):1202–11.
49. Sagnelli E, Macera M, Russo A, et al. Epidemiological and etiological variations in hepatocellular carcinoma. Infection 2020;48(1):7–17.
50. Blach S, Zeuzem S, Manns M, et al. Global prevalence and genotype distribution of hepatitis C virus infection in 2015: a modelling study. Lancet Gastroenterol Hepatol 2017;2(3):161–76.

51. Fried MW, Shiffman ML, Reddy KR, et al. Peginterferon alfa-2a plus ribavirin for chronic hepatitis C virus infection. N Engl J Med 2002;347(13):975–82.
52. Morgan RL, Baack B, Smith BD, et al. Eradication of hepatitis C virus infection and the development of hepatocellular carcinoma: a meta-analysis of observational studies. Ann Intern Med 2013;158(5 Pt 1):329–37.
53. Kanwal F, Kramer J, Asch SM, et al. Risk of hepatocellular cancer in HCV patients treated with direct-acting antiviral agents. Gastroenterology 2017;153(4):996–1005.e1.
54. Okeke E, Davwar PM, Roberts L, et al. Epidemiology of Liver Cancer in Africa: Current and Future Trends. Semin Liver Dis 2020;40(2):111–23.
55. Li DK, Ren Y, Fierer DS, et al. The short-term incidence of hepatocellular carcinoma is not increased after hepatitis C treatment with direct-acting antivirals: an ERCHIVES study. Hepatology 2018;67(6):2244–53.
56. Singal AG, Rich NE, Mehta N, et al. Direct-acting antiviral therapy for hepatitis C virus infection is associated with increased survival in patients with a history of hepatocellular carcinoma. Gastroenterology 2019;157(5):1253–63.e2.
57. Lok AS, Seeff LB, Morgan TR, et al. Incidence of hepatocellular carcinoma and associated risk factors in hepatitis C-related advanced liver disease. Gastroenterology 2009;136(1):138–48.
58. Morgan TR, Ghany MG, Kim HY, et al. Outcome of sustained virological responders with histologically advanced chronic hepatitis C. Hepatology 2010;52(3):833–44.
59. Heimbach JK, Kulik LM, Finn RS, et al. AASLD guidelines for the treatment of hepatocellular carcinoma. Hepatology 2018;67(1):358–80.
60. European Association for the Study of the Liver. EASL clinical practice guidelines: management of hepatocellular carcinoma. J Hepatol 2018;69(1):182–236.
61. Vogel A, Cervantes A, Chau I, et al. Hepatocellular carcinoma: ESMO Clinical Practice Guidelines for diagnosis, treatment and follow-up. Ann Oncol 2018;29(Suppl 4):iv238–55.
62. Farhang Zangneh H, Wong WWL, Sander B, et al. Cost effectiveness of hepatocellular carcinoma surveillance after a sustained virologic response to therapy in patients with hepatitis C virus infection and advanced fibrosis. Clin Gastroenterol Hepatol 2019;17(9):1840–9.e6.
63. Kanwal F, Kramer JR, Asch SM, et al. Long-term risk of hepatocellular carcinoma in HCV patients treated with direct acting antiviral agents. Hepatology 2020;71(1):44–55.
64. Centers for Disease Control and Prevention (CDC). Vital signs: overdoses of prescription opioid pain relievers—United States, 1999–2008. MMWR Morb Mortal Wkly Rep 2011;60(43):1487.
65. Dart RC, Surratt HL, Cicero TJ, et al. Trends in opioid analgesic abuse and mortality in the United States. N Engl J Med 2015;372(3):241–8.
66. Gonzalez SA, Trotter JF. The rise of the opioid epidemic and hepatitis C-positive organs: a new era in liver transplantation. Hepatology 2018;67(4):1600–8.
67. Ghany MG, Morgan TR. Hepatitis C guidance 2019 update: American Association for the Study of Liver Diseases-Infectious Diseases Society of America recommendations for testing, managing, and treating hepatitis C virus infection. Hepatology 2020;71(2):686–721.
68. Tsui JI, Williams EC, Green PK, et al. Alcohol use and hepatitis C virus treatment outcomes among patients receiving direct antiviral agents. Drug Alcohol Depend 2016;169:101–9.

69. Blanc J-F, Doussau A, Picat M-Q, et al. Diabetes, HBV infection and smoking are independent risk factors for developing hepatocellular carcinoma on non-fibrotic liver in the NoFLIC French multicenter case-control study. Hepatology 2015; 62:132.

70. Seitz HK, Stickel F. Molecular mechanisms of alcohol-mediated carcinogenesis. Nat Rev Cancer 2007;7(8):599–612.

Lifestyle and Environmental Approaches for the Primary Prevention of Hepatocellular Carcinoma

Tracey G. Simon, MD, MPH[a,b,c], Andrew T. Chan, MD, MPH[a,b,c,d,e,f],*

KEYWORDS

- Cancer prevention • Hepatocellular carcinoma • Chemoprevention • Lifestyle
- Modifiable risk factor

KEY POINTS

- Cancer chemoprevention approaches can include primordial, primary, or secondary prevention strategies; primary prevention strategies include modification of behaviors or high-risk exposures in order to eliminate risk factors for chronic liver disease.
- Epidemiologic data show that modifiable lifestyle factors contribute to the pathogenesis of hepatocellular carcinoma (HCC), including an unhealthy diet, alcohol use, obesity, type 2 diabetes, and nonuse of certain medications, including aspirin and statins.
- Lifestyle modification or the repurposing of medications used for other conditions, including statins, aspirin, and metformin, represent novel and important strategies for the primary prevention of HCC.
- Research to define the molecular determinants of HCC could help elucidate much-needed prognostic biomarkers and thereby facilitate the design of more efficient, biomarker-driven HCC chemoprevention trials.

INTRODUCTION

Hepatocellular carcinoma (HCC) represents the third leading cause of cancer-related mortality worldwide, and is a major cause of death among patients with cirrhosis.[1] In

Grant support: NIH K24 DK098311 (A.T. Chan), NIH K23 DK122104 (T.G. Simon). Dr T.G. Simon is supported by the Harvard University Center for AIDS Research (Career Development Award). Dr A.T. Chan is a Stuart and Suzanne Steele MGH Research Scholar.
a Division of Gastroenterology, GRJ-825C, Massachusetts General Hospital, 55 Fruit Street, Boston, MA 02114, USA; b Harvard Medical School, Boston, MA, USA; c Clinical and Translational Epidemiology Unit, Massachusetts General Hospital, Boston, MA, USA; d Channing Division of Network Medicine, Department of Medicine, Brigham and Women's Hospital, Boston, MA, USA; e Broad Institute, Boston, MA, USA; f Department of Immunology and Infectious Diseases, Harvard T.H. Chan School of Public Health, Boston, MA, USA
* Corresponding author. Division of Gastroenterology, GRJ-825C, Massachusetts General Hospital, 55 Fruit Street, Boston, MA 02114.
E-mail address: achan@mgh.harvard.edu

Clin Liver Dis 24 (2020) 549–576
https://doi.org/10.1016/j.cld.2020.06.002
1089-3261/20/© 2020 Elsevier Inc. All rights reserved.

the United States, the incidence of HCC has tripled over the past 30 years, and mortalities from HCC are increasing at an alarming pace.[2,3] At present, it is recommended that patients at high risk for developing HCC undergo regular surveillance ultrasonography with assessment of alpha fetoprotein.[4] This approach has a sensitivity of 84% (95% confidence interval [CI], 76%–92%) for the detection of any-stage HCC; however, the sensitivity of ultrasonography for detecting early-stage HCC is only 47% (95% CI, 33%–61%).[5] Moreover, the accuracy of ultrasonography varies widely with body habitus and operator expertise,[6] and it is underused among high-risk populations.[7] Thus, HCC is often diagnosed at a late stage, when treatment options are limited and prognosis is poor.[8] Despite recent advances in treatment, patients diagnosed with HCC have a 5-year survival rate of less than 15%, and 70% of patients experience tumor recurrence within 5 years.[1,3] Given these alarming trends, an urgent need remains to develop effective primary prevention strategies that improve patient outcomes by preventing the development of HCC.

HCC risk varies according to the underlying cause of chronic liver disease, the severity of liver fibrosis, and individual clinical and demographic factors. Major risk factors for HCC include chronic hepatitis B virus (HBV) infection, chronic hepatitis C virus (HCV) infection, alcohol-related liver disease, and nonalcoholic fatty liver disease (NAFLD).[9,10] Most HCC tumors arise within cirrhotic livers; however, HCC may also arise in the absence of cirrhosis, particularly in patients with chronic HBV infection and NAFLD.[11–13] There are also well-established disparities in the incidence of HCC, with the highest rates observed in men and in racial and ethnic minorities.[14,15] In addition, patients with HCC are often clustered in areas of high poverty and unemployment, relative to the general population.[16] In addition, an increasing body of literature now shows that environmental and lifestyle factors play a key role in the pathogenesis of HCC, including diabetes, obesity, diet, and use of certain medications[17–21] (Fig. 1). Thus, developing comprehensive strategies for HCC prevention requires a thorough assessment of risk, based on these diverse clinical, demographic, lifestyle, and environmental factors.

Given the limited treatment options and poor prognosis of HCC, strategies focused on preventing the development of HCC would likely carry the most impact. This article outlines recent advances in understanding of modifiable HCC risk factors that could inform the development of much-needed biomarker-based strategies for HCC prevention.

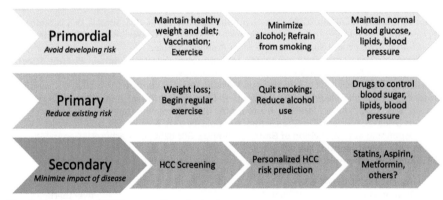

Fig. 1. Overview of HCC prevention strategies.

OVERVIEW OF HEPATOCELLULAR CARCINOMA PREVENTION STRATEGIES

HCC prevention strategies can be applied before or during the natural history of chronic liver disease, and may be categorized as primordial, primary, secondary, and tertiary prevention strategies. Primordial prevention includes behaviors and actions that maintain overall health and thereby prevent the development of risk factors for liver disease. Primary prevention is defined as the modification of behaviors or high-risk exposures in order to reduce risk factors for liver disease. Secondary and tertiary prevention includes screening and surveillance procedures that accurately identify and diagnose existing disease, facilitate early detection and timely interventions for HCC, or that minimize risk of HCC recurrence, among patients with established disease (**Fig. 2**).

When this framework is applied to HCC prevention, primordial prevention involves maintenance of a healthy body weight, eating a healthy diet with minimization of alcohol use, vaccination against HBV infection, avoiding smoking, and maintaining normal circulating blood glucose and cholesterol levels. Primary prevention of HCC includes lifestyle and behavioral modification, including making changes to adopt a healthy diet; quit smoking or reduce alcohol consumption; weight loss; or taking medications to control or reduce risk factors, including diabetes, obesity, hypertension, and/or dyslipidemia. Among patients with HBV or chronic HCV infection, the initiation of antiviral therapy is also considered primary prevention, because the control of HBV DNA or the eradication of HCV infection can control these risk factors and thereby reduce long-term HCC risk. In addition, secondary prevention for patients with high-risk disease or cirrhosis includes engagement in regular HCC surveillance, every 6 months.

HCC risk can be reduced with cause-specific treatments, which include the use of antiviral therapy to suppress HBV DNA levels or to eradicate HCV infection, among patients with chronic viral hepatitis. These cause-specific strategies have been reviewed in detail elsewhere.[22] However, even with such therapies, excess HCC risk may nevertheless persist, particularly in high-risk patients or in those with cirrhosis.[9,23] Furthermore, as the prevalence of lifestyle-related liver diseases grows, it is increasingly recognized that primary prevention strategies focused on lifestyle modification are likely to provide the most impactful benefits.[11,22] However, to date, the optimal strategy for primary HCC prevention remains undefined.

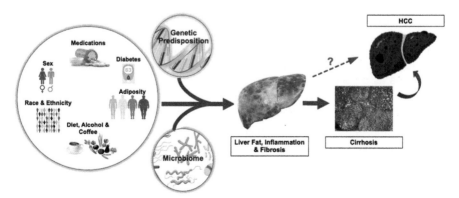

Fig. 2. Emerging risk factors for hepatocellular carcinoma (HCC).

ESTABLISHED AND EMERGING LIFESTYLE RISK FACTORS FOR HEPATOCELLULAR CARCINOMA

Accumulating preclinical, clinical, and epidemiologic evidence shows that modifiable environmental and lifestyle factors play a key role in the pathogenesis of HCC, including diet, alcohol use, obesity, type 2 diabetes, and medications (**Table 1**). Accordingly, lifestyle modification has emerged as an important strategy for the primary prevention of HCC.

Alcohol

Alcohol use represents a major underlying cause of HCC. Worldwide, approximately one-third of incident HCC cases are attributable to alcohol, although these rates vary markedly between regions.[24,25] For example, the proportion of HCC cases attributable to alcohol is estimated to be 6% in the Middle East, 14% in northern Africa, 20% in southern Europe, and as high as 63% in some eastern European countries.[26] According to the Global Burden of Disease study, approximately 854,000 new primary liver cancers were diagnosed in 2015, and there were 815,000 liver cancer–related deaths.[26] Of these recorded cases of new primary liver cancer, 245,000 cases (30%) were attributable to alcohol use, with a strong male predominance (204,000 cases).[26] In longitudinal cohort studies from France, Spain, Belgium, and Japan, the annual incidence of HCC among adults with alcoholic cirrhosis ranged between 2.1% and 5.6%.[27–30] Although prior studies have developed strategies to predict future HCC risk in this population,[27,28] large-scale validation studies are still needed. This topic represents a research area of important unmet need, for it is projected that the proportion of HCC cases attributable to alcohol is likely to increase in the coming decades, because of the improved efficacy of antiviral therapies for chronic viral hepatitis, HBV vaccination strategies, and the increasing per capita consumption of alcohol that has been recorded in regions of northern Europe, eastern Europe, and in the United States.[24,31]

Epidemiologic studies show that heavy alcohol use is independently associated with a 1.2-fold higher risk of developing incident HCC, compared with nondrinking.[32] In a meta-analysis of 19 cohorts and 4445 incident cases of HCC, alcohol consumption contributed to HCC risk in a dose-dependent manner, with 46% higher risk observed with 50 g of alcohol consumption per day, and 66% higher risk with 100 g of alcohol consumption per day.[32] This excess risk is compounded in patients with underlying liver fibrosis,[24,33,34] and alcohol contributes synergistically to the development of HCC in patients with obesity, diabetes,[33,34] and chronic HCV infection.[34] Notably, even after alcohol cessation, the excess observed HCC risk related to alcohol use seems to last for many years.[35] In a meta-analysis of 4 studies, HCC risk declined by approximately 6% per year with abstinence from alcohol; the investigators found that, for patients with cirrhosis, it takes approximately 23 years before an individual achieves the same HCC incidence rates as a nondrinker.[35]

NONALCOHOLIC FATTY LIVER DISEASE, OBESITY, AND DIABETES

Worldwide, approximately 25% of adults are affected by nonalcoholic fatty liver disease (NAFLD).[17] Closely linked to obesity and diabetes, NAFLD is thought to represent the hepatic manifestation of the metabolic syndrome. Although most patients with NAFLD have nonprogressive disease, nearly 30% of adults with NAFLD develop nonalcoholic steatohepatitis (NASH) and fibrosis, and, among those patients, between 10% and 20% progress to cirrhosis.[36] NAFLD represents the most rapidly growing

Table 1
Summary of prior studies relating lifestyle factors with hepatocellular carcinoma risk

Risk Factor	Relative Risk Estimates[a]	Proposed Mechanisms for HCC Prevention
Obesity	HR 1.95, 95% CI 1.46–2.46 for BMI >30 (vs BMI <25)[38]; HR 1.59, 95% CI 1.38–1.83 for increased WC vs normal WC[193]	Hyperinsulinemia; lipotoxicity; adipokine disruption; alterations in the gut microbiome and gut-derived metabolites[47,194–196]
Diabetes	RR 2.01, 95% CI 1.61–2.51 for diabetes (vs no diabetes)[39]	Insulin resistance, hyperglycemia cause ROS formation, lipotoxicity and increased IGF-I and IGF-II levels, which activate Wnt signaling through PI3K/B-catenin pathways[197,198]
Alcohol use	HR 1.16, 95% CI 1.01–1.34 for 3 or more drinks/d (vs nondrinking)[32]	DNA adducts alter DNA repair mechanisms and change protein structure and function; induction of the CYP2E1 enzyme, mitochondrial dysfunction, and ROS lead to cellular toxicity[199]
Diet	HR 0.68, 95% CI 0.51–0.90 for the highest quintile of the AMED score (vs the lowest quintile)[56]	Healthy diet reduces ROS formation and lipotoxicity, inhibits synthesis of proinflammatory cytokines and blocks B-catenin and COX-2 signaling pathways[75,200]
Coffee	RR 0.71 for consumption of >2 cups of coffee/d (vs none)[66]	Induction of UDP glucuronosyltransferase genes may have antioxidant and cytoprotective effects; caffeine inhibits CTGF and TGF-β[201,202]
Aspirin	HR 0.69, 95%CI 0.62–0.76 for low-dose (<163 mg/d) aspirin use (vs nonuse)[166]	Inhibition of COX-2 and proinflammatory prostaglandins may reduce angiogenesis and tumor cell proliferation,[137] by blocking protein kinase 3 and NF-kB pathways[140,141]
Statins	OR 0.63, 95%CI 0.52–0.76 for statin use (vs nonuse)[120]	Blockade of diverse carcinogenic pathways governed by Myc, PI3K-Akt, integrins, Rho-dependent kinase, NF-kB, and the Hippo signaling pathway[102–109]
Metformin	OR 0.52, 95%CI 0.40–0.68[170] for metformin use (vs nonuse)	AMPK-mediated inhibition of VEGF and HIF1A, preventing angiogenesis and cell signaling,[167,203] and suppression of hepatic progenitor cells[168]

Abbreviations: Akt, protein kinase B; AMED, Alternative Mediterranean Diet; AMPK, adenosine monophosphate-activated protein kinase; BMI, body mass index; COX-2, cyclooxygenase-2; CTGF, connective tissue growth factor; CYP2E1, cytochrome P450 2E1; HIF1A, hypoxia-inducible factor 1-alpha; HR, hazard ratio; IGF, insulinlike growth factor; NF-kB, nuclear factor kappa B; OR, odds ratio; PI3K, phosphatidylinositol 3 kinase; ROS, reactive oxygen species; RR, relative risk; TGF, transforming growth factor; UDP, uridine 5'-diphospho; VEGF, vascular endothelial growth factor; WC, waist circumference.

[a] Relative risk estimates were selected from meta-analyses (if available) or from the largest published cohort studies to date.

cause of cirrhosis in the United States, and it is also the fastest growing indication for liver transplant, among adults with HCC.[37]

Obesity and diabetes are present in 51% and 23% of patients with NAFLD,[17] and both conditions represent independent risk factors for the development of HCC. Epidemiologic studies have linked excess adiposity (defined by total body weight, body mass index [BMI], waist circumference, and so forth) to an increased risk of incident HCC,[18–20] and to a nearly 2-fold higher risk of HCC-related mortality.[38] Similarly, type 2 diabetes is significantly and independently associated with excess HCC risk.[20,39–42] In a meta-analysis of 23 cohort studies, diabetes was associated with a 2-fold higher pooled relative risk of incident HCC.[39] Furthermore, recent evidence shows that this risk increases with longer duration of type 2 diabetes,[42] with additional metabolic comorbidities,[32,42] and also that diabetes compounds HCC risk among patients with chronic viral hepatitis.[43]

There is increasing awareness of a link between NAFLD and HCC; however, clinical data are limited and conflicting regarding the precise magnitude of this risk. In a 2011 meta-analysis, the 5-year to 10-year risk estimates of HCC incidence ranged from 0% to 38% and showed marked heterogeneity, caused by the small sample sizes and limited numbers of cases of incident HCC, among the included studies.[44] This limitation was partially addressed by a 2018 retrospective cohort study of 296,707 US veterans with NAFLD and matched non-NAFLD controls, which found that a diagnosis of NAFLD was associated with a modest but statistically significant increased risk of developing HCC (incidence rate difference, 0.02 per 1000 person-years), and the highest excess risk was observed with NAFLD cirrhosis (incidence rate difference, 10.6 per 1000 person-years).[12] However, this cohort was primarily male (94%), with NAFLD and cirrhosis identified by administrative codes and/or by surrogate serum fibrosis scores; thus, future studies are still needed in unselected, population-based cohorts, including those with NAFLD histology, to establish more precise and generalizable estimates of HCC risk across the complete NAFLD histologic spectrum.

Recent evidence has also suggested that HCC risk might be increased in patients with NAFLD who do not have cirrhosis.[45] Although prospective studies are still needed to fully define this relationship, it suggests that the mechanisms that underpin NAFLD-related hepatocarcinogenesis may depend less on liver fibrosis, compared with other causes of liver disease. It has been hypothesized that these mechanisms might relate to gut microbial dysbiosis, changes in circulating gut microbiota-derived metabolites (ie, secondary bile acids or short-chain fatty acids), oxidative stress, disruption of circadian rhythms, or dysregulation of circulating and hepatic adipokines and proinflammatory cytokines.[46–50] Further research is needed in animal models and in human studies to more precisely characterize these pathways and to translate these findings to novel preventive therapies.

DIETARY PATTERNS

A growing body of clinical and epidemiologic evidence suggests that dietary patterns may influence HCC risk. Dietary patterns reflect complex combinations of nutrients and individual compounds that act synergistically within whole foods and across combinations of foods to exert biological effects, which may affect long-term health outcomes.[51] In one of the earliest observational studies of dietary patterns and incident HCC risk, male and female participants in the Shanghai Men's and Women's Health Studies who adhered to a vegetable-based dietary pattern had a significantly reduced risk of developing incident HCC.[52]

More recently, the National Cancer Institute launched the Dietary Patterns Methods Project, which compares validated indices of overall diet quality in relation to incident cancers.[53] These indices were selected based on their established associations with cancer and cardiovascular disease,[54] and include the Alternative Healthy Eating Index (AHEI), the Healthy Eating Index, the Dietary Approaches to Stop Hypertension (DASH), and the Alternate Mediterranean Diet (AMED). Since that time, 3 observational cohort studies have evaluated index-based dietary patterns in relation to HCC incidence.[21,55,56] Two of those studies were conducted in 3 large, prospective US cohort studies (the National Institutes of Health [NIH]/AARP Diet and Health Study, the Nurses' Health Study, and the Health Professionals Follow-up Study), and these found significantly lower HCC risk in participants with higher AHEI-2010 and AMED dietary scores.[21,55] The third study included 169,806 adults enrolled in the prospective Multiethnic Cohort study, and found that higher AMED dietary scores were associated with significantly lower risk of incident HCC (adjusted hazard ratio for the highest quintile vs the lowest quintile, 0.68; 95% CI, 0.51–0.90).[56] However, published evidence is not yet sufficiently robust to recommend 1 particular diet for HCC primary prevention.

INDIVIDUAL FOODS, NUTRIENTS, AND DIETARY COMPOUNDS
Fruit, Vegetables, Meat, and Fat

Consumption of fruits and vegetables has also been studied in relation to HCC incidence. In a 2014 meta-analysis of 19 studies (1.29 million subjects and 3912 cases of incident HCC), each 100-g increase in daily vegetable intake was associated with an 8% lower risk of incident HCC, among the included cohort studies (OR, 0.92; 95%CI, 0.88–0.95).[57] In contrast, a null association was found for fruit consumption and incident HCC risk.[57] Observational cohort studies and case-control studies have also evaluated the intake of red meat, white meat, and fish, in relation to incident HCC. In a meta-analysis pooling results from 9 studies, the highest category of daily red meat intake was not significantly associated with increased HCC incidence, compared with the lowest category (pooled OR, 1.10; 95% CI, 0.85–1.42).[58] In contrast, both white meat and fish consumption were significantly associated with reduced HCC risk, when the highest versus the lowest categories of consumption were compared (pooled OR for white meat and fish, 0.69; 95% CI, 0.58–0.81).[58]

Although human data regarding dietary fat intake and HCC risk are more limited, a notable study included 495,006 older adults enrolled in the prospective NIH-AARP cohort, and observed that a higher daily intake of saturated fat at baseline was associated with a significant, 1.9-fold increased risk of incident HCC (hazard ratio [HR], 1.87; 95% CI, 1.23–2.85).[59] In contrast, the prospective European Prospective Investigation into Cancer and Nutrition (EPIC) cohort study did not find a significant association between saturated fats and incident HCC risk (HR, 1.08; 95% CI, 0.88–1.34), whereas monounsaturated fats were inversely associated with HCC risk (per each 5 g/d: HR, 0.71; 95% CI, 0.55–0.92).[60]

Coffee

Coffee contains well-described antiinflammatory, antioxidant, and antifibrotic properties, and it has been observed that coffee drinkers tend to have lower risk of developing advanced liver disease, including liver fibrosis,[61] cirrhosis, and incident HCC.[62,63] Both the World Cancer Research Fund and the International Agency for Research on Cancer have also published reports supporting the beneficial effects of coffee for the prevention of HCC.[64,65]

A recent meta-analysis of 26 studies and 1825 incident HCC cases showed that consumption of at least 2 cups/d of coffee was associated with significantly reduced risk of incident HCC, with a pooled relative risk of 0.71.[66] Per each additional 2 cups of coffee consumed per day, the magnitude of observed benefit was significantly greater with caffeinated coffee (27% relative risk reduction) than with decaffeinated coffee (14% relative risk reduction).[66] Overall, the strength and consistency of the epidemiologic associations for coffee have led to recommendations for moderate coffee consumption for HCC prevention in the 2018 guidelines from the European Association for the Study of the Liver (EASL).[67] However, several important questions remain unanswered, including the optimal "dose" and preparation of coffee (ie, espresso vs drip coffee, type of coffee bean, or roasting process), the optimal timing of initiation, and the necessary duration of consumption during the natural history of liver disease to achieve meaningful risk reduction. Thus, high-quality, prospective studies are needed in well-phenotyped populations that include more specific details regarding coffee consumption.

Green Tea

Two meta-analyses have evaluated green tea consumption in relation to HCC incidence.[68,69] The most recent 2016 meta-analysis included 11 Asian cohort studies of more than 460,000 individuals and 3694 cases of liver cancer, and showed a pooled relative risk for incident HCC of 0.88 (95% CI, 0.81–0.97) when the highest category of green tea intake was compared with the lowest category.[68] In a dose-response analysis, each additional 1 cup of daily green tea was associated with a 3% reduction in HCC risk (95% CI, 0.95–1.00). In contrast, data from European cohort studies have been mixed: in the EPIC cohort, persons in the highest quintile of green tea consumption had a 59% lower risk of developing HCC (adjusted HR, 0.41; 95% CI, 0.22–0.78) compared with the lowest quintile,[70] whereas 2 prior Italian case-control studies found null associations.[71,72]

Green tea is produced by heating or steaming fresh tea leaves at high temperatures, in processes that result in minimal oxidation and thus preservation of the polyphenols (ie, catechins) within the tea. Between 50% and 75% of the primary catechins in green tea are epigallocatechin-3-gallate (EGCG), whereas the remainder include epigallocatechin, epicatechin-3-gallate, and epicatechin. In preclinical studies, EGCG inhibits carcinogenesis at numerous sites, including within the liver, albeit with potential risk of hepatotoxicity at high levels.[73] However, in an epidemiologic cohort study, higher levels of urinary catechins were associated with increased HCC risk among subjects with positive HBV surface antigens, and this excess risk was magnified in patients with low circulating retinol levels (adjusted odds ratio, 2.62; 95% CI, 1.25–5.51).[74] Given that green tea is the primary source of catechins, these data indicate that further research is needed to understand the relationship between green tea consumption and HCC risk, particularly among patients with chronic HBV infection.

Omega-3 Polyunsaturated Fatty Acids

Preclinical data suggest that intake of the omega-3 (n-3) polyunsaturated fatty acids (PUFAs), eicosapentaenoic acid (EPA), docosapentaenoic acid (DPA), and docosahexanoic acid (DHA), could prevent hepatocarcinogenesis by inhibiting the proinflammatory cyclooxygenase (COX)-2 enzyme, which in turn inhibits endogenous biosynthesis of prostaglandins and β-catenin signaling pathways,[75] while simultaneously stimulating the endogenous biosynthesis of proresolution lipid mediators. When fat-1 transgenic mice (which endogenously form n-3 PUFAs) were compared with wild-type pairs, both the size and number of hepatic tumors was reduced after diethylnitrosamine treatment, and hepatic COX-2 expression was significantly reduced, whereas levels of circulating n-3 PUFA–derived proresolution lipid mediators were significantly increased.[76] These proresolution lipid mediators, which include lipoxins, resolvins, maresins, and protectins, are also stimulated by aspirin and have been shown in murine models to mediate antitumor activity (**Fig. 3**).[77]

In a large, prospective, cohort study of 90,296 Japanese adults, consumption of an n-3 PUFA–rich diet and individual n-3 PUFA supplements was significantly and inversely associated with reduced HCC risk, in a dose-dependent manner.[78] Specifically, compared with the lowest quintiles of n-3 PUFA intake, the adjusted HRs in the highest quintiles were 0.64 for n-3 PUFA–rich fish, 0.56 for EPA, 0.64 for DPA, and 0.56 for DHA.[78] These findings are also supported by prior cohort studies that have similarly shown significant inverse associations between intake of diets rich in n-3 PUFA–rich fish or white meat, and reduced HCC risk.[79–81]

Vitamin D

Both preclinical and clinical studies have linked higher levels of vitamin D (25-hydroxyvitamin D [25(OH)D]), to reduced HCC incidence. In vitro, administration of 1-alpha,25(OH)$_2$D has proapoptotic and antiproliferative effects on numerous cancer cells,[82–84] and inhibits growth of HCC cell lines,[85] by modulating cell cycle growth via induction of p21 and p27 tumor suppressor genes and suppression of cyclins and cyclin-dependent kinases.[86,87] In humans, higher 25(OH)D levels have been associated with reduced HCC risk, with a relative risk of 0.51[88]; in contrast, low 25(OH)D$_3$ levels have been linked to excess HCC risk in patients with chronic HBV infection (adjusted HR, 1.90).[89]

Several carcinogenic signaling pathways are hypothesized to be responsive to vitamin D and its metabolites. First, 1-alpha,25(OH)$_2$D has been shown to downregulate epidermal growth factor receptor expression, which inhibits cell growth and promotes cell division, through mitogen-activated protein kinase (MAPK)–dependent pathways.[90] Second, vitamin D$_3$ might inhibit vascular endothelial growth factor–mediated endothelial cell proliferation and angiogenesis.[91,92] In addition, it has been

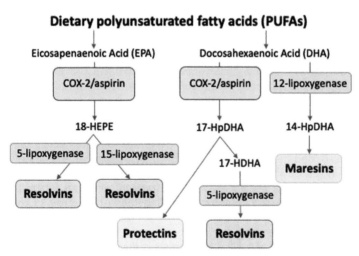

Fig. 3. Polyunsaturated fatty acids promote the endogenous biosynthesis of antiinflammatory, proresolution lipid mediators. HDHA, hydroxydocosahexanoic acid; HEPE, hydroxyeicosapentaenoic acid; HpDHA, hydroperoxydocosahexanoic acid.

posited that vitamin D might act on insulinlike growth factor (IGF) I and II signaling pathways,[93] which may in turn affect liver cancer cell proliferation.

Branched-Chain Amino Acids

Preclinical data suggest that increased circulating branched-chain amino acid (BCAA) levels might protect against hepatocarcinogenesis. In vivo, BCAA treatment enhances mammalian target of rapamycin (mTOR) signaling, which reduces both liver fibrosis and HCC.[94,95] In HCV-transgenic mice, BCAA administration reduces hepatic iron deposition and decreases reactive oxygen species (ROS) formation,[96] and, in high-fat diet–fed mice with NASH, BCAA therapy represses profibrogenic gene expression in hepatic stellate cells and protects hepatocytes from apoptosis.[97] Furthermore, in vivo, BCAA therapy suppresses expression of interleukin (IL)-6, IL-1b, IL-18, and tumor necrosis factor, reducing inflammation in both the liver and white adipose tissues, and inhibiting spontaneous HCC development.[98]

BCAA therapy has historically been used as a treatment of hepatic encephalopathy, and clinical evidence linking BCAA supplementation to HCC incidence is sparse. In a prospective study of 299 Japanese patients with cirrhosis, those provided with BCAA supplementation (5.5–12.0 g/d) had a significantly lower risk of developing incident HCC (relative risk, 0.45)[99] compared with controls. In a meta-analysis of 11 studies, oral BCAA supplementation in patients with established HCC was associated with improved mortality among Child-Pugh class B patients and among those with higher levels of albumin (standardized mean difference, 0.234), and lower rates of ascites (relative risk, 0.55).[100] More recently, in an observational study of 166 patients undergoing evaluation for liver transplant, reduced plasma levels of valine and the valine to phenylalanine ratio were significantly associated with increased overall mortality.[101]

Other Dietary Compounds

Numerous additional dietary components and phytochemicals have been examined for their potential role in HCC chemoprevention, including curcumin, resveratrol, flavonoids (including silymarin), and carotenoids. However, to date, robust clinical evidence supporting HCC preventive effects from these compounds in humans is still lacking.

STATINS

Statins, or 3-hydroxy-3-methyl-glutaryl-coenzyme A (HMG-CoA) reductase inhibitors, are prescribed for the reduction of low-density lipoprotein cholesterol levels. Beyond their cholesterol-lowering effects, statins also exert a diverse array of pleiotropic anti-inflammatory and antineoplastic effects. Both in vitro and in vivo studies show that statins block numerous carcinogenic signaling pathways, including those governed by Myc, protein kinase B (Akt), integrins, Rho-dependent kinase, nuclear factor kappa B (NF-kB), IL-6, and the Hippo pathway.[102–109] By curtailing mevalonate synthesis, statins also inhibit downstream posttranslational modification of Ras/Rho signaling proteins, which regulate cellular survival and growth, and they inhibit the cellular breakdown of p21 and p27, thereby permitting these molecules to exert potent growth-inhibitory effects.[106,110]

Statins also seem to exert direct antifibrotic actions within the liver, which may potentiate their anti-HCC benefits. Liver fibrosis is driven by the activation of hepatic stellate cells (HSCs), which undergo a phenotypic change from a quiescent state to become proliferative myofibroblasts. In preclinical studies, statins inhibit the activation and proliferation of HSCs[111–113] by upregulating Kruppel-like factor 2, a transcription factor that promotes HSC quiescence and thereby limits collagen production.[114] The administration of statins has also been shown to reduce pressures in the portal circulation, which may further limit hepatic fibrogenesis,[115] potentially through noncanonical Hedgehog signaling pathways.[116]

Observational studies largely support a link between statin use and reduced HCC risk. The authors observed a dose-dependent, inverse association between statin use and reduced risk of cirrhosis and incident HCC among US veterans with chronic HCV infection,[117] and also in a posthoc analysis of a randomized controlled trial.[118] Kaplan and colleagues[119] studied a different cohort of US veterans with new diagnoses of cirrhosis and found significant HCC risk reduction with statin use for at least 90 days, compared with nonuse. These findings have been confirmed in several large meta-analyses,[120–122] which have shown a significant, inverse association between statin use and reduced HCC risk. The observed benefits of statins were most apparent among observational studies, whereas, in contrast, posthoc analyses of prior randomized controlled trials (RCTs) of statins for cardiovascular disease have failed to show significant HCC risk reduction. However, those prior RCTs were not designed or powered to evaluate the long-term effect of statins on HCC incidence. Further, because they excluded patients with cirrhosis, they comprised study populations at very low risk for developing incident HCC.[120,121]

Emerging evidence further suggests that statin class may also influence HCC risk. Specifically, statins can be broadly divided into lipophilic and hydrophilic subclasses, and it has been hypothesized that lipophilic statins (ie, atorvastatin, simvastatin, fluvastatin, and lovastatin) may confer more potent anti-HCC effects than hydrophilic statins (ie, pravastatin, rosuvastatin). This hypothesis based on 4 lines of evidence. First, in preclinical studies, lipophilic statins suppress viral replication, potentiate antiviral therapy, and stimulate antitumor immunity to a greater degree than is observed with hydrophilic statins.[123–126] Second, in the setting of progressive liver fibrosis, the expression of organic anion transporter proteins on the surface of hepatocytes is markedly reduced, and this may prevent hydrophilic statins from entering hepatocytes, whereas lipophilic statins can passively diffuse across cell membranes.[127,128] Third, lipophilic statins limit cell growth and promote cellular apoptosis by inducing cell cycle arrest via regulation of Ras/Raf/MEK/ERK signaling.[108] Further, administration of simvastatin to hepatocyte cell lines enhances expression of the proapoptotic BAX gene and suppresses expression of the antiapoptotic BCL-2 gene, indicating that lipophilic statins can induce apoptosis by acting at the pretranslational level, as well.[129]

Epidemiologic data comparing lipophilic and hydrophilic statins are both limited and conflicting. Specifically, 2 prior studies did not identify differences in HCC risk with use of lipophilic compared with hydrophilic statins[121,130]; however, in a large, population-based cohort study of Swedish adults, the authors recently showed significantly reduced HCC risk among lipophilic statin users, compared with nonusers, whereas the relationship between hydrophilic statin use and incident HCC risk was null.[131] Although future studies are still needed to confirm these findings, such data suggest that the observed benefits associated with statin use in prior studies may have been driven by the unique, class-specific benefits of lipophilic statins.

To date, evidence supporting the use of statins for HCC chemoprevention is not yet sufficient to be incorporated into guidelines. First, published data derive primarily from observational studies, which lack the benefits of randomization and are prone to selection or confounding by indication bias. Among prior studies, only a few have appropriately balanced the prevalence of underlying HCC risk factors (such as HBV and HCV infection, alcohol-related liver disease, diabetes, obesity, and smoking status) between exposure groups.[119,131] Such imbalances could introduce confounding by indication, particularly because physicians historically have avoided prescribing statins to patients with liver disease out of concern for hepatotoxicity. Second, high-quality, prospective data are scarce regarding the optimal statin type, necessary duration of use, and the durability of statin-related treatment response, nor are sufficient data available regarding the impact of statins in patients with NAFLD or alcohol-related liver disease. In addition, it remains unknown whether there might be potential additive benefits from the concomitant use of statins together with other medications with putative anti-HCC effects, such as aspirin or metformin. Although some prior data suggest that the relationship between statin use and reduced HCC risk is not significantly modified by concurrent aspirin or antidiabetic medication use,[131] confirmatory studies are needed to validate these findings.

ASPIRIN

Preclinical evidence supports a role for aspirin in the prevention of HCC. Although the precise mechanisms remain undefined, both COX-dependent and COX-independent actions have been proposed. Specifically, the inducible, proinflammatory COX-2 enzyme is overexpressed in many cancers associated with obesity and chronic inflammation,[132,133] including HCC,[134,135] and aspirin irreversibly inhibits COX-2 expression in a dose-dependent manner.[136] COX-2 expression in hepatocytes promotes the spontaneous development of HCC in mice, by reducing tet methylcytosinedioxygenase 1 (TET1) expression, silencing tumor suppressor genes, and activating oncogenic pathways.[134] Hepatocarcinogenesis has also been linked to hepatic translocation of 2 gut microbial metabolites, lipoteichoic acid and deoxycholic acid, which promote cellular senescence and upregulate COX-2 expression, driving the production of prostaglandin E2 and suppressing antitumor immunity.[47] Moreover, by stimulating production of prostaglandins, COX-2 overexpression also promotes angiogenesis and cellular proliferation,[137–139] by activating the proinflammatory protein kinase 3, mTOR, and NF-kB signaling cascades.[134] In contrast, aspirin inhibits NF-kB activation and protein kinase 3 signaling,[140–142] and, in preclinical models, pharmacologic inhibition of COX-2 or prostaglandin E2 prevents the proliferation of liver cancer cells[135] and promotes the resolution of liver fibrosis.[143–145]

The benefits of aspirin in the liver may also derive from the inhibition of platelet activity, which has been shown to limit hepatic inflammation, fibrosis, and hepatocarcinogenesis.[146] Platelets play a central role in promoting accumulation of CD8+ T cells in the liver during chronic viral infection. They also generate platelet-derived growth factor-beta, which activates HSCs and promotes fibrosis progression in rodent models.[147] Recently, Malehmir and colleagues[148] showed in murine models that antiplatelet therapy with aspirin prevented the development of NASH and subsequent HCC via inhibition of platelet-derived glycoprotein 1b alpha, which subsequently reduced intrahepatic platelet accumulation, activation, and immune cell trafficking. Together, these lines of evidence provide additional promising mechanistic explanations for the observed hepatoprotective effects of aspirin.

Clinical evidence regarding the impact of aspirin use on HCC incidence derives exclusively from observational studies.[149–166] Although some investigators have reported conflicting results, most of these observational studies have found a significant, inverse association between aspirin use and reduced risk of incident HCC (**Table 2**). For example, within 2 prospective cohorts of US women and men, the authors showed that regular aspirin use was associated with a significant, 49% lower risk of developing incident HCC (adjusted HR, 0.51; 95% CI, 0.34–0.77), and these

Table 2
Observational studies of aspirin use and risk of hepatocellular carcinoma

Study (Author, Year)	Region	Study Design	HCC Cases (N)	Aspirin Users (N)	Total (N)	HCC Risk (OR, RR, HR; 95% CI)
Simon et al,[149] 2020	Sweden	Retrospective cohort	1612	14,205	50,275	0.69 (0.62–0.76)
Du et al,[161] 2019	China	Retrospective cohort	41	59	264	0.16 (0.04–0.71)
Lee et al,[150] 2019	Korea	Retrospective cohort	697	2123	10, 615	0.70 (0.58–0.86)
Tsoi et al,[151] 2019	Hong Kong	Retrospective cohort	9370	204,170	612,509	0.49 (0.45–0.53)
Hwang et al,[152] 2018	Korea	Prospective cohort	2336	64,782	460,755	0.87 (0.77–0.98)
Simon et al,[165] 2018	United States	Prospective cohort	108	58,855	133,371	0.51 (0.34–0.77)
Lin et al,[154] 2018	Taiwan	Retrospective cohort	110	3576	18,243	0.67 (0.42–1.08)
Tseng et al,[155] 2018	Taiwan	Retrospective cohort	1750	23,112	43,800	0.83 (0.69–0.99)
Lee et al,[157] 2017	Korea	Retrospective cohort[a]	63	343	14,392	0.34 (0.15–0.77)
Lee et al,[156] 2017	Taiwan	Retrospective cohort	NR	5602	18,080	0.70 (0.37–1.36)
Kim et al,[153] 2017	Korea	Case control	229	390	1374	0.34 (0.15–0.78)
Yang et al,[162] 2016	United Kingdom	Case control	1195	1670	5835	1.11 (0.86–1.44)
Petrick et al,[164] 2015	United States	Prospective cohort	679	477,470	1,084,133	0.68 (0.57–0.81)
Sahasrabuddhe et al,[163] 2012	United States	Prospective cohort	250	89,585	300,504	0.51 (0.35–0.75)
Chiu et al,[158] 2011	Taiwan	Case control	1166	162	2332	1.0 (0.73–1.38)
Friis et al,[160] 2003	Denmark	Retrospective cohort	21	29,470	29,470	1.0 (0.60–1.50)
Coogan et al,[159] 2000	United States	Case control	51	491	7101	0.90 (0.30–2.90)

[a] Estimates provided are from the propensity score-matched cohort.

benefits were both dose and duration dependent.[165] More recently, we confirmed these associations in a nationwide, unselected population of Swedish adults with chronic HBV or HCV infection, in whom low-dose aspirin use (<163 mg) was associated with significant, duration-dependent reductions in risk of developing incident HCC (adjusted HR, 0.69; 95% CI, 0.62–0.76) and in the risk of liver-related mortality (adjusted HR, 0.73; 95% CI, 0.67–0.81).[166] Similarly, a pooled analysis of 10 US-based prospective cohorts (with nearly 1.1 million adults, and 679 incident HCC cases) reported a pooled HR for incident HCC of 0.68 with aspirin use, compared with nonuse.[164] Although these lines of evidence are promising, additional prospective data are still needed to more fully characterize the potential benefits of aspirin across the complete spectrum of chronic liver disease, and also to quantify the potential risks of bleeding associated with aspirin use.

METFORMIN

Antidiabetic medications have also been explored as potential agents for HCC chemoprevention. Among them, the best studied is metformin, a biguanide derivative that blocks gluconeogenesis and enhances peripheral insulin sensitivity. Metformin exerts diverse antiangiogenic, antiinflammatory, and antineoplastic effects; by activating adenosine monophosphate-activated protein kinase (AMPK), metformin inhibits hypoxia-inducible factor 1 alpha and vascular endothelial growth factor signaling, which serve to block angiogenesis.[167] Metformin also suppresses hepatic progenitor cell activation[168] and can inhibit cellular proliferation by suppressing NF-kB and reducing the expression of cyclin D1.[167] Furthermore, in murine models, metformin prevents HSC activation and attenuates fibrosis,[169] and it also seems to reduce HCC development, particularly when it is initiated before the development of cirrhosis.[168]

In humans, several prior meta-analyses have shown that metformin use is associated with reduced HCC incidence. The most recent meta-analysis included 19 studies and more than 550,000 patients with diabetes, and found a 48% lower risk of incident HCC with metformin use, compared with nonuse (pooled OR, 0.52; 95% CI, 0.40–0.68).[170] Notably, the investigators found no significant reduction in HCC incidence in a subanalysis of 2 posthoc studies of prior RCTs of metformin use among patients with diabetes (pooled OR, 0.84 with metformin use vs nonuse; 95% CI, 0.10–6.83); however, those 2 prior RCTs were limited by very few cases of liver cancer, and they were not designed or powered to assess HCC end points, thus their findings should be interpreted with caution.[171]

Pioglitazone, which stimulates the nuclear receptor peroxisome proliferator-activated receptor gamma, has shown efficacy for reducing liver fat levels and inflammation in patients with established NASH[172]; however, whether this translates to reduced HCC risk is still unknown. To date, 1 case-control study reported significantly reduced HCC risk with use of pioglitazone, compared with nonuse (OR, 0.83; 95% CI, 0.72–0.95),[173] and 2 studies have found significant risk reduction with use of any thiazolidinedione medication, compared with nonuse,[174,175] although others have shown null associations.[176,177] In addition, although glucagonlike peptide-1 (GLP-1) receptor agonists have shown short-term efficacy for the resolution of NASH,[178] little is currently known about the long-term impact of GLP-1 receptor agonists or dipeptidyl peptidase-4 (DPP-4) inhibitors on HCC incidence.

OTHER POTENTIAL CHEMOPREVENTIVE DRUGS

Although published data are limited, several other medications could represent plausible agents for HCC chemoprevention, including angiotensin-converting enzyme inhibitors and menopausal hormone therapy. The renin-angiotensin axis participates in liver fibrogenesis and hepatocarcinogenesis,[179] and, by activating NF-kB, angiotensin II can promote the survival of hepatic myofibroblasts, but this effect is reversed with captopril treatment.[180] Moreover, telmisartan, an angiotensin II type 1 receptor blocker (ARB), can prevent fibrosis and HCC development in rodents.[181] In addition, it is well established that there are marked sex disparities in the incidence of HCC, with men being affected more frequently than women, leading to the hypothesis that estrogen may protect against HCC incidence. In support of this, a case-control study of 234 women with treated HCC and 282 healthy controls showed that menopausal hormone therapy use was associated with reduced odds of developing HCC.[182] A meta-analysis of 87 studies also found that variants in the estrogen receptor 1 (ESR1) gene were associated with excess HCC risk.[183] Moreover, in a large consortium of prospective US cohort studies, bilateral oophorectomy was significantly associated with increased HCC incidence (HR, 2.67; 95% CI, 1.22–5.85), after accounting for other lifestyle and clinical factors and duration of exposure to exogenous hormone therapy.[184,185]

THE POTENTIAL IMPACT OF LIFESTYLE MODIFICATION FOR HEPATOCELLULAR CARCINOMA RISK REDUCTION

Given the growing prevalence of chronic liver disease attributable to an unhealthy lifestyle, and the significant associations between high-risk lifestyle factors and excess HCC risk, HCC prevention strategies focused on adopting a low-risk lifestyle would likely offer substantial benefits. However, in order to identify priorities for public health interventions, it is important to quantify the magnitude of contribution of lifestyle factors to HCC risk. Using 2 nationwide, prospective US cohort studies, the authors recently showed that more than 80% of HCC cases could theoretically have been prevented with adherence to low-risk lifestyles. Such data underscore the enormous potential impact of primary HCC prevention efforts focused on lifestyle modification. Nevertheless, important knowledge gaps still remain. In order to translate such data into meaningful recommendations, well-designed, prospective studies are needed to define the optimal approaches to lifestyle modification to achieve clinically meaningful and durable HCC risk reduction in patients who are at high risk of developing incident HCC.

CHALLENGES AND FUTURE DIRECTIONS

Progress in the development and clinical translation of HCC prevention strategies has thus far been limited by 4 important barriers. First, despite promising associations between low-risk lifestyle factors and reduced HCC risk, data are lacking regarding the optimal approaches to lifestyle modification that might translate to effective and durable HCC risk reduction in high-risk populations. Second, the molecular mechanisms of hepatocarcinogenesis remain largely uncharacterized[11,186] because of the genetic heterogeneity of HCC tumors[187] and also suboptimal animal models,[188] which limit the ability to translate hypotheses from preclinical studies to humans. Third, research into other cancers benefits from ready access to tumor biospecimens, precursor lesions, and adjacent normal tissues, which facilitates the discovery and validation of targeted, molecular chemoprevention strategies.[189] In contrast, access to HCC specimens is more difficult, because HCC tumors may be diagnosed without confirmatory pathologic specimens. Although there have been promising recent developments in molecular tools for HCC risk prediction and in the use of liquid biopsy, the clinical utility of these approaches is not yet established.[11]

In addition, a major challenge has been the need for large numbers of subjects and prolonged follow-up times in HCC chemoprevention trials. It has been hypothesized that these requirements for large populations and prolonged follow-up are caused by the inclusion of heterogeneous study populations, which dilute potential treatment effects. For example, 2 large chemoprevention trials of low-dose interferon therapy for patients with advanced fibrosis or cirrhosis failed to show significant HCC risk reduction with treatment.[189–191] However, among patients with cirrhosis (the subgroup at highest risk of developing HCC), a significant treatment benefit was found. Thus, it is plausible that enrollment of an enriched, high-risk study population might maximize the potential to detect a treatment effect, which in turn would enable the design of more feasible and efficient clinical trials, requiring smaller numbers of patients and shorter follow-up times.[186]

In addition to risk-stratified enrollment, biomarker-based HCC chemoprevention trials are needed. To achieve this goal, such biomarkers must (1) predict future risk of HCC development, (2) predict response to chemoprevention therapy, and (3) provide insight into drug pharmacokinetics. Recently, molecular biomarkers of HCC risk have been developed and are undergoing rigorous validation for these purposes.[11] For example, liver tissue–derived transcriptomic signatures have been validated for predicting incident HCC risk among patients with cirrhosis of any cause, including chronic HBV or HCV infection, alcohol-related liver disease, and NAFLD.[192] Based on these results, enrollment was recently completed for a phase I/II clinical trial of erlotinib for the prevention of HCC in patients with cirrhosis (NCT02273362); this trial used a liver tissue transcriptomic prognostic signature as a selection factor for study enrollment and as a surrogate, biomarker-based end point. Showing that a high-risk transcriptomic signature predicts meaningful HCC risk reduction with erlotinib would form a strong scientific rationale for future biomarker-driven HCC chemoprevention trials that use molecular-based risk-stratified enrollment procedures and validated, surrogate biomarker end points for HCC.[186] Such trials would have enhanced feasibility, overcoming many of the barriers outlined earlier, and would therefore enable more rapid translation of preclinical discoveries to humans.

SUMMARY

Given the diversity of HCC and its underlying risk factors, strategies for primordial and primary HCC prevention are likely to have broad clinical applicability for patients with chronic liver disease. Lifestyle modification or the repurposing of medications such as statins, aspirin, or metformin could be readily combined with cause-specific HCC prevention strategies and might offer synergistic benefits. In parallel, research to better characterize the molecular determinants of HCC will help elucidate much-needed prognostic biomarkers and thereby enable the design of more efficient, biomarker-based HCC chemoprevention trials. Ultimately, combining lifestyle modification strategies with the use of safe, generic compounds and targeted biomarkers for predicting HCC risk could provide a robust and cost-effective strategy for HCC chemoprevention among at-risk patients with chronic liver disease.

DISCLOSURES AND CONFLICTS OF INTEREST

Dr A.T. Chan has previously served as a consultant for Bayer Pharma AG, Janssen Pharmaceuticals, Pfizer Inc, and Boehringer Ingelheim for unrelated work. Dr T.G. Simon has no disclosures and no conflicts of interest to disclose.

REFERENCES

1. Bertuccio P, Turati F, Carioli G, et al. Global trends and predictions in hepatocellular carcinoma mortality. J Hepatol 2017;67:302–9.
2. Mokdad AH, Dwyer-Lindgren L, Fitzmaurice C, et al. Trends and patterns of disparities in cancer mortality among US Counties, 1980-2014. JAMA 2017;317: 388–406.
3. Ferlay J, Colombet M, Soerjomataram I, et al. Estimating the global cancer incidence and mortality in 2018: GLOBOCAN sources and methods. Int J Cancer 2019;144:1941–53.
4. Heimbach JK, Kulik LM, Finn RS, et al. AASLD guidelines for the treatment of hepatocellular carcinoma. Hepatology 2018;67:358–80.
5. Tzartzeva K, Obi J, Rich NE, et al. Surveillance imaging and alpha fetoprotein for early detection of hepatocellular carcinoma in patients with cirrhosis: a meta-analysis. Gastroenterology 2018;154:1706–1718 e1.
6. Simmons O, Fetzer DT, Yokoo T, et al. Predictors of adequate ultrasound quality for hepatocellular carcinoma surveillance in patients with cirrhosis. Aliment Pharmacol Ther 2017;45:169–77.
7. Singal AG, Yopp AC, Gupta S, et al. Failure rates in the hepatocellular carcinoma surveillance process. Cancer Prev Res (Phila) 2012;5:1124–30.
8. Parikh ND, Singal AG, Hutton DW. Cost effectiveness of regorafenib as second-line therapy for patients with advanced hepatocellular carcinoma. Cancer 2017; 123:3725–31.
9. Schuppan D, Afdhal NH. Liver cirrhosis. Lancet 2008;371:838–51.
10. Mittal S, El-Serag HB. Epidemiology of hepatocellular carcinoma: consider the population. J Clin Gastroenterol 2013;47(Suppl):S2–6.
11. Fujiwara N, Friedman SL, Goossens N, et al. Risk factors and prevention of hepatocellular carcinoma in the era of precision medicine. J Hepatol 2018;68: 526–49.
12. Kanwal F, Kramer JR, Mapakshi S, et al. Risk of hepatocellular cancer in patients with non-alcoholic fatty liver disease. Gastroenterology 2018;155:1828–37.e2.
13. Lim J, Singal AG. Surveillance and diagnosis of hepatocellular carcinoma. Clin Liver Dis (Hoboken) 2019;13:2–5.
14. Kim AK, Singal AG. Health disparities in diagnosis and treatment of hepatocellular carcinoma. Clin Liver Dis (Hoboken) 2014;4:143–5.
15. Yu L, Sloane DA, Guo C, et al. Risk factors for primary hepatocellular carcinoma in black and white Americans in 2000. Clin Gastroenterol Hepatol 2006;4: 355–60.
16. Shebl FM, Capo-Ramos DE, Graubard BI, et al. Socioeconomic status and hepatocellular carcinoma in the United States. Cancer Epidemiol Biomarkers Prev 2012;21:1330–5.
17. Younossi ZM, Koenig AB, Abdelatif D, et al. Global epidemiology of nonalcoholic fatty liver disease-Meta-analytic assessment of prevalence, incidence, and outcomes. Hepatology 2016;64:73–84.
18. Hagstrom H, Tynelius P, Rasmussen F. High BMI in late adolescence predicts future severe liver disease and hepatocellular carcinoma: a national, population-based cohort study in 1.2 million men. Gut 2018;67:1536–42.
19. Hassan MM, Abdel-Wahab R, Kaseb A, et al. Obesity early in adulthood increases risk but does not affect outcomes of hepatocellular carcinoma. Gastroenterology 2015;149:119–29.

20. Campbell PT, Newton CC, Freedman ND, et al. Body mass index, waist circumference, diabetes, and risk of liver cancer for U.S. Adults. Cancer Res 2016;76: 6076–83.
21. Ma Y, Yang W, Simon TG, et al. Dietary patterns and risk of hepatocellular carcinoma among U.S. men and women. Hepatology 2019;70:577–86.
22. Singh S, Singh PP, Roberts LR, et al. Chemopreventive strategies in hepatocellular carcinoma. Nat Rev Gastroenterol Hepatol 2014;11:45–54.
23. Loomba R, Yang HI, Su J, et al. Synergism between obesity and alcohol in increasing the risk of hepatocellular carcinoma: a prospective cohort study. Am J Epidemiol 2013;177:333–42.
24. Pimpin L, Cortez-Pinto H, Negro F, et al. Burden of liver disease in Europe: epidemiology and analysis of risk factors to identify prevention policies. J Hepatol 2018;69:718–35.
25. Schutze M, Boeing H, Pischon T, et al. Alcohol attributable burden of incidence of cancer in eight European countries based on results from prospective cohort study. BMJ 2011;342:d1584.
26. Global Burden of Disease Liver Cancer Collaboration, Akinyemiju T, Abera S, et al. The burden of primary liver cancer and underlying etiologies from 1990 to 2015 at the global, regional, and national level: results from the global burden of disease study 2015. JAMA Oncol 2017;3:1683–91.
27. Mancebo A, Gonzalez-Dieguez ML, Cadahia V, et al. Annual incidence of hepatocellular carcinoma among patients with alcoholic cirrhosis and identification of risk groups. Clin Gastroenterol Hepatol 2013;11:95–101.
28. Ganne-Carrie N, Chaffaut C, Bourcier V, et al. Estimate of hepatocellular carcinoma incidence in patients with alcoholic cirrhosis. J Hepatol 2018;69:1274–83.
29. Kodama K, Tokushige K, Hashimoto E, et al. Hepatic and extrahepatic malignancies in cirrhosis caused by nonalcoholic steatohepatitis and alcoholic liver disease. Alcohol Clin Exp Res 2013;37(Suppl 1):E247–52.
30. Torisu Y, Ikeda K, Kobayashi M, et al. Diabetes mellitus increases the risk of hepatocarcinogenesis in patients with alcoholic cirrhosis: a preliminary report. Hepatol Res 2007;37:517–23.
31. Haughwout Sarah P, Slater ME. Apparent per capita alcohol consumption: national S, and regional trends, 1977-2016; national Institute on alcohol abuse and alcoholism, surveillance report #110. Available at: https://pubs.niaaa.nih.gov/publications/surveillance110/CONS16.htm. Accessed May 17, 2020.
32. Turati F, Galeone C, Rota M, et al. Alcohol and liver cancer: a systematic review and meta-analysis of prospective studies. Ann Oncol 2014;25:1526–35.
33. Grewal P, Viswanathen VA. Liver cancer and alcohol. Clin Liver Dis 2012;16: 839–50.
34. Hassan MM, Hwang LY, Hatten CJ, et al. Risk factors for hepatocellular carcinoma: synergism of alcohol with viral hepatitis and diabetes mellitus. Hepatology 2002;36:1206–13.
35. Heckley GA, Jarl J, Asamoah BO, et al. How the risk of liver cancer changes after alcohol cessation: a review and meta-analysis of the current literature. BMC Cancer 2011;11:446.
36. Vernon G, Baranova A, Younossi ZM. Systematic review: the epidemiology and natural history of non-alcoholic fatty liver disease and non-alcoholic steatohepatitis in adults. Aliment Pharmacol Ther 2011;34:274–85.
37. Wong RJ, Cheung R, Ahmed A. Nonalcoholic steatohepatitis is the most rapidly growing indication for liver transplantation in patients with hepatocellular carcinoma in the U.S. Hepatology 2014;59:2188–95.

38. Gupta A, Das A, Majumder K, et al. Obesity is independently associated with increased risk of hepatocellular cancer-related mortality: a systematic review and meta-analysis. Am J Clin Oncol 2018;41:874–81.

39. Wang C, Wang X, Gong G, et al. Increased risk of hepatocellular carcinoma in patients with diabetes mellitus: a systematic review and meta-analysis of cohort studies. Int J Cancer 2012;130:1639–48.

40. Lai SW, Chen PC, Liao KF, et al. Risk of hepatocellular carcinoma in diabetic patients and risk reduction associated with anti-diabetic therapy: a population-based cohort study. Am J Gastroenterol 2012;107:46–52.

41. Chen HF, Chen P, Li CY. Risk of malignant neoplasms of liver and biliary tract in diabetic patients with different age and sex stratifications. Hepatology 2010;52:155–63.

42. Simon TG, King LY, Chong DQ, et al. Diabetes, metabolic comorbidities, and risk of hepatocellular carcinoma: results from two prospective cohort studies. Hepatology 2018;67:1797–806.

43. Tan Y, Zhang X, Zhang W, et al. The influence of metabolic syndrome on the risk of hepatocellular carcinoma in patients with chronic hepatitis B infection in mainland China. Cancer Epidemiol Biomarkers Prev 2019;28:2038–46.

44. White DL, Kanwal F, El-Serag HB. Association between nonalcoholic fatty liver disease and risk for hepatocellular cancer, based on systematic review. Clin Gastroenterol Hepatol 2012;10:1342–1359 e2.

45. Mittal S, El-Serag HB, Sada YH, et al. Hepatocellular carcinoma in the absence of cirrhosis in United States veterans is associated with nonalcoholic fatty liver disease. Clin Gastroenterol Hepatol 2016;14:124–131 e1.

46. Loo TM, Kamachi F, Watanabe Y, et al. Gut microbiota promotes obesity-associated liver cancer through PGE2-mediated suppression of antitumor immunity. Cancer Discov 2017;7:522–38.

47. Yoshimoto S, Loo TM, Atarashi K, et al. Obesity-induced gut microbial metabolite promotes liver cancer through senescence secretome. Nature 2013;499:97–101.

48. Kettner NM, Voicu H, Finegold MJ, et al. Circadian homeostasis of liver metabolism suppresses hepatocarcinogenesis. Cancer Cell 2016;30:909–24.

49. Park EJ, Lee JH, Yu GY, et al. Dietary and genetic obesity promote liver inflammation and tumorigenesis by enhancing IL-6 and TNF expression. Cell 2010;140:197–208.

50. Gomes AL, Teijeiro A, Buren S, et al. Metabolic inflammation-associated IL-17A causes non-alcoholic steatohepatitis and hepatocellular carcinoma. Cancer Cell 2016;30:161–75.

51. Tapsell LC, Neale EP, Satija A, et al. Foods, nutrients, and dietary patterns: interconnections and implications for dietary guidelines. Adv Nutr 2016;7:445–54.

52. Zhang W, Xiang YB, Li HL, et al. Vegetable-based dietary pattern and liver cancer risk: results from the Shanghai women's and men's health studies. Cancer Sci 2013;104:1353–61.

53. National Cancer Institute. Applied research: cancer control and population sciences. Dietary patterns methods Project. Rockville (MD): MNCI; 2018.

54. Chiuve SE, Fung TT, Rimm EB, et al. Alternative dietary indices both strongly predict risk of chronic disease. J Nutr 2012;142:1009–18.

55. Li WQ, Park Y, McGlynn KA, et al. Index-based dietary patterns and risk of incident hepatocellular carcinoma and mortality from chronic liver disease in a prospective study. Hepatology 2014;60:588–97.

56. Bogumil D, Park SY, Le Marchand L, et al. High-quality diets are associated with reduced risk of hepatocellular carcinoma and chronic liver disease: the multiethnic cohort. Hepatol Commun 2019;3:437–47.

57. Yang Y, Zhang D, Feng N, et al. Increased intake of vegetables, but not fruit, reduces risk for hepatocellular carcinoma: a meta-analysis. Gastroenterology 2014;147:1031–42.

58. Luo J, Yang Y, Liu J, et al. Systematic review with meta-analysis: meat consumption and the risk of hepatocellular carcinoma. Aliment Pharmacol Ther 2014;39: 913–22.

59. Freedman ND, Cross AJ, McGlynn KA, et al. Association of meat and fat intake with liver disease and hepatocellular carcinoma in the NIH-AARP cohort. J Natl Cancer Inst 2010;102:1354–65.

60. Duarte-Salles T, Fedirko V, Stepien M, et al. Dietary fat, fat subtypes and hepatocellular carcinoma in a large European cohort. Int J Cancer 2015;137: 2715–28.

61. Alferink LJM, Fittipaldi J, Kiefte-de Jong JC, et al. Coffee and herbal tea consumption is associated with lower liver stiffness in the general population: the Rotterdam study. J Hepatol 2017;67:339–48.

62. Saab S, Mallam D, Cox GA 2nd, et al. Impact of coffee on liver diseases: a systematic review. Liver Int 2014;34:495–504.

63. Bravi F, Tavani A, Bosetti C, et al. Coffee and the risk of hepatocellular carcinoma and chronic liver disease: a systematic review and meta-analysis of prospective studies. Eur J Cancer Prev 2017;26:368–77.

64. Loomis D, Guyton KZ, Grosse Y, et al. Carcinogenicity of drinking coffee, mate, and very hot beverages. Lancet Oncol 2016;17:877–8.

65. World Cancer Research Fund International/American Institute for Cancer Research. Continuous update Project report: diet N, physical activity and liver cancer 2015. Available at: https://wcrf.org/sites/default/files/Liver-Cancer-2015-Report.pdf. Accessed May01, 2020.

66. Kennedy OJ, Roderick P, Buchanan R, et al. Coffee, including caffeinated and decaffeinated coffee, and the risk of hepatocellular carcinoma: a systematic review and dose-response meta-analysis. BMJ Open 2017;7:e013739.

67. European Association for the Study of the Liver. EASL clinical practice guidelines: management of hepatocellular carcinoma. J Hepatol 2018;69:182–236.

68. Huang YQ, Lu X, Min H, et al. Green tea and liver cancer risk: a meta-analysis of prospective cohort studies in Asian populations. Nutrition 2016;32:3–8.

69. Fon Sing M, Yang WS, Gao S, et al. Epidemiological studies of the association between tea drinking and primary liver cancer: a meta-analysis. Eur J Cancer Prev 2011;20:157–65.

70. Bamia C, Lagiou P, Jenab M, et al. Coffee, tea and decaffeinated coffee in relation to hepatocellular carcinoma in a European population: multicentre, prospective cohort study. Int J Cancer 2015;136:1899–908.

71. Montella M, Polesel J, La Vecchia C, et al. Coffee and tea consumption and risk of hepatocellular carcinoma in Italy. Int J Cancer 2007;120:1555–9.

72. La Vecchia C, Negri E, Franceschi S, et al. Tea consumption and cancer risk. Nutr Cancer 1992;17:27–31.

73. Lambert JD, Kennett MJ, Sang S, et al. Hepatotoxicity of high oral dose (-)-epigallocatechin-3-gallate in mice. Food Chem Toxicol 2010;48:409–16.

74. Butler LM, Huang JY, Wang R, et al. Urinary biomarkers of catechins and risk of hepatocellular carcinoma in the Shanghai Cohort Study. Am J Epidemiol 2015; 181:397–405.

75. Lim K, Han C, Dai Y, et al. Omega-3 polyunsaturated fatty acids inhibit hepato-cellular carcinoma cell growth through blocking beta-catenin and cyclooxyge-nase-2. Mol Cancer Ther 2009;8:3046–55.

76. Weylandt KH, Krause LF, Gomolka B, et al. Suppressed liver tumorigenesis in fat-1 mice with elevated omega-3 fatty acids is associated with increased omega-3 derived lipid mediators and reduced TNF-alpha. Carcinogenesis 2011;32:897–903.

77. Gilligan MM, Gartung A, Sulciner ML, et al. Aspirin-triggered proresolving medi-ators stimulate resolution in cancer. Proc Natl Acad Sci U S A 2019;116:6292–7.

78. Sawada N, Inoue M, Iwasaki M, et al. Consumption of n-3 fatty acids and fish reduces risk of hepatocellular carcinoma. Gastroenterology 2012;142:1468–75.

79. Yu SZ, Huang XE, Koide T, et al. Hepatitis B and C viruses infection, lifestyle and genetic polymorphisms as risk factors for hepatocellular carcinoma in Haimen, China. Jpn J Cancer Res 2002;93:1287–92.

80. Wang MP, Thomas GN, Ho SY, et al. Fish consumption and mortality in Hong Kong Chinese–the LIMOR study. Ann Epidemiol 2011;21:164–9.

81. Talamini R, Polesel J, Montella M, et al. Food groups and risk of hepatocellular carcinoma: a multicenter case-control study in Italy. Int J Cancer 2006;119: 2916–21.

82. Chiang KC, Chen TC. Vitamin D for the prevention and treatment of pancreatic cancer. World J Gastroenterol 2009;15:3349–54.

83. Chiang KC, Persons KS, Istfan NW, et al. Fish oil enhances the antiproliferative effect of 1alpha,25-dihydroxyvitamin D3 on liver cancer cells. Anticancer Res 2009;29:3591–6.

84. Flanagan JN, Zheng S, Chiang KC, et al. Evaluation of 19-nor-2alpha-(3-hydrox-ypropyl)-1alpha,25-dihydroxyvitamin D3 as a therapeutic agent for androgen-dependent prostate cancer. Anticancer Res 2009;29:3547–53.

85. Pourgholami MH, Akhter J, Lu Y, et al. In vitro and in vivo inhibition of liver cancer cells by 1,25-dihydroxyvitamin D3. Cancer Lett 2000;151:97–102.

86. Caputo A, Pourgholami MH, Akhter J, et al. 1,25-Dihydroxyvitamin D(3) induced cell cycle arrest in the human primary liver cancer cell line HepG2. Hepatol Res 2003;26:34–9.

87. Hager G, Formanek M, Gedlicka C, et al. 1,25(OH)2 vitamin D3 induces elevated expression of the cell cycle-regulating genes P21 and P27 in squa-mous carcinoma cell lines of the head and neck. Acta Otolaryngol 2001;121: 103–9.

88. Fedirko V, Duarte-Salles T, Bamia C, et al. Prediagnostic circulating vitamin D levels and risk of hepatocellular carcinoma in European populations: a nested case-control study. Hepatology 2014;60:1222–30.

89. Wong GL, Chan HL, Chan HY, et al. Adverse effects of vitamin D deficiency on outcomes of patients with chronic hepatitis B. Clin Gastroenterol Hepatol 2015; 13:783–790 e1.

90. Deeb KK, Trump DL, Johnson CS. Vitamin D signalling pathways in cancer: po-tential for anticancer therapeutics. Nat Rev Cancer 2007;7:684–700.

91. Chung I, Wong MK, Flynn G, et al. Differential antiproliferative effects of calcitriol on tumor-derived and matrigel-derived endothelial cells. Cancer Res 2006;66: 8565–73.

92. Iseki K, Tatsuta M, Uehara H, et al. Inhibition of angiogenesis as a mechanism for inhibition by 1alpha-hydroxyvitamin D3 and 1,25-dihydroxyvitamin D3 of co-lon carcinogenesis induced by azoxymethane in Wistar rats. Int J Cancer 1999; 81:730–3.

93. Scharf JG, Dombrowski F, Ramadori G. The IGF axis and hepatocarcinogenesis. Mol Pathol 2001;54:138–44.
94. Cha JH, Bae SH, Kim HL, et al. Branched-chain amino acids ameliorate fibrosis and suppress tumor growth in a rat model of hepatocellular carcinoma with liver cirrhosis. PLoS One 2013;8:e77899.
95. Nakano M, Nakashima A, Nagano T, et al. Branched-chain amino acids enhance premature senescence through mammalian target of rapamycin complex I-mediated upregulation of p21 protein. PLoS One 2013;8:e80411.
96. Korenaga M, Nishina S, Korenaga K, et al. Branched-chain amino acids reduce hepatic iron accumulation and oxidative stress in hepatitis C virus polyprotein-expressing mice. Liver Int 2015;35:1303–14.
97. Takegoshi K, Honda M, Okada H, et al. Branched-chain amino acids prevent hepatic fibrosis and development of hepatocellular carcinoma in a non-alcoholic steatohepatitis mouse model. Oncotarget 2017;8:18191–205.
98. Terakura D, Shimizu M, Iwasa J, et al. Preventive effects of branched-chain amino acid supplementation on the spontaneous development of hepatic preneoplastic lesions in C57BL/KsJ-db/db obese mice. Carcinogenesis 2012;33:2499–506.
99. Kawaguchi T, Shiraishi K, Ito T, et al. Branched-chain amino acids prevent hepatocarcinogenesis and prolong survival of patients with cirrhosis. Clin Gastroenterol Hepatol 2014;12:1012–1018 e1.
100. Chen L, Chen Y, Wang X, et al. Efficacy and safety of oral branched-chain amino acid supplementation in patients undergoing interventions for hepatocellular carcinoma: a meta-analysis. Nutr J 2015;14:67.
101. Kinny-Koster B, Bartels M, Becker S, et al. Plasma amino acid concentrations predict mortality in patients with end-stage liver disease. PLoS One 2016;11:e0159205.
102. Higashi T, Hayashi H, Kitano Y, et al. Statin attenuates cell proliferative ability via TAZ (WWTR1) in hepatocellular carcinoma. Med Oncol 2016;33:123.
103. Wang J, Tokoro T, Higa S, et al. Anti-inflammatory effect of pitavastatin on NF-kappaB activated by TNF-alpha in hepatocellular carcinoma cells. Biol Pharm Bull 2006;29:634–9.
104. Relja B, Meder F, Wang M, et al. Simvastatin modulates the adhesion and growth of hepatocellular carcinoma cells via decrease of integrin expression and ROCK. Int J Oncol 2011;38:879–85.
105. Roudier E, Mistafa O, Stenius U. Statins induce mammalian target of rapamycin (mTOR)-mediated inhibition of Akt signaling and sensitize p53-deficient cells to cytostatic drugs. Mol Cancer Ther 2006;5:2706–15.
106. Cao Z, Fan-Minogue H, Bellovin DI, et al. MYC phosphorylation, activation, and tumorigenic potential in hepatocellular carcinoma are regulated by HMG-CoA reductase. Cancer Res 2011;71:2286–97.
107. Yang PM, Liu YL, Lin YC, et al. Inhibition of autophagy enhances anticancer effects of atorvastatin in digestive malignancies. Cancer Res 2010;70:7699–709.
108. Sutter AP, Maaser K, Hopfner M, et al. Cell cycle arrest and apoptosis induction in hepatocellular carcinoma cells by HMG-CoA reductase inhibitors. Synergistic antiproliferative action with ligands of the peripheral benzodiazepine receptor. J Hepatol 2005;43:808–16.
109. Kah J, Wustenberg A, Keller AD, et al. Selective induction of apoptosis by HMG-CoA reductase inhibitors in hepatoma cells and dependence on p53 expression. Oncol Rep 2012;28:1077–83.

110. Rao S, Porter DC, Chen X, et al. Lovastatin-mediated G1 arrest is through inhibition of the proteasome, independent of hydroxymethyl glutaryl-CoA reductase. Proc Natl Acad Sci U S A 1999;96:7797–802.

111. Trebicka J, Hennenberg M, Odenthal M, et al. Atorvastatin attenuates hepatic fibrosis in rats after bile duct ligation via decreased turnover of hepatic stellate cells. J Hepatol 2010;53:702–12.

112. Miyaki T, Nojiri S, Shinkai N, et al. Pitavastatin inhibits hepatic steatosis and fibrosis in non-alcoholic steatohepatitis model rats. Hepatol Res 2011;41: 375–85.

113. Wang W, Zhao C, Zhou J, et al. Simvastatin ameliorates liver fibrosis via mediating nitric oxide synthase in rats with non-alcoholic steatohepatitis-related liver fibrosis. PLoS One 2013;8:e76538.

114. Marrone G, Maeso-Diaz R, Garcia-Cardena G, et al. KLF2 exerts antifibrotic and vasoprotective effects in cirrhotic rat livers: behind the molecular mechanisms of statins. Gut 2014;64(9):1434–43.

115. Abraldes JG, Albillos A, Banares R, et al. Simvastatin lowers portal pressure in patients with cirrhosis and portal hypertension: a randomized controlled trial. Gastroenterology 2009;136:1651–8.

116. Uschner FE, Ranabhat G, Choi SS, et al. Statins activate the canonical hedgehog-signaling and aggravate non-cirrhotic portal hypertension, but inhibit the non-canonical hedgehog signaling and cirrhotic portal hypertension. Sci Rep 2015;5:14573.

117. Simon TG, Bonilla H, Yan P, et al. Atorvastatin and fluvastatin are associated with dose-dependent reductions in cirrhosis and hepatocellular carcinoma, among patients with hepatitis C virus: results from ERCHIVES. Hepatology 2016;64: 47–57.

118. Simon TG, King LY, Zheng H, et al. Statin use is associated with a reduced risk of fibrosis progression in chronic hepatitis C. J Hepatol 2015;62:18–23.

119. Kaplan DE, Serper MA, Mehta R, et al. Effects of hypercholesterolemia and statin exposure on survival in a large national cohort of patients with cirrhosis. Gastroenterology 2019;156:1693–1706 e12.

120. Singh S, Singh PP, Singh AG, et al. Statins are associated with a reduced risk of hepatocellular cancer: a systematic review and meta-analysis. Gastroenterology 2013;144:323–32.

121. Shi M, Zheng H, Nie B, et al. Statin use and risk of liver cancer: an update meta-analysis. BMJ Open 2014;4:e005399.

122. Pradelli D, Soranna D, Scotti L, et al. Statins and primary liver cancer: a meta-analysis of observational studies. Eur J Cancer Prev 2013;22:229–34.

123. Syed GH, Amako Y, Siddiqui A. Hepatitis C virus hijacks host lipid metabolism. Trends Endocrinol Metab 2010;21:33–40.

124. Kapadia SB, Chisari FV. Hepatitis C virus RNA replication is regulated by host geranylgeranylation and fatty acids. Proc Natl Acad Sci U S A 2005;102:2561–6.

125. Xia Y, Xie Y, Yu Z, et al. The mevalonate pathway is a druggable target for vaccine adjuvant discovery. Cell 2018;175:1059–73.e21.

126. Bader T, Korba B. Simvastatin potentiates the anti-hepatitis B virus activity of FDA-approved nucleoside analogue inhibitors in vitro. Antiviral Res 2010;86: 241–5.

127. Kato S, Smalley S, Sadarangani A, et al. Lipophilic but not hydrophilic statins selectively induce cell death in gynaecological cancers expressing high levels of HMGCoA reductase. J Cell Mol Med 2010;14:1180–93.

128. Thakkar N, Slizgi JR, Brouwer KLR. Effect of liver disease on hepatic transporter expression and function. J Pharm Sci 2017;106:2282–94.

129. Spampanato C, De Maria S, Sarnataro M, et al. Simvastatin inhibits cancer cell growth by inducing apoptosis correlated to activation of Bax and down-regulation of BCL-2 gene expression. Int J Oncol 2012;40:935–41.

130. Tsan YT, Lee CH, Wang JD, et al. Statins and the risk of hepatocellular carcinoma in patients with hepatitis B virus infection. J Clin Oncol 2012;30:623–30.

131. Simon TG, Duberg AS, Aleman S, et al. Lipophilic statins and risk for hepatocellular carcinoma and death in patients with chronic viral hepatitis: results from a nationwide Swedish population. Ann Intern Med 2019;171:318–27.

132. Chan AT, Ogino S, Fuchs CS. Aspirin and the risk of colorectal cancer in relation to the expression of COX-2. N Engl J Med 2007;356:2131–42.

133. Singh B, Berry JA, Shoher A, et al. COX-2 overexpression increases motility and invasion of breast cancer cells. Int J Oncol 2005;26:1393–9.

134. Chen H, Cai W, Chu ESH, et al. Hepatic cyclooxygenase-2 overexpression induced spontaneous hepatocellular carcinoma formation in mice. Oncogene 2017;36:4415–26.

135. Kern MA, Schubert D, Sahi D, et al. Proapoptotic and antiproliferative potential of selective cyclooxygenase-2 inhibitors in human liver tumor cells. Hepatology 2002;36:885–94.

136. Patrono C, Garcia Rodriguez LA, Landolfi R, et al. Low-dose aspirin for the prevention of atherothrombosis. N Engl J Med 2005;353:2373–83.

137. Kim AK, Dziura J, Strazzabosco M. Nonsteroidal anti-inflammatory drug use, chronic liver disease, and hepatocellular carcinoma: the egg of columbus or another illusion? Hepatology 2013;58:819–21.

138. Hossain MA, Kim DH, Jang JY, et al. Aspirin enhances doxorubicin-induced apoptosis and reduces tumor growth in human hepatocellular carcinoma cells in vitro and in vivo. Int J Oncol 2012;40:1636–42.

139. Fajardo AM, Piazza GA. Chemoprevention in gastrointestinal physiology and disease. Anti-inflammatory approaches for colorectal cancer chemoprevention. Am J Physiol Gastrointest Liver Physiol 2015;309:G59–70.

140. Chan TA, Morin PJ, Vogelstein B, et al. Mechanisms underlying nonsteroidal antiinflammatory drug-mediated apoptosis. Proc Natl Acad Sci U S A 1998; 95:681–6.

141. Leng J, Han C, Demetris AJ, et al. Cyclooxygenase-2 promotes hepatocellular carcinoma cell growth through Akt activation: evidence for Akt inhibition in celecoxib-induced apoptosis. Hepatology 2003;38:756–68.

142. Fodera D, D'Alessandro N, Cusimano A, et al. Induction of apoptosis and inhibition of cell growth in human hepatocellular carcinoma cells by COX-2 inhibitors. Ann N Y Acad Sci 2004;1028:440–9.

143. Kanai S, Ishihara K, Kawashita E, et al. ASB14780, an Orally Active Inhibitor of Group IVA phospholipase A2, is a pharmacotherapeutic candidate for nonalcoholic fatty liver disease. J Pharmacol Exp Ther 2016;356:604–14.

144. Hu X, Cifarelli V, Sun S, et al. Major role of adipocyte prostaglandin E2 in lipolysis-induced macrophage recruitment. J Lipid Res 2016;57:663–73.

145. Paik YH, Kim JK, Lee JI, et al. Celecoxib induces hepatic stellate cell apoptosis through inhibition of Akt activation and suppresses hepatic fibrosis in rats. Gut 2009;58:1517–27.

146. Sitia G, Aiolfi R, Di Lucia P, et al. Antiplatelet therapy prevents hepatocellular carcinoma and improves survival in a mouse model of chronic hepatitis B. Proc Natl Acad Sci U S A 2012;109:E2165–72.

147. Yoshida S, Ikenaga N, Liu SB, et al. Extrahepatic platelet-derived growth factor-beta, delivered by platelets, promotes activation of hepatic stellate cells and biliary fibrosis in mice. Gastroenterology 2014;147:1378–92.

148. Malehmir M, Pfister D, Gallage S, et al. Platelet GPIbalpha is a mediator and potential interventional target for NASH and subsequent liver cancer. Nat Med 2019;25:641–55.

149. Simon TG, Duberg A, Aleman S, et al. Association of Aspirin with Hepatocellular Carcinoma and Liver-Related Mortality. N Engl J Med 2020;382(11):1018–28.

150. Lee TY, Hsu YC, Tseng HC, et al. Association of daily aspirin therapy with risk of hepatocellular carcinoma in patients with chronic hepatitis B. JAMA Intern Med 2019;179:633–40.

151. Tsoi KKF, Ho JMW, Chan FCH, et al. Long-term use of low-dose aspirin for cancer prevention: a 10-year population cohort study in Hong Kong. Int J Cancer 2019;145:267–73.

152. Hwang IC, Chang J, Kim K, et al. Aspirin Use and risk of hepatocellular carcinoma in a national cohort study of Korean adults. Sci Rep 2018;8:4968.

153. Kim G, Jang SY, Han E, et al. Effect of statin on hepatocellular carcinoma in patients with type 2 diabetes: a nationwide nested case-control study. Int J Cancer 2017;140:798–806.

154. Lin YS, Yeh CC, Huang SF, et al. Aspirin associated with risk reduction of secondary primary cancer for patients with head and neck cancer: a population-based analysis. PLoS One 2018;13:e0199014.

155. Tseng CH. Metformin and risk of hepatocellular carcinoma in patients with type 2 diabetes. Liver Int 2018;38:2018–27.

156. Lee TY, Wu JC, Yu SH, et al. The occurrence of hepatocellular carcinoma in different risk stratifications of clinically noncirrhotic nonalcoholic fatty liver disease. Int J Cancer 2017;141:1307–14.

157. Lee M, Chung GE, Lee JH, et al. Antiplatelet therapy and the risk of hepatocellular carcinoma in chronic hepatitis B patients on antiviral treatment. Hepatology 2017;66:1556–69.

158. Chiu HF, Ho SC, Chen CC, et al. Statin use and the risk of liver cancer: a population-based case–control study. Am J Gastroenterol 2011;106:894–8.

159. Coogan PF, Rosenberg L, Palmer JR, et al. Nonsteroidal anti-inflammatory drugs and risk of digestive cancers at sites other than the large bowel. Cancer Epidemiol Biomarkers Prev 2000;9:119–23.

160. Friis S, Sørensen HT, McLaughlin JK, et al. A population-based cohort study of the risk of colorectal and other cancers among users of low-dose aspirin. Br J Cancer 2003;88:684–8.

161. Du ZQ, Zhao JZ, Dong J, et al. Effect of low-dose aspirin administration on long-term survival of cirrhotic patients after splenectomy: a retrospective single-center study. World J Gastroenterol 2019;25:3798–807.

162. Yang B, Petrick JL, Chen J, et al. Associations of NSAID and paracetamol use with risk of primary liver cancer in the Clinical Practice Research Datalink. Cancer Epidemiol 2016;43:105–11.

163. Sahasrabuddhe VV, Gunja MZ, Graubard BI, et al. Nonsteroidal anti-inflammatory drug use, chronic liver disease, and hepatocellular carcinoma. J Natl Cancer Inst 2012;104:1808–14.

164. Petrick JL, Sahasrabuddhe VV, Chan AT, et al. NSAID use and risk of hepatocellular carcinoma and intrahepatic cholangiocarcinoma: the liver cancer pooling project. Cancer Prev Res (Phila) 2015;8:1156–62.

165. Simon TG, Ma Y, Ludvigsson JF, et al. Association between aspirin use and risk of hepatocellular carcinoma. JAMA Oncol 2018;4:1683–90.

166. Simon TG, Duberg AS, Aleman S, et al. Association of aspirin with hepatocellular carcinoma and liver-related mortality. N Engl J Med 2020;382:1018–28.

167. Zheng L, Yang W, Wu F, et al. Prognostic significance of AMPK activation and therapeutic effects of metformin in hepatocellular carcinoma. Clin Cancer Res 2013;19:5372–80.

168. DePeralta DK, Wei L, Ghoshal S, et al. Metformin prevents hepatocellular carcinoma development by suppressing hepatic progenitor cell activation in a rat model of cirrhosis. Cancer 2016;122:1216–27.

169. Shankaraiah RC, Callegari E, Guerriero P, et al. Metformin prevents liver tumourigenesis by attenuating fibrosis in a transgenic mouse model of hepatocellular carcinoma. Oncogene 2019;38:7035–45.

170. Ma S, Zheng Y, Xiao Y, et al. Meta-analysis of studies using metformin as a reducer for liver cancer risk in diabetic patients. Medicine (Baltimore) 2017; 96:e6888.

171. Home PD, Kahn SE, Jones NP, et al. Experience of malignancies with oral glucose-lowering drugs in the randomised controlled ADOPT (A diabetes outcome progression trial) and RECORD (rosiglitazone evaluated for cardiovascular outcomes and regulation of glycaemia in diabetes) clinical trials. Diabetologia 2010;53:1838–45.

172. Belfort R, Harrison SA, Brown K, et al. A placebo-controlled trial of pioglitazone in subjects with nonalcoholic steatohepatitis. N Engl J Med 2006;355:2297–307.

173. Chang CH, Lin JW, Wu LC, et al. Association of thiazolidinediones with liver cancer and colorectal cancer in type 2 diabetes mellitus. Hepatology 2012;55: 1462–72.

174. Hassan MM, Curley SA, Li D, et al. Association of diabetes duration and diabetes treatment with the risk of hepatocellular carcinoma. Cancer 2010;116: 1938–46.

175. Huang MY, Chung CH, Chang WK, et al. The role of thiazolidinediones in hepatocellular carcinoma risk reduction: a population-based cohort study in Taiwan. Am J Cancer Res 2017;7:1606–16.

176. Kasmari AJ, Welch A, Liu G, et al. Independent of cirrhosis, hepatocellular carcinoma risk is increased with diabetes and metabolic syndrome. Am J Med 2017;130:746 e1–7.

177. Kawaguchi T, Taniguchi E, Morita Y, et al. Association of exogenous insulin or sulphonylurea treatment with an increased incidence of hepatoma in patients with hepatitis C virus infection. Liver Int 2010;30:479–86.

178. Armstrong MJ, Gaunt P, Aithal GP, et al. Liraglutide safety and efficacy in patients with non-alcoholic steatohepatitis (LEAN): a multicentre, double-blind, randomised, placebo-controlled phase 2 study. Lancet 2016;387:679–90.

179. Hoshida Y, Fuchs BC, Tanabe KK. Prevention of hepatocellular carcinoma: potential targets, experimental models, and clinical challenges. Curr Cancer Drug Targets 2012;12:1129–59.

180. Oakley F, Teoh V, Ching ASG, et al. Angiotensin II activates I kappaB kinase phosphorylation of RelA at Ser 536 to promote myofibroblast survival and liver fibrosis. Gastroenterology 2009;136:2334–2344 e1.

181. Tamaki Y, Nakade Y, Yamauchi T, et al. Angiotensin II type 1 receptor antagonist prevents hepatic carcinoma in rats with nonalcoholic steatohepatitis. J Gastroenterol 2013;48:491–503.

182. Hassan MM, Botrus G, Abdel-Wahab R, et al. Estrogen replacement reduces risk and increases survival times of women with hepatocellular carcinoma. Clin Gastroenterol Hepatol 2017;15:1791–9.
183. Sun H, Deng Q, Pan Y, et al. Association between estrogen receptor 1 (ESR1) genetic variations and cancer risk: a meta-analysis. J BUON 2015;20:296–308.
184. McGlynn KA, Sahasrabuddhe VV, Campbell PT, et al. Reproductive factors, exogenous hormone use and risk of hepatocellular carcinoma among US women: results from the Liver Cancer Pooling Project. Br J Cancer 2015;112: 1266–72.
185. Chen HP, Shieh JJ, Chang CC, et al. Metformin decreases hepatocellular carcinoma risk in a dose-dependent manner: population-based and in vitro studies. Gut 2013;62:606–15.
186. Bode AM, Dong Z. Cancer prevention research - then and now. Nat Rev Cancer 2009;9:508–16.
187. Cancer Genome Atlas Research Network. Comprehensive and integrative genomic characterization of hepatocellular carcinoma. Cell 2017;169: 1327–41.e23.
188. Le Magnen C, Dutta A, Abate-Shen C. Optimizing mouse models for precision cancer prevention. Nat Rev Cancer 2016;16:187–96.
189. Maresso KC, Tsai KY, Brown PH, et al. Molecular cancer prevention: current status and future directions. CA Cancer J Clin 2015;65:345–83.
190. Bruix J, Poynard T, Colombo M, et al. Maintenance therapy with peginterferon alfa-2b does not prevent hepatocellular carcinoma in cirrhotic patients with chronic hepatitis C. Gastroenterology 2011;140:1990–9.
191. Lok AS, Everhart JE, Wright EC, et al. Maintenance peginterferon therapy and other factors associated with hepatocellular carcinoma in patients with advanced hepatitis C. Gastroenterology 2011;140:840–9 [quiz: e12].
192. Nakagawa S, Wei L, Song WM, et al. Molecular liver cancer prevention in cirrhosis by organ transcriptome analysis and lysophosphatidic acid pathway inhibition. Cancer Cell 2016;30:879–90.
193. Rahmani J, Kord Varkaneh H, Kontogiannis V, et al. Waist circumference and risk of liver cancer: a systematic review and meta-analysis of over 2 million cohort study participants. Liver Cancer 2020;9:6–14.
194. Esposito K, Capuano A, Giugliano D. Metabolic syndrome and cancer: holistic or reductionist? Endocrine 2014;45:362–4.
195. Vanni E, Bugianesi E. Obesity and liver cancer. Clin Liver Dis 2014;18:191–203.
196. Farrell G. Insulin resistance, obesity, and liver cancer. Clin Gastroenterol Hepatol 2014;12:117–9.
197. Michelotti GA, Machado MV, Diehl AM. NAFLD, NASH and liver cancer. Nat Rev Gastroenterol Hepatol 2013;10:656–65.
198. Gehmert S, Sadat S, Song YH, et al. The anti-apoptotic effect of IGF-1 on tissue resident stem cells is mediated via PI3-kinase dependent secreted frizzled related protein 2 (Sfrp2) release. Biochem Biophys Res Commun 2008;371: 752–5.
199. Sidharthan S, Kottilil S. Mechanisms of alcohol-induced hepatocellular carcinoma. Hepatol Int 2014;8:452–7.
200. Endres S, Ghorbani R, Kelley VE, et al. The effect of dietary supplementation with n-3 polyunsaturated fatty acids on the synthesis of interleukin-1 and tumor necrosis factor by mononuclear cells. N Engl J Med 1989;320:265–71.
201. Gressner OA, Lahme B, Rehbein K, et al. Pharmacological application of caffeine inhibits TGF-beta-stimulated connective tissue growth factor

expression in hepatocytes via PPARgamma and SMAD2/3-dependent pathways. J Hepatol 2008;49:758–67.

202. Kalthoff S, Ehmer U, Freiberg N, et al. Coffee induces expression of glucuronosyltransferases by the aryl hydrocarbon receptor and Nrf2 in liver and stomach. Gastroenterology 2010;139:1699–710, 1710.e1-2.

203. Zhou X, Chen J, Yi G, et al. Metformin suppresses hypoxia-induced stabilization of HIF-1alpha through reprogramming of oxygen metabolism in hepatocellular carcinoma. Oncotarget 2016;7:873–84.

Role of Biomarkers and Biopsy in Hepatocellular Carcinoma

Vincent L. Chen, MD, MS, Pratima Sharma, MD, MS*

KEYWORDS

- AFP • AFP-L3 • DCP • PIVKA-II • Liquid biopsy • Sequencing

KEY POINTS

- Hepatocellular surveillance with alpha-fetoprotein and ultrasound has substantially greater sensitivity for early stage hepatocellular carcinoma (HCC) than with ultrasound alone.
- Combining alpha-fetoprotein with other biomarkers (eg, GALAD score) may further improve early detection.
- Biopsy of hepatocellular carcinoma lesions is associated with risk, and there is little evidence that tumor sequencing can be used to determine systemic therapy decisions in HCC.
- More frequent use of biopsy in a research setting may improve our understanding of HCC biology and assist with development of targeted therapy in the future.

INTRODUCTION

Hepatocellular carcinoma (HCC) is the third leading cause of cancer death worldwide.[1] HCC prevalence and attributable mortality in the United States are increasing rapidly,[2,3] driven largely by increasing prevalence in alcoholic liver disease and nonalcoholic fatty liver disease, as well as peaking hepatitis C virus prevalence.[4,5]

HCC usually arises in the setting of cirrhosis, and international liver societies recommend screening for HCC in at-risk patients using biannual ultrasound (US) with or without alpha-fetoprotein (AFP) measurement.[6–8] The motivation behind these guidelines is to increase the probability of detection of early stage HCC that is amenable to curative therapy.[9,10] However, commonly used methods of HCC screening have inadequate sensitivity, especially for early stage cancer: the combination of US and AFP results in only a 63% sensitivity for detection of early stage HCC.[11] Given this

Division of Gastroenterology and Hepatology, Department of Internal Medicine, University of Michigan, 3912 Taubman Center, 1500 East Medical Center Drive, Ann Arbor, MI 48109, USA
* Corresponding author.
E-mail address: pratimas@med.umich.edu

Clin Liver Dis 24 (2020) 577–590
https://doi.org/10.1016/j.cld.2020.07.001
1089-3261/20/Published by Elsevier Inc.

liver.theclinics.com

limitation, there has been interest in developing and validating improved biomarkers for early detection of HCC, prognostication, and management.

Unlike other common malignancies, HCC can be diagnosed based on imaging characteristics without a biopsy, which reduces risks of biopsy-related complications such as tumor seeding and bleeding.[12] However, this practice may result in some limitations. First, greater than 5% of MRI-diagnosed HCC may be false positive or non-HCC lesions.[13] Second, the lack of routine liver biopsies has resulted in limited understanding of HCC at a molecular level that has hampered drug development.[14]

The purpose of this article is to review the utility of serum biomarkers in HCC detection and prognostication and potential use of liver biopsy to guide therapy decisions in HCC.

HEPATOCELLULAR CARCINOMA BIOMARKERS

HCC biomarkers include AFP, Lens culinaris agglutinin-reactive fraction of AFP (AFP-L3), and des-gamma-carboxyprothrombin (DCP).

Diagnosis and Detection

The role of AFP in HCC diagnosis has evolved over time. In early American and European HCC guidelines, high AFP levels were used as an adjunct to imaging for HCC diagnosis.[12,15] With advances in imaging methods, AFP is no longer used for HCC diagnosis but may have a role in HCC detection in conjunction with US.[6–8] There has been some controversy on the role of AFP in HCC screening. Recent American, European, and Asia-Pacific HCC guidelines are agnostic as to whether AFP should be included in HCC surveillance programs.[6–8] AFP concentration elevations greater than 20 ng/mL have been reported in up to 10% to 20% of patients with viral hepatitis or cirrhosis and may be more common with active hepatitis.[16,17] Conversely, the sensitivity of AFP alone is relatively low in early stage HCC.[17] The cost-effectiveness of AFP in addition to US-only surveillance has also been questioned,[18] although, of note, the study used estimates of sensitivity/specificity that were not restricted to early stage HCC.

More recent studies have supported the use of AFP in HCC surveillance. A recent meta-analysis found that AFP greatly increased sensitivity for early HCC over US alone from 45% to 63%, and this increase in sensitivity was robust across several subgroups including prospective studies, post-2000 studies, and studies only including patients with cirrhosis.[11] Although screening strategies with US plus AFP had lower specificity for early HCC than did US alone (84% vs 92%),[11] this relatively small decrease in specificity would likely be offset by increased probability of early detection. Trends in AFP over time may also be informative in HCC detection. One recent study of 1050 patients with hepatitis C found that an empirical Bayes model incorporating not only US and absolute AFP level but also the average of prior AFP values in that same patient had superior performance characteristics for identifying patients who went on to develop HCC than did US and AFP alone.[19] AFP is frequently incorporated into HCC surveillance in real-world cohorts,[20–24] suggesting that despite the controversy over the utility of AFP in HCC surveillance, many providers consider it useful in clinical practice.

Two other commonly used biomarkers are AFP-L3 and DCP, also known as protein induced by vitamin K absence or antagonist II. AFP comprises 3 glycoforms with distinct binding affinity to Lens culinaris agglutinin. The glycoform with the greatest affinity, AFP-L3, is upregulated in HCC compared with nonmalignant liver disease.[25] DCP is an abnormal form of prothrombin that does not undergo posttranslational modification with gamma-carboxylation. DCP levels are higher levels in patients with HCC than in those with nonmalignant liver disease. The most commonly used cut-offs are greater than 40 mAU/mL for DCP and greater than 5% to 10% for AFP-L3.[26] One meta-analysis found that for distinguishing early stage HCC from controls, AFP and DCP had similar area under the receiver operating characteristic curve (AUC) (0.75 vs 0.70), whereas that of AFP-L3 was marginally lower (0.67).[26] Notably, though, AFP-L3 and DCP are complementary to AFP, as they may be abnormal even when AFP is not.[27] In one study, AFP-L3 and DCP demonstrated similar predictive power for distinguishing HCC from chronic liver disease in patients with HCC and AFP less than 20 ng/mL (AUC 0.63 and 0.74, respectively) compared with that in all patients with HCC, and the combination of AFP, AFP-L3, and DCP had greater predictive power than did any individual marker.[26] Note that similar to prothrombin time, DCP is affected by vitamin K antagonists and cannot be used as an HCC biomarker in patients taking warfarin.

The fact that AFP-L3 and DCP provide information beyond AFP alone suggests that scores combining multiple patient characteristics and biomarkers may have greater sensitivity than individual markers in early detection of HCC. One notable recent score that has combined multiple markers with demographics is the GALAD score (*gender, age, AFP-L3%, AFP,* and *DCP*). Overall, GALAD has been shown to have excellent performance characteristics with AUC greater than 0.90 at distinguishing HCC from nonmalignant liver disease (**Table 1**).[28–32] Importantly, most of the studies on GALAD for HCC detection specifically evaluated the most clinically relevant problems of detection at an early stage and/or whether GALAD offers incremental benefit to the most commonly used HCC biomarker, AFP. In addition, GALAD scores seem to increase months or even years before clinically apparent HCC is present,[30,31] so trends in GALAD scores rather than merely absolute scores may be useful in HCC detection, similar to what has been demonstrated for AFP.[19] GALAD has shown excellent promise in large phase 2 studies (case-control) and to an extent in phase 3 (retrospective longitudinal) studies, but further validation in larger phase 3 and phase 4 (prospective screening) studies is required.[33] The Roche Elecsys GALAD score recently received Breakthrough Device Designation by the US Food and Drug Administration, allowing for streamlined market clearance/approval.

Prognosis

AFP has value both as a prognostic marker (ie, impacts survival regardless of treatment type) and predictive marker (ie, predicts response to therapy). This finding may be related to differences in cancer biology: AFP-secreting HCC tumors are more often associated with *TP53* mutations and poor differentiation.[34–36] Elevated AFP is associated with poorer outcomes in patients receiving resection,[37] liver transplantation,[38] tumor ablation,[39] transarterial chemoembolization,[40] and sorafenib.[41] In addition, AFP trends have been used to monitor response to treatments including systemic chemotherapy and ablation, and improvement in AFP has been associated with improved outcomes.[42,43]

Perhaps the best-established use of AFP as a predictive marker is with ramucirumab, a VEGFR2 inhibitor. In a randomized controlled trial, ramucirumab did not improve survival over placebo as second-line therapy in the overall cohort but on subgroup analysis and in a subsequent study led to a survival advantage (and is approved for use solely) in patients with AFP greater than 400 ng/mL.[44,45] Likewise, survival benefit to cabozantinib was greater in patients with HCC with serum AFP greater than or equal to 200 ng/mL.[46]

Table 1
Selected studies validating the GALAD score

Study, Ref	Location	HCC Patients	Controls	Results
Johnson et al,[28] 2014	UK: Birmingham and Newcastle	N = 394 27% alcohol, 11% HCV, 8% HBV	N = 439 17% HCV, 16% alcohol, 13% HBV	Birmingham: AUC 0.97 overall and 0.96 for early stage Newcastle: AUC 0.95
Berhane et al,[29] 2016	UK, Germany, Japan, Hong Kong	N = 2430 49% HCV, 21% HBV	N = 4404 40% HCV, 26% HBV, 34% other liver disease, 5% non-HCC cancer, 2% healthy	All patients: AUC 0.97/0.93/0.94 in UK/Japan/Germany Early HCC: AUC 0.93/0.91 in UK/Japan
Berhane et al,[30] 2017	Japan	N = 119	N = 2128	2247 patients under surveillance. Increase in GALAD score preceded HCC development
Best et al,[31] 2019	Germany, Japan	N = 126 (Germany) N = 26 (Japan) 100% NAFLD	N = 231 (Germany) N = 363 (Japan) 100% NAFLD	Germany: AUC 0.92 (early stage HCC), 0.93 (cirrhosis only), 0.85 (early stage HCC and cirrhosis) Japan: increase in GALAD score preceded HCC development
Yang et al,[32] 2019	US	N = 111 43% HCV, 27% NAFLD, 13% alcohol, 10% HBV	N = 180 27% NAFLD, 21% alcohol, 18% HCV, 15% HBV	AUC 0.95 overall, 0.92 for BCLC stage 0/A, 0.90 for AFP <20 ng/mL

More recently, the BALAD and BALAD-2 scores, which incorporate bilirubin, albumin, AFP-L3, AFP, and DCP, have also been used for prognostication in HCC (**Table 2**).[29,47–51] BALAD and BALAD-2 include the same variables, but BALAD considers them as either normal or abnormal, whereas BALAD-2 uses them as continuous variables. Most studies on BALAD and BALAD-2 have been conducted in patients with chronic hepatitis C in Japan, although it has been studied internationally as well. BALAD and BALAD-2 may add information beyond treatment type and conventional staging alone,[29,49–51] although this benefit is likely to be small.[48]

Other novel protein and nonprotein biomarkers

Identifying non-AFP biomarkers to predict response to systemic therapy has been challenging. The SHARP study did not identify any serum biomarkers predictive of treatment response to sorafenib.[52] Similarly, neither AFP nor c-Met were associated with response to regorafenib treatment.[53] A recent study identified a set of microRNAs and plasma proteins associated with response to regorafenib, although this requires further validation.[54]

Table 2
Selected studies validating the BALAD and BALAD 2 scores

Study, Ref	Location	HCC Patients	Results
Toyoda et al,[47] 2006	Japan, 5 institutions	N = 2600 75% HCV, 14% HBV, 2% HBV + HCV, 9% nonviral	Patients with high BALAD score were less likely to receive resection or ablation and more likely to receive systemic or no therapy. Similar prognostic significance as TNM staging
Kitai et al,[48] 2008	Japan, 5 institutions	N = 1173 75% HCV, 13% HBV, 2% HBV + HCV	BALAD was inferior to conventional and biomarker-combined Japan Integrated Staging scores
Chan et al,[49] 2015	Hong Kong, 1 institution	N = 198 100% HBV	BALAD added additional prognostic information to BCLC stage
Berhane et al,[29] 2016	UK, Germany, Japan, Hong Kong	N = 2430 49% HCV, 21% HBV	Higher BALAD-2 score associated with poorer prognosis in all countries and treatment types
Toyoda et al,[50] 2017	Japan, >750 institutions	N = 24,029 70% HCV, 16% HBV	Both BALAD and BALAD-2 associated with prognosis in multivariable analysis. BALAD-2 had predictive power across treatment types and disease causes
Wongjarupong et al,[51] 2018	US, 1 institution	N = 113 58% HCV, 12% alcohol, 12% NAFLD/cryptogenic, 10% HBV 100% liver transplant recipients	Both BALAD and BALAD-2 associated with recurrence and survival posttransplant. Tumor size plus BALAD/2 showed the best test characteristic.

Glycoprotein biomarkers, other than AFP, AFP-L3 and DCP, are also under investigation as HCC biomarkers. Glycosylation of proteins is altered in malignant transformation, including in HCC, and there has been interest in evaluating them as biomarkers for HCC detection. In a study of 42 patients with HCC and 53 patients with viral hepatitis, multifucosylated alpha-1-acid glycoprotein has been shown to have very high predictive power for HCC (AUC 0.93 for HCC vs hepatitis B).[55] Altered N-glycosylation and fucosylation of haptoglobin has been noted in HCC compared with chronic liver disease controls.[56,57] Multimarker studies are also possible in glycoproteomics. One group collected serum from 8 patients with HCC and 14 healthy controls, performed affinity chromatography followed by liquid chromatography/mass spectrometry, and identified 21 liver-expressed candidate biomarkers that were mostly found in higher levels in HCC.[58] Existing studies on glycoprotein markers in HCC have been limited in scope and require external validation before they can be recommended for clinical use.

Finally, the authors briefly discuss nonprotein biomarkers.[59] Neutrophil-lymphocyte ratio reflects systemic inflammation, which is thought to play an important role in carcinogenesis by inhibiting apoptosis and promoting angiogenesis.[60] Elevated neutrophil-lymphocyte ratio has been associated with poorer overall survival and disease-free survival in patients treated with surgical therapy and is also associated with poorer overall survival in patients receiving palliative therapy or ablation.[61] Circulating tumor cells are malignant cells that have been detached from the primary tumors and released into the circulation and can be found in most solid tumors.[62] Cell-free DNA is released into the circulation by cells and can be quantified or sequenced.[59] Extracellular vesicles are formed when cell membranes, apoptotic bodies, or lysosomes bud off and can be isolated from serum/plasma.[63] Circulating tumor cells have only modest sensitivity (70%) for HCC detection. The literature on extracellular vesicles for early HCC detection is limited by heterogeneity on which property of extracellular vesicles is evaluated: most studies investigated microRNAs, but there has been little consistency in which microRNAs were studied.[64,65] In comparison, cell-free DNA methylation profiles have demonstrated greater potential: 2 large studies from China and the United States found sensitivity and specificity of greater than 90% for distinguishing HCC from chronic liver disease and sensitivity greater than 75% in identifying early stage HCC.[66,67] Whether these methylation scores can be validated across disease causes and ethnicities remains to be seen.

ROLE OF BIOPSY IN HEPATOCELLULAR CARCINOMA
Diagnosis

Biopsy is not needed to establish the diagnosis of HCC because of high specificity of dynamic imaging (computed tomography and MRI) in identifying HCC greater than or equal to 2 cm.[6–8] In addition, patients with cirrhosis and coagulopathy are at increased risk of developing biopsy-related complications such as bleeding,[14] and tumor seeding after biopsy has been reported to be as high as 2.7%.[68] A recent meta-analysis reported a pooled specificity of both computed tomography and MRI of 91% to 92%, implying a greater than 5% false-positive rate of HCC diagnosis with imaging alone.[69]

The Liver Reporting and Data System (LIRADS) represents an attempt to standardize liver imaging and may result in a lower rate of false positives.[70,71] However, entities such as combined HCC-intrahepatic cholangiocarcinoma, metastatic lesions, and dysplastic nodules may be difficult to distinguish from HCC radiographically.[72,73] Routinely conducting liver biopsy to reduce false-positive rates has not been well studied; however, the authors acknowledge that a greater than 5% false-positive HCC diagnosis rate is significant. The standard of care in many tertiary care centers is to review most patients with a new HCC diagnosis in a multidisciplinary tumor board setting and only obtain biopsies of lesions that are not definitely HCC based on LIR-ADS criteria.

Biopsy and Precision Medicine

Precision oncology has attracted major interest recently and is a bedrock of several other cancer types. Her2/neu inhibitors improve survival in patients with Her2/neu-amplified breast cancer, alectinib and erlotinib are used for lung cancer with *EGFR* mutations and *EML4-ALK* fusions, and pembrolizumab is approved for any microsatellite instability-high or mismatch repair–deficient solid tumors.[74–77] Unfortunately, precision therapy for HCC is comparatively lacking, in part because of nonavailability of tissue to study tumor mutations and biology, as it is not standard of care to biopsy HCC, as detailed earlier.[12,14,78] Only recently has deep sequencing of human HCC tissue identified molecular subtypes with distinct prognoses.[34,79,80] Commercially available sequencing platforms such as Foundation One are frequently used in oncology to determine tissue of origin and even guide therapy or clinical trial eligibility.[81,82] Although there are comparatively few data on this topic in HCC, small sequencing studies have suggested that next-generation sequencing may yield additional insights into cancer biology.[83]

Molecular characterization of HCC has yielded substantial insight into driver mutations in HCC.[80,84–88] **Fig. 1** shows the frequency of common gene mutations in HCC. Genes consistently shown to be mutated in HCC include those involved in telomere maintenance (*TERT* promoter), WNT/beta-catenin pathways (*CTNNB1*, *AXIN1*), tumor suppressor genes (*TP53*, *TSC2*), cell cycle (*CDKN2A*), chromatin remodeling (*ARID1A*, *ARID2*), oxidative stress (*NFE2L2*), MAP kinase (*RPS6KA3*), and normal liver function (*ALB*, *APOB*).[80,84–88] Mutational profiles may differ based on disease cause. *TERT* promoter mutations may be more frequently found in NAFLD or alcohol-related HCC.[80,89] HBV-related HCC is associated with *TP53*-inactivating mutations[80,85] and

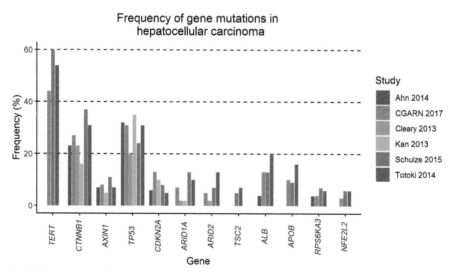

Fig. 1. Frequency of common gene mutations in HCC.

more frequently has *RB1* and less frequently has *CTNNB1* mutations compared with HCC of other causes.[87]

Recently, investigators have divided HCC into subgroups based on a combination of driver mutations and histology.[34] One subgroup is characterized by *TP53* mutations, poorly differentiated histology, and elevated AFP and carries a poorer prognosis, whereas another more often involves *CTNNB1* mutations and well-differentiated histology, with more favorable prognosis. One large recent study evaluated mutations in 801 tumors from 720 patients and found that presence of a high-risk gene expression profile was associated with poorer survival in patients undergoing resection, ablation, or noncurative therapy.[90]

Whether mutational profiles are useful in guiding therapy is an emerging topic of investigation. In one study, patients receiving sorafenib whose tumors carried *PI3K-mTOR* pathway mutations had shorter progression-free and overall survival, whereas WNT/beta-catenin mutations were also associated with poorer prognosis among patients receiving checkpoint inhibitors.[91] *FGF19* copy number amplification may also be associated with improved response to sorafenib in HCC.[92] These findings require external validation but (if patients have undergone molecular characterization of tumors) may help guide therapy, as the list of systemic therapeutics against HCC becomes increasingly diverse. Although it has been reported that greater than 20% of early stage HCC have mutations potentially targetable by Food and Drugs Administration–approved medications,[80] phase 2 studies for several of these medications in overall HCC populations have already been unsuccessful.[93–95] Whether these medications are effective among individuals carrying specific mutations remains to be determined, and ongoing studies are evaluating this possibility.[96]

SUMMARY

AFP is the oldest biomarker still in use for HCC detection and prognostication, and we support its use in HCC surveillance given the improvement in early detection sensitivity with AFP plus US over US alone. The GALAD score that combines AFP, AFP-L3, DCP, age, and sex may be an even more promising surveillance tool, although validation in larger phase 3 and 4 studies is still required. Recent research on sequencing HCC tumors has yielded substantial insights into HCC tumor biology and has raised the possibility of precision oncology in which therapy decisions are guided by cancer genetics. At this point, though, no mutational profile has been convincingly shown to predict response to HCC therapy. Given this, it has been believed that routine biopsy with sequencing of HCC is unlikely to change patient management in the short term. However, biopsy in a research setting to expand the understanding of HCC tumor genetics may assist in development of future, more effective systemic therapy for HCC.

DISCLOSURE

V.L. Chen and P. Sharma: No conflicts of interest.

REFERENCES

1. Bertuccio P, Turati F, Carioli G, et al. Global trends and predictions in hepatocellular carcinoma mortality. J Hepatol 2017;67(2):302–9.

2. Njei B, Rotman Y, Ditah I, et al. Emerging trends in hepatocellular carcinoma incidence and mortality. Hepatology 2015;61(1):191–9.

3. Tapper EB, Parikh ND. Mortality due to cirrhosis and liver cancer in the United States, 1999-2016: observational study. BMJ 2018;362:k2817.

4. Thrift AP, El-Serag HB, Kanwal F. Global epidemiology and burden of HCV infection and HCV-related disease. Nat Rev Gastroenterol Hepatol 2017;14(2):122–32.

5. Kim D, Li AA, Perumpail BJ, et al. Changing trends in etiology-based and ethnicity-based annual mortality rates of cirrhosis and hepatocellular carcinoma in the United States. Hepatology 2019;69(3):1064–74.

6. Omata M, Cheng AL, Kokudo N, et al. Asia-Pacific clinical practice guidelines on the management of hepatocellular carcinoma: a 2017 update. Hepatol Int 2017; 11(4):317–70.

7. Heimbach JK, Kulik LM, Finn RS, et al. AASLD guidelines for the treatment of hepatocellular carcinoma. Hepatology 2018;67(1):358–80.

8. Galle PR, Forner A, Llovet JM, et al. EASL clinical practice guidelines: management of hepatocellular carcinoma. J Hepatol 2018;69(1):182–236.

9. Singal AG, Mittal S, Yerokun OA, et al. Hepatocellular carcinoma screening associated with early tumor detection and improved survival among patients with cirrhosis in the US. Am J Med 2017;130(9):1099–106.e1.

10. Chen VL, Singal AG, Tapper EB, et al. Hepatocellular carcinoma surveillance, early detection, and survival in a privately-insured US cohort. Liver Int 2020; 40(4):947–55.

11. Tzartzeva K, Obi J, Rich NE, et al. Surveillance imaging and alpha fetoprotein for early detection of hepatocellular carcinoma in patients with cirrhosis: a meta-analysis. Gastroenterology 2018;154(6):1706–18.e1.

12. Bruix J, Sherman M. Management of hepatocellular carcinoma. Hepatology 2005; 42(5):1208–36.

13. Lee YJ, Lee JM, Lee JS, et al. Hepatocellular carcinoma: diagnostic performance of multidetector CT and MR imaging—a systematic review and meta-analysis. Radiology 2015;275(1):97–109.

14. Tapper EB, Lok AS. Use of liver imaging and biopsy in clinical practice. N Engl J Med 2017;377(8):756–68.

15. Bruix J, Sherman M, Llovet JM, et al. Clinical management of hepatocellular carcinoma. Conclusions of the Barcelona-2000 EASL conference. J Hepatol 2001; 35(3):421–30.

16. Fabris C, Basso DA, Leandro G, et al. Serum CA 19-9 and alpha-fetoprotein levels in primary hepatocellular carcinoma and liver cirrhosis. Cancer 1991; 68(8):1795–8.

17. Trevisani F, D'Intino PE, Morselli-Labate AM, et al. Serum α-fetoprotein for diagnosis of hepatocellular carcinoma in patients with chronic liver disease: influence of HBsAg and anti-HCV status. J Hepatol 2001;34(4):570–5.

18. Andersson KL, Salomon JA, Goldie SJ, et al. Cost effectiveness of alternative surveillance strategies for hepatocellular carcinoma in patients with cirrhosis. Clin Gastroenterol Hepatol 2008;6(12):1418–24.

19. Tayob N, Lok AS, Do KA, et al. Improved detection of hepatocellular carcinoma by using a longitudinal alpha-fetoprotein screening algorithm. Clin Gastroenterol Hepatol 2016;14(3):469–75.e2.

20. Zhao C, Jin M, Le RH, et al. Poor adherence to hepatocellular carcinoma surveillance: a systematic review and meta-analysis of a complex issue. Liver Int 2018; 38(3):503–14.

21. Farvardin S, Patel J, Khambaty M, et al. Patient-reported barriers are associated with lower hepatocellular carcinoma surveillance rates in patients with cirrhosis. Hepatology 2017;65(3):875–84.

22. Chalasani N, Said A, Ness R, et al. Screening for hepatocellular carcinoma in patients with cirrhosis in the United States: results of a national survey. Am J Gastroenterol 1999;94(8):2224–9.

23. Singal AG, Conjeevaram HS, Volk ML, et al. Effectiveness of hepatocellular carcinoma surveillance in patients with cirrhosis. Cancer Epidemiol Biomarkers Prev 2012;21(5):793–9.

24. Lun Yau AH, Galorport C, Coffin CS, et al. Hepatocellular carcinoma screening practices among patients with chronic hepatitis B by Canadian gastroenterologists and hepatologists: an online survey. Can Liver J 2019;2(4):199–209.

25. Li D, Mallory T, Satomura S. AFP-L3: a new generation of tumor marker for hepatocellular carcinoma. Clin Chim Acta 2001;313(1):15–9.

26. Lim TS, Kim DY, Han KH, et al. Combined use of AFP, PIVKA-II, and AFP-L3 as tumor markers enhances diagnostic accuracy for hepatocellular carcinoma in cirrhotic patients. Scand J Gastroenterol 2016;51(3):344–53.

27. Choi JY, Jung SW, Kim HY, et al. Diagnostic value of AFP-L3 and PIVKA-II in hepatocellular carcinoma according to total-AFP. World J Gastroenterol 2013;19(3):339–46.

28. Johnson PJ, Pirrie SJ, Cox TF, et al. The detection of hepatocellular carcinoma using a prospectively developed and validated model based on serological biomarkers. Cancer Epidemiol Biomarkers Prev 2014;23(1):144–53.

29. Berhane S, Toyoda H, Tada T, et al. Role of the GALAD and BALAD-2 serologic models in diagnosis of hepatocellular carcinoma and prediction of survival in patients. Clin Gastroenterol Hepatol 2016;14(6):875–86.e8.

30. Berhane S, Johnson PJ, Tada T, et al. Serial changes in serum biomarkers (GALAD model) prior to detection of HCC by ultrasound surveillance; application of statistical process control methodology. J Hepatol 2017;66(1):S628.

31. Best J, Bechmann LP, Sowa JP, et al. GALAD score detects early hepatocellular carcinoma in an international cohort of patients with nonalcoholic steatohepatitis. Clin Gastroenterol Hepatol 2019;18(3):728–35.e4.

32. Yang JD, Addissie BD, Mara KC, et al. GALAD score for hepatocellular carcinoma detection in comparison with liver ultrasound and proposal of GALADUS score. Cancer Epidemiol Biomarkers Prev 2019;28(3):531–8.

33. Pepe MS, Etzioni R, Feng Z, et al. Phases of biomarker development for early detection of cancer. J Natl Cancer Inst 2001;93(14):1054–61.

34. Calderaro J, Couchy G, Imbeaud S, et al. Histological subtypes of hepatocellular carcinoma are related to gene mutations and molecular tumour classification. J Hepatol 2017;67(4):727–38.

35. Yamashita T, Forgues M, Wang W, et al. EpCAM and alpha-fetoprotein expression defines novel prognostic subtypes of hepatocellular carcinoma. Cancer Res 2008;68(5):1451–61.

36. Hoshida Y, Nijman SM, Kobayashi M, et al. Integrative transcriptome analysis reveals common molecular subclasses of human hepatocellular carcinoma. Cancer Res 2009;69(18):7385–92.

37. Ma W-j, Wang H-y, Teng L-s. Correlation analysis of preoperative serum alpha-fetoprotein (AFP) level and prognosis of hepatocellular carcinoma (HCC) after hepatectomy. World J Surg Oncol 2013;11(1):212.

38. Hakeem AR, Young RS, Marangoni G, et al. Systematic review: the prognostic role of alpha-fetoprotein following liver transplantation for hepatocellular carcinoma. Aliment Pharmacol Ther 2012;35(9):987–99.

39. Thomasset SC, Dennison AR, Garcea G. Ablation for recurrent hepatocellular carcinoma: a systematic review of clinical efficacy and prognostic factors. World J Surg 2015;39(5):1150–60.

40. Wang Y, Chen Y, Ge N, et al. Prognostic significance of alpha-fetoprotein status in the outcome of hepatocellular carcinoma after treatment of transarterial chemoembolization. Ann Surg Oncol 2012;19(11):3540–6.

41. Bruix J, Cheng AL, Meinhardt G, et al. Prognostic factors and predictors of sorafenib benefit in patients with hepatocellular carcinoma: analysis of two phase III studies. J Hepatol 2017;67(5):999–1008.

42. Chan SL, Mo FK, Johnson PJ, et al. New utility of an old marker: serial alpha-fetoprotein measurement in predicting radiologic response and survival of patients with hepatocellular carcinoma undergoing systemic chemotherapy. J Clin Oncol 2009;27(3):446–52.

43. Tateishi R, Shiina S, Yoshida H, et al. Prediction of recurrence of hepatocellular carcinoma after curative ablation using three tumor markers. Hepatology 2006; 44(6):1518–27.

44. Zhu AX, Park JO, Ryoo B-Y, et al. Ramucirumab versus placebo as second-line treatment in patients with advanced hepatocellular carcinoma following first-line therapy with sorafenib (REACH): a randomised, double-blind, multicentre, phase 3 trial. Lancet Oncol 2015;16(7):859–70.

45. Zhu AX, Kang Y-K, Yen C-J, et al. Ramucirumab after sorafenib in patients with advanced hepatocellular carcinoma and increased α-fetoprotein concentrations (REACH-2): a randomised, double-blind, placebo-controlled, phase 3 trial. Lancet Oncol 2019;20(2):282–96.

46. Kelley RK, El-Khoueiry AB, Meyer T, et al. Outcomes By Baseline Alpha-Fetoprotein (AFP) Levels in the Phase 3 Celestial Trial of Cabozantinib (C) Versus Placebo (P) in Previously Treated Advanced Hepatocellular Carcinoma (HCC). Annals of Oncology 2018;29(8Supple);205-70.

47. Toyoda H, Kumada T, Osaki Y, et al. Staging hepatocellular carcinoma by a novel scoring system (BALAD score) based on serum markers. Clin Gastroenterol Hepatol 2006;4(12):1528–36.

48. Kitai S, Kudo M, Minami Y, et al. Validation of a new prognostic staging system for hepatocellular carcinoma: a comparison of the biomarker-combined Japan Integrated Staging Score, the conventional Japan Integrated Staging Score and the BALAD Score. Oncology 2008;75(Suppl 1):83–90.

49. Chan SL, Mo F, Johnson P, et al. Applicability of BALAD score in prognostication of hepatitis B-related hepatocellular carcinoma. J Gastroenterol Hepatol 2015; 30(10):1529–35.

50. Toyoda H, Tada T, Johnson PJ, et al. Validation of serological models for staging and prognostication of HCC in patients from a Japanese nationwide survey. J Gastroenterol 2017;52(10):1112–21.

51. Wongjarupong N, Negron-Ocasio GM, Chaiteerakij R, et al. Model combining pre-transplant tumor biomarkers and tumor size shows more utility in predicting hepatocellular carcinoma recurrence and survival than the BALAD models. World J Gastroenterol 2018;24(12):1321–31.

52. Llovet JM, Pena CE, Lathia CD, et al. Plasma biomarkers as predictors of outcome in patients with advanced hepatocellular carcinoma. Clin Cancer Res 2012;18(8):2290–300.

53. Teufel M, Köchert K, Meinhardt G, et al. Efficacy of regorafenib (REG) in patients with hepatocellular carcinoma (HCC) in the phase III RESORCE trial according to

alpha-fetoprotein (AFP) and c-Met levels as predictors of poor prognosis. J Clin Oncol 2017;35(15_suppl):4078.

54. Teufel M, Seidel H, Kochert K, et al. Biomarkers associated with response to regorafenib in patients with hepatocellular carcinoma. Gastroenterology 2019; 156(6):1731–41.

55. Tanabe K, Kitagawa K, Kojima N, et al. Multifucosylated alpha-1-acid glycoprotein as a novel marker for hepatocellular carcinoma. J Proteome Res 2016; 15(9):2935–44.

56. Zhu J, Lin Z, Wu J, et al. Analysis of serum haptoglobin fucosylation in hepatocellular carcinoma and liver cirrhosis of different etiologies. J Proteome Res 2014; 13(6):2986–97.

57. Zhu J, Chen Z, Zhang J, et al. Differential quantitative determination of site-specific intact n-glycopeptides in serum haptoglobin between hepatocellular carcinoma and cirrhosis using LC-EThcD-MS/MS. J Proteome Res 2019;18(1): 359–71.

58. Kaji H, Ocho M, Togayachi A, et al. Glycoproteomic discovery of serological biomarker candidates for HCV/HBV infection-associated liver fibrosis and hepatocellular carcinoma. J Proteome Res 2013;12(6):2630–40.

59. Chen VL, Parikh ND. Liquid biopsy for hepatocellular carcinoma. Curr Hepatol Rep 2019;18(4):390–9.

60. Halazun KJ, Hardy MA, Rana AA, et al. Negative impact of neutrophil-lymphocyte ratio on outcome after liver transplantation for hepatocellular carcinoma. Ann Surg 2009;250(1):141–51.

61. Xiao W-K, Chen D, Li S-Q, et al. Prognostic significance of neutrophil-lymphocyte ratio in hepatocellular carcinoma: a meta-analysis. BMC Cancer 2014;14(1):117.

62. Allard WJ, Matera J, Miller MC, et al. Tumor cells circulate in the peripheral blood of all major carcinomas but not in healthy subjects or patients with nonmalignant diseases. Clin Cancer Res 2004;10(20):6897–904.

63. EL Andaloussi S, Mager I, Breakefield XO, et al. Extracellular vesicles: biology and emerging therapeutic opportunities. Nat Rev Drug Discov 2013;12(5): 347–57.

64. Chen VL, Xu D, Wicha MS, et al. Utility of liquid biopsy analysis in detection of hepatocellular carcinoma, determination of prognosis, and disease monitoring: a systematic review. Clin Gastroenterol Hepatol 2020. https://doi.org/10.1016/j. cgh.2020.04.019.

65. Chen VL, Xu D, Harouaka R, et al. Liquid biopsy for diagnosis and prognosis in hepatocellular carcinoma: a systematic review and metaanalysis. Chicago: International Liver Cancer Association; 2019.

66. Xu RH, Wei W, Krawczyk M, et al. Circulating tumour DNA methylation markers for diagnosis and prognosis of hepatocellular carcinoma. Nat Mater 2017;16(11): 1155–61.

67. Kisiel JB, Dukek BA, Kanipakam R VSR, et al. Hepatocellular carcinoma detection by plasma methylated DNA: discovery, phase I Pilot, and Phase II clinical validation. Hepatology 2018;69(3):1180–92.

68. Silva MA, Hegab B, Hyde C, et al. Needle track seeding following biopsy of liver lesions in the diagnosis of hepatocellular cancer: a systematic review and meta-analysis. Gut 2008;57(11):1592–6.

69. Roberts LR, Sirlin CB, Zaiem F, et al. Imaging for the diagnosis of hepatocellular carcinoma: a systematic review and meta-analysis. Hepatology 2018;67(1): 401–21.

70. Chernyak V, Fowler KJ, Kamaya A, et al. Liver imaging reporting and data system (LI-RADS) Version 2018: imaging of hepatocellular carcinoma in at-risk patients. Radiology 2018;289(3):816–30.
71. van der Pol CB, Lim CS, Sirlin CB, et al. Accuracy of the liver imaging reporting and data system in computed tomography and magnetic resonance image analysis of hepatocellular carcinoma or overall malignancy-a systematic review. Gastroenterology 2019;156(4):976–86.
72. Lee H, Yoon JH, Kim H, et al. False positive diagnosis of hepatocellular carcinoma in liver resection patients. J Korean Med Sci 2017;32(2):315–20.
73. Kim MJ, Lee S, An C. Problematic lesions in cirrhotic liver mimicking hepatocellular carcinoma. Eur Radiol 2019;29(9):5101–10.
74. Romond EH, Perez EA, Bryant J, et al. Trastuzumab plus adjuvant chemotherapy for operable HER2-positive breast cancer. N Engl J Med 2005;353(16):1673–84.
75. Piccart-Gebhart MJ, Procter M, Leyland-Jones B, et al. Trastuzumab after adjuvant chemotherapy in HER2-positive breast cancer. N Engl J Med 2005; 353(16):1659–72.
76. Peters S, Camidge DR, Shaw AT, et al. Alectinib versus Crizotinib in Untreated ALK-positive non–small-cell lung cancer. N Engl J Med 2017;377(9):829–38.
77. Diaz LA, Marabelle A, Delord J-P, et al. Pembrolizumab therapy for microsatellite instability high (MSI-H) colorectal cancer (CRC) and non-CRC. J Clin Oncol 2017; 35(15_suppl):3071.
78. Bruix J, Sherman M. Management of hepatocellular carcinoma: an update. Hepatology 2011;53(3):1020–2.
79. Hoshida Y, Villanueva A, Kobayashi M, et al. Gene expression in fixed tissues and outcome in hepatocellular carcinoma. N Engl J Med 2008;359(19):1995–2004.
80. Schulze K, Imbeaud S, Letouze E, et al. Exome sequencing of hepatocellular carcinomas identifies new mutational signatures and potential therapeutic targets. Nat Genet 2015;47(5):505–11.
81. Strom SP. Current practices and guidelines for clinical next-generation sequencing oncology testing. Cancer Biol Med 2016;13(1):3–11.
82. Roychowdhury S, Iyer MK, Robinson DR, et al. Personalized oncology through integrative high-throughput sequencing: a pilot study. Sci Transl Med 2011; 3(111):111ra121.
83. Janku F, Kaseb AO, Tsimberidou AM, et al. Identification of novel therapeutic targets in the PI3K/AKT/mTOR pathway in hepatocellular carcinoma using targeted next generation sequencing. Oncotarget 2014;5(10):3012–22.
84. Cleary SP, Jeck WR, Zhao X, et al. Identification of driver genes in hepatocellular carcinoma by exome sequencing. Hepatology 2013;58(5):1693–702.
85. Kan Z, Zheng H, Liu X, et al. Whole-genome sequencing identifies recurrent mutations in hepatocellular carcinoma. Genome Res 2013;23(9):1422–33.
86. Totoki Y, Tatsuno K, Covington KR, et al. Trans-ancestry mutational landscape of hepatocellular carcinoma genomes. Nat Genet 2014;46(12):1267–73.
87. Ahn SM, Jang SJ, Shim JH, et al. Genomic portrait of resectable hepatocellular carcinomas: implications of RB1 and FGF19 aberrations for patient stratification. Hepatology 2014;60(6):1972–82.
88. Cancer Genome Atlas Research Network, Electronic address wbe, Cancer Genome Atlas Research Network. Comprehensive and integrative genomic characterization of hepatocellular carcinoma. Cell 2017;169(7):1327–41.e1.
89. Ki Kim S, Ueda Y, Hatano E, et al. TERT promoter mutations and chromosome 8p loss are characteristic of nonalcoholic fatty liver disease-related hepatocellular carcinoma. Int J Cancer 2016;139(11):2512–8.

90. Nault JC, Martin Y, Caruso S, et al. Clinical impact of genomic diversity from early to advanced hepatocellular carcinoma. Hepatology 2020;71(1):164–82.
91. Harding JJ, Nandakumar S, Armenia J, et al. Prospective genotyping of hepatocellular carcinoma: clinical implications of next-generation sequencing for matching patients to targeted and immune therapies. Clin Cancer Res 2019;25(7): 2116–26.
92. Kaibori M, Sakai K, Ishizaki M, et al. Increased FGF19 copy number is frequently detected in hepatocellular carcinoma with a complete response after sorafenib treatment. Oncotarget 2016;7(31):49091–8.
93. Zhu AX, Stuart K, Blaszkowsky LS, et al. Phase 2 study of cetuximab in patients with advanced hepatocellular carcinoma. Cancer 2007;110(3):581–9.
94. Thomas MB, Chadha R, Glover K, et al. Phase 2 study of erlotinib in patients with unresectable hepatocellular carcinoma. Cancer 2007;110(5):1059–67.
95. Zhu AX, Kudo M, Assenat E, et al. Effect of everolimus on survival in advanced hepatocellular carcinoma after failure of sorafenib: the EVOLVE-1 randomized clinical trial. JAMA 2014;312(1):57–67.
96. Lim HY, Merle P, Weiss KH, et al. Phase II studies with Refametinib or Refametinib plus sorafenib in patients with RAS-mutated hepatocellular carcinoma. Clin Cancer Res 2018;24(19):4650–61.

Hepatocellular Carcinoma

Role of Pathology in the Era of Precision Medicine

Monika Vyas, MBBS[a], Xuchen Zhang, MD, PhD[b],*

KEYWORDS

- Liver cancer • Hepatocellular carcinoma • Subtypes • Classification • Pathology

KEY POINTS

- Precise diagnosis of hepatocellular carcinoma (HCC) requires clinical, radiological, and histologic correlation.
- Ancillary tests should be used cautiously while establishing a diagnosis of HCC.
- Certain subtypes of HCC have molecular correlates that have an impact on prognosis and treatment.

INTRODUCTION

Our understanding of hepatocellular carcinoma (HCC) has evolved over the past few decades. Several new histologic variants of HCC have been identified in recent years and new underlying molecular alterations have been described. Although our prior understanding of histologic features of HCC was based on more advanced carcinoma, increasing recognition of early HCC and precursor lesions has enabled us to refine our morphologic diagnosis. Immunohistochemistry (IHC) is routinely used in the diagnosis of HCC and we have learned to interpret immunohistochemical stains with increasing caution for potential pitfalls. Molecular tests are sometimes used for diagnostic purpose (eg, in fibrolamellar HCC) but more often for finding molecular alterations for targeted therapy. Role of ancillary testing for prediction of response to immunotherapy is also being evaluated. All these advances have propelled the role of pathology from diagnosis to patient management and personalized therapy.

[a] Department of Pathology, Beth Israel Deaconess Medical Center, Harvard Medical School, 303 Brookline Avenue, Boston, MA 02215, USA; [b] Department of Pathology, Yale School of Medicine, 310 Cedar Street, PO Box 208023, New Haven, CT 06520-8023, USA
* Corresponding author.
E-mail address: xuchen.zhang@yale.edu

Clin Liver Dis 24 (2020) 591–610
https://doi.org/10.1016/j.cld.2020.07.010
1089-3261/20/© 2020 Elsevier Inc. All rights reserved.

DIAGNOSIS OF HEPATOCELLULAR CARCINOMA

Knowledge of clinical and radiologic findings is paramount for the pathologist while making the diagnosis of HCC. Clinical information, especially age, is very helpful and can point to certain diagnoses. Presence of risk factors, such as metabolic disorders, nonalcoholic steatohepatitis (NASH), and viral hepatitis, increases the likelihood of detecting abnormality in the pathology specimen. Similarly, the importance of radiologic impression cannot be overemphasized. In many instances when the radiologic impression is diagnostic, a biopsy is not deemed necessary for diagnosis and treatment. However, in presence of atypical features on imaging, a confirmation of diagnosis via biopsy is sought.[1] Biopsy diagnosis of HCC in a cirrhotic liver can be challenging not only due to limited tissue but also presence of premalignant changes. Although tissue diagnosis is considered gold standard for diagnosis of HCC, being invasive, it is less suitable for close monitoring of patients. The advent of liquid biopsy or cell free DNA is very promising, not only for surveillance of early hepatocellular lesions but also for therapeutic monitoring, detection of recurrent disease and changes in molecular profile of tumors that can be used to direct targeted therapy.[2] Attempts have been made to analyze circulating tumor cells, microRNA, cell free DNA for mutated genes (such as *RAS, TP53, CTNNB1,* and *TERT*) and DNA methylation patterns.[3] Large-scale studies will be required before liquid biopsy finds real-time applications in surveillance and management of HCC.[4]

Premalignant Lesions

What are sampled as "atypical" nodules based on imaging appearance, can represent a multitude of entities on histologic examination. Varying degrees of hepatocellular atypia has been recognized in the context of liver cirrhosis. These lesions can range from regenerative nodules to HCC, with an array of intermediate lesions, including dysplastic foci and dysplastic nodules. The diagnosis of hepatocellular neoplasia depends on identification of architectural and cytologic atypia. Normal hepatocellular architecture consists of polygonal hepatocyte lobules with a hepatic vein in the center and hepatocytes arranged in radiating cell plates of 1 to 2 cell thickness separated by sinusoids and evenly spaced portal tracts. Disturbance of the hepatocyte cell plates, plate thickening (>3 cell nuclei thick), acinar arrangement and absence of normal portal structures are suggestive of neoplasia. In addition, hepatocellular neoplasms demonstrate features of neoangiogenesis in the form of arteriolization of the sinusoids and unpaired arterioles in the lobules.[5] The concept of liver cell dysplasia is central to recognition of precancerous lesions.[6] The cytologic atypia/dysplasia can be in the form of small cell change or large cell change.[7] Small cell change is seen as foci of nuclear crowding as the cells have smaller volume, higher nuclear:cytoplasmic (N:C) ratio with mild nuclear pleomorphism. Large cell change is described as enlargement of hepatocyte and nucleus with preservation of N:C ratio, nuclear pleomorphism, hyperchromasia, or sometimes multinucleation.[6,8] Large cell change is often seen in association with regenerating hepatocytes and studies suggest that small cell change is a true form of dysplasia with higher malignant potential.[6,8]

Dysplastic foci usually measure smaller than 1 mm, identified incidentally within a regenerative nodule as these are too small to produce an independent radiologic abnormality. These are foci of hepatocellular dysplasia that do not meet the threshold for neoplasia. The nature of dysplasia can be similar to that observed in dysplastic nodules, small or large cell change, or focal iron free area.[7] There is no consensus if these incidentally identified dysplastic foci to be reported or not. However, the identification of focal iron free area in hemochromatosis or small cell change in viral chronic hepatitis often indicate higher potential to develop HCC.

Dysplastic nodules (DNs) stand out among the cirrhotic nodules because of their distinct color, texture, size, or bulging cut surface.[6] DNs are usually 5 to 15 mm in size and are, but not always, detected in cirrhotic livers. The International Consensus Group for Hepatocellular Neoplasia (ICGHN) classified nodular lesions in cirrhotic livers into macroregenerative nodule (MRN), low-grade DN (LGDN), and high-grade DN (HGDN).[9] LGDNs are often distinct from surrounding liver because of fibrous tissue around the nodule. They show mild increase in cell density (<1.3 times) and lack cytologic atypia (small cell change), although they may show large cell change.[10] They may show accumulation of iron or copper.[6] Non-triadal (unpaired) arteries are sometimes present and indicate the clonal nature of the lesion.[5,7,9] LGDN may be very difficult to distinguish from MRNs. MRNs represent cirrhotic nodules that are greater than 5 mm and stand out prominently on imaging or gross examination. On microscopic examination, they are devoid of any cytologic or architectural atypia.[7,9] Although reproducible and widely accepted criteria have not been achieved, any nodule demonstrating unpaired arteries or cytologic or architectural atypia greater than background liver that is insufficient for a diagnosis of HGDN or HCC, is considered to be a DN.[7]

HGDNs show higher degree of cytologic atypia (usually in the form of small cell change) and increased cell density (1.3–2 times), but the features are insufficient to diagnose HCC.[10] More features of neoangiogenesis (partial sinusoidal arteriolization and few non-triadal unpaired arterioles) can be seen in HGDN. Mild architectural atypia, such as thickened cell plates and rare acini, can be seen in HGDN.[6] Foci of iron loss in otherwise siderotic nodules also likely represent HGDN.[6] Sometimes foci of higher cytologic atypia are present within an HGDN, giving rise to a "nodule in nodule" appearance and most likely represent HCC arising in HGDN.[7,9] The presence of any stromal invasion in to portal tracts or fibrous septae qualifies for a diagnosis of HCC over HGDN; however, these features may not be appreciated in biopsy specimens.[7,9] HGDN has a higher risk of malignant transformation and hence, this diagnosis assumes more significance than MRN/LGDN.[6,7] Recent genetic and molecular data suggest that LGDN, HGDN, "nodule in nodule" early HCC and HCC is the likely sequence of carcinogenesis in HCC.[8,10]

Hepatocellular Carcinoma

As mentioned earlier, HCC larger than 2 cm can be diagnosed solely on radiology, if classic features are present. This 2-cm cutoff is also used to classify HCC as small HCC (≤2 cm) and conventional HCC (>2 cm). Small HCCs have been further classified into early (vaguely nodular) HCC and progressed (distinctly nodular) HCC, based on morphologic features.[9] Early HCC has well-differentiated morphology, a vaguely nodular appearance without a well-defined fibrous capsule.[11] On microscopy, early HCC may show stromal invasion, but not vascular invasion. It may have a few portal tracts and the non-triadal unpaired arterioles are often not well developed. The cell density is often at least twice the adjacent background liver. Progressed HCC have clear features of malignancy with distinct nodular architecture, destructive or pushing growth, and sometimes vascular invasion.[11] Although it is believed that progressed HCC arises from early HCC, they can also arise de novo or from preexisting HGDN.[12] Although identification of early HCC has prognostic implications, this distinction is rarely made on histologic grounds.

Conventional HCCs (>2 cm) can be well, moderately, or poorly differentiated, based on the morphology comparing with a mature, benign hepatocytes. In well and moderately differentiated HCC, the tumor cells are clearly hepatocytic in nature, and demonstrate obvious cytologic atypia, nuclear pleomorphism, thick hepatic cords (>3 cell plates thick), pseudo-acini and loss of reticulin fibers. Cells may have eosinophilic, steatotic, or sometimes clear cytoplasm. A variety of intra-hepatocytic inclusions may be seen that include Mallory-Denk bodies, bile, diastase-resistant periodic acid–Schiff positive eosinophilic globules, and pale bodies. HCC may show several cytoarchitectural patterns and morphologic subtypes, as discussed later in this article. Usually, well to moderately differentiated HCCs in a background of cirrhosis usually do not require any IHC stains to confirm their hepatocytic differentiation but may need IHC markers to make a distinction between benign and malignant nodules. Reticulin stain also helps by delineating the thick trabeculae and loss of reticulin network. Poorly differentiated HCC may show a trabecular or solid growth pattern with marked cellular pleomorphism and generally do not need IHC support for malignancy; however, may need support to prove hepatocellular lineage and distinction from other poorly differentiated epithelioid tumors.

Ancillary Tests in the Pathologic Diagnosis of Hepatocellular Carcinoma

Ancillary tests, such as immunohistochemical stains, are often used in the diagnostic workup of hepatocellular lesions (**Table 1**). Role of ancillary tests in diagnosis includes differentiation of benign versus malignant, confirmation of hepatocytic lineage and companion diagnostics for therapeutic/prognostic purposes.

Differentiation of benign versus malignant hepatic lesions

The distinction between HDN and HCC can be tricky in some cases, especially on biopsies. Reticulin stain is deemed most useful for making this distinction. Although expanded hepatic cell plates or loss of reticulin framework is diagnostic when identified, this feature may not be very well developed in early HCC.[7] Even though stromal invasion is the most reliable feature of small HCC, it is not always evident. Absence of ductular reaction in HCC can be highlighted with a CK7 and/or CK19 stain and helps differentiate it from MRNs and DNs.[13] Similarly demonstration of neoarteriolization may also be a useful feature in the diagnosis of a neoplastic hepatocellular lesion. Diffuse endothelial staining for CD34, signifying arteriolization of the sinusoids, is indicative of HCC[14]; however, this feature alone may not be reliable because vascularization can at times be seen in HDN, hepatic adenoma, and even cirrhotic nodules.

A panel of 3 immunohistochemical stains, namely, glypican 3 (GPC3), glutamine synthetase (GS), and heat shock protein 70 (HSP70), has been studied to differentiate early HCC from other benign or dysplastic hepatic nodules.[15–17] GPC3 is a cell surface heparan sulfate proteoglycan that is expressed in HCC in a diffuse cytoplasmic, membranous or Golgi pattern, but it is not expressed in normal liver or benign hepatocellular lesions such as hepatocellular adenoma or focal nodular hyperplasia (FNH).[7,14] HSP70 is a stress protein with antiapoptotic properties and is expressed in the nucleus and cytoplasm. The expression of HSP70 is found to be upregulated in HCC and hence, serves as a useful marker.[18] GS is a target of beta-catenin and increased expression has been observed not only in beta-catenin mutated HCCs but also in hepatic adenomas. Perivenular staining is normally observed in non-neoplastic livers, hence, diffuse staining in at least 50% of the tumor cells is necessary.[14] Convincing staining with at least 2 of 3 markers is considered supportive of a diagnosis of HCC; however, the sensitivity of 3 marker combination is up to 70% with specificity of 100%.[15,16] Some studies have shown that the diagnostic accuracy of the 3-marker panel (GPC3, GS, and HSP70) can be increased by addition of a fourth stain, clathrin heavy chain, especially in cases of small HCCs.[19]

Table 1
Ancillary tests used in the diagnosis of HCC

Ancillary Test or IHC	Functional Correlates	Additional Comments
Markers of hepatocellular differentiation		
Hepatocyte Paraffin-1 (Hep Par-1)	Carbamoyl phosphate synthase − 1 in urea cycle	Sensitivity and specificity >80%. Lower sensitivity in poorly differentiated and scirrhous HCC
Arginase −1	Manganese metalloproteinase enzyme in urea cycle	Sensitivity and specificity >90%
Albumin (by RNA-ISH)	Protein synthesized only in the liver	Sensitivity >90% and highly specific
Polyclonal CEA	Glycoprotein in the glycocalyx of the cells	Canalicular staining pattern specific for liver, overall sensitivity is low and positivity can be seen in other adenocarcinomas
CD10	Membrane metalloendopeptidase	Canalicular staining pattern is specific for liver
Bile salt export protein (BSEP)	ATP-binding transmembrane protein in the canalicular membrane	Canalicular staining pattern in hepatic parenchyma
Markers used for distinguishing benign from malignant		
Glypican-3 (GPC-3)	Heparan sulfate proteoglycan present in fetal liver, oncofetal protein	Sensitivity −50%−80% Also expressed in other tumors including germ cell tumors
Alpha fetoprotein	Oncofetal protein (produced by primitive liver and yolk sac)	Low sensitivity −25%−50% Not specific, positive in yolk sac tumors and other fetal type tumors
Heat shock protein (HSP)-70	Antiapoptotic stress protein	Used in conjunction with GPC-3 and GS
Glutamine synthetase (GS)	Enzyme of nitrogen metabolism. Overexpression is seen with beta-catenin mutations	Pericentral staining- Normal liver "Geographic" staining - focal nodular hyperplasia Diffuse (>50%) staining- HCC and beta-catenin mutated hepatocellular adenoma
CD34	Marker of endothelial differentiation	Positive staining in HCC sinusoids (capillarization/ arterialization) signifies neoangiogenesis and hence higher rate of malignant transformation
Reticulin	Constituent of the supporting framework of hepatic parenchyma	Disturbance/expansion of trabeculae (>3 cell thickness) signifies malignancy

Abbreviations: CEA, carcinoembryonic antigen; HCC, hepatocellular carcinoma; IHC, immunohistochemistry.

Confirmation hepatocytic lineage

Confirmation of hepatocellular phenotype is not generally necessary in well-differentiated hepatic neoplasms; however, the differential diagnosis of moderately to poorly differentiated hepatic neoplasms is broad and includes a host of neoplasms that exhibit epithelioid morphology. The markers that are useful in this context are Arginase, HepPar-1, polyclonal carcinoembryonic antigen (pCEA)/CD10 (canalicular pattern), alpha-fetal protein (AFP), and recently described albumin RNA by in situ hybridization (ISH).

Aginase-1 has been touted to be the most sensitive and specific marker of hepatocellular differentiation.[20] It is an enzyme involved in urea cycle and it displays diffuse cytoplasmic staining with variable nuclear reactivity. Interestingly, it is also positive in hepatoid neoplasms found elsewhere in the body or positive in adenocarcinomas of pancreatic, colorectal, and breast origin.[21,22] It is important to remember that it can be negative in a subset of well-differentiated hepatocellular carcinomas.[23,24] HepPar-1 is a monoclonal antibody that recognizes carbamyl phosphatase 1, an enzyme in the urea cycle. IHC stain is typically seen as a diffuse cytoplasmic granular pattern. HepPar-1 is a useful marker for diagnosis HCC and is positive in about 80% HCCs.[14] HepPar-1 has low sensitivity in poorly differentiated (50%–60%) and scirrhous subtype (20%–30%) HCCs.[25,26] Although most adenocarcinomas are negative, HepPar-1 can be positive in hepatoid carcinomas, and carcinomas of esophageal, lung, pancreatic, urothelial, adrenocortical, colorectal, duodenal, prostatic, and uterine cervical origins.[14,27,28] The polyclonal CEA cross-reacts with biliary glycoprotein and yields a typical canalicular pattern, which is seen in 80% to 90% of well-differentiated to moderately differentiated HCCs.[25] However, the canalicular pattern can be misinterpreted as adenocarcinoma when weak canalicular or luminal staining occurs, and can be confused with the luminal or membranous staining seen in adenocarcinomas when there is intense canalicular staining.[29] The sensitivity of pCEA is low in poorly differentiated HCC (25%–50%) and scirrhous HCC (37%).[25,26,30] CD10 IHC shows similar canalicular staining pattern as that of pCEA.[29] Although AFP, an oncofetal protein produced by liver is a marker of hepatocellular differentiation, it has a low sensitivity of 25% to 50% for HCC, and its staining tends to be patchy with high background staining.[10,14,31]

Albumin RNA in situ hybridization has been shown to be a highly sensitive maker for hepatocellular differentiation with sensitivity near 100%.[32–34] Although albumin is quite sensitive, it lacks the specificity for pure hepatocellular origin and can be expressed in tumors showing hepatocellular differentiation such as hepatoid carcinomas of various organs, intrahepatic cholangiocarcinoma (iCCA), yolk sac tumor, acinar cell carcinoma, and also in tumors of lung, gallbladder, pancreas, breast origins.[32–35]

Companion diagnostics for therapeutic/prognostic purposes

As in neoplasms of other sites, the need for biomarkers for prediction of response to therapeutic agents has led to exploration of avenues for companion diagnostics. Although microsatellite instibility (MSI) status is deemed predictive of response to immunotherapy across all solid tumors, there has been increasing interest in evaluation of DNA mismatch repair protein IHC as a surrogate to predict treatment response. In addition, IHC for PD-L1 is also being evaluated for this purpose. Large-scale studies of tumor mutational burden and next-generation sequencing of HCCs have shown that MSI is not a hallmark for HCC and is only observed in about 3% HCCs.[36,37] PD-L1 IHC is used as a predictor of response to immune checkpoint blockade in several organ systems; however, has failed to show much promise in management of HCC.[38] However, studies have shown that lymphocyte-rich subtype HCCs demonstrated high level of PD-L1 expressing inflammatory cells and this is being touted as a potential candidate likely benefit from immune checkpoint blockade.[39]

Another promising target for potential therapy is GPC3. A novel anti-GPC3 antibody, codrituzumab, has shown promising results and the expression of GPC3 on the tumor cells by IHC can be used as a biomarker to predict response to therapy.[40] This application is gaining attention not only in treatment of HCC but also in management of other GPC-3 expressing tumors, especially pediatric embryonal tumors.[41] Last, expression of CK19 has been associated with aggressive behavior and dual expression of CK19 and glypican-3 is associated with worse prognosis.[42-44]

MAJOR HEPATOCELLULAR CARCINOMA SUBTYPES

Many architectural growth patterns and histologic subtypes of HCC have been recognized. It is important to identify the morphologic spectrum of HCC not only to enable accurate diagnosis but also for prognostication. Histologic subtypes should not be confused with architectural growth patterns. Although there are 4 major architectural growth patterns, there can be many histologic subtypes (**Table 2**). The 4 major architectural growth patterns include trabecular, solid/compact, pseudoglandular/acinar, and macrotrabecular (**Fig. 1**). In contrast, distinct histologic subtypes are characterized by distinct histologic morphology, supported by specific immunohistochemical profile or molecular alterations and have specific clinical correlates.[45] For example, the steatohepatic subtype is frequently seen in association with metabolic syndrome and NASH, and fibrolamellar HCC is associated with a specific translocation involving *DNAJB1* and *PRKACA* genes. Approximately 35% of HCC can be classified into distinct histologic subtypes.[10] Because many of these histologic subtypes have prognostic significance, it is important to know and report these when possible. At the same time, it is also important to know that HCC can exhibit significant intratumoral heterogeneity and overinterpretation on small biopsy specimens can lead to erroneous misclassification of the tumor. Of note, although some HCCs, such as cirrhotomimetic HCC or fibronodular HCC have no distinct histology, they sometimes are still categorized as HCC subtypes based on their specific appearance and clinical features.

Fibrolamellar Hepatocellular Carcinoma

Fibrolamellar (FL)-HCC is a distinct subtype of HCC that typically arises in younger individuals without any background liver cirrhosis.[11] This entity has gained a lot of attention in recent years due to the identification of a specific molecular alteration associated with this neoplasm. Grossly, these tumors are larger than conventional HCCs and often show a central scar with calcifications. The tumor cells are polygonal, large with abundant eosinophilic granular cytoplasm, show conspicuous eosinophilic macronucleoli, and are invested within abundant collagenous stroma that has a lamellar appearance (**Fig. 2**A). These features though diagnostic of FL-HCC, may not all be seen in every case. Pale bodies are frequently present, but are not specific. These tumors are positive for HepPar-1, pCEA (canalicular pattern) and arginase.[46] Granular cytoplasmic staining with CD68 is sensitive but not specific[47] and the cells frequently express CK7 and CK19.[48] The novel *DNAJB1-PRKACA* fusion was considered sine-que-non of FL-HCC[49,50]; however, recently this fusion gene has also been identified in a set of pancreaticobiliary neoplasms with distinct oncocytic morphology, and is not unique to FL-HCC.[51,52] However, when in question, demonstration of this gene fusion is still considered the gold standard for making the diagnosis.[50] The

Table 2
Key histologic and molecular features of specific hepatocellular carcinoma subtypes

Subtype	Histologic Criteria/Key Features	Specific Molecular Alteration
Fibrolamellar	Bands of lamellar fibrosis, Neoplastic cells are large, eosinophilic with prominent nucleoli. Pale bodies/hyaline globules +/−	*PRKACA* activation; most commonly due to *DNAJB1-PRKACA* fusion
Scirrhous	>50% tumor shows dense fibrosis, pericellular fibrosis +	*TSC1/2* mutations; *TGF-β* signaling activation
Steatohepatitic	>50% tumor shows steatohepatitic features; background liver steatohepatitis	*IL-6/JAK/STAT* activation
Macrotrabecular	Thickened trabecular (≥6–10 cell plate thickness) involving >50% of the tumor	*TP53* mutations and *FGF19* amplifications
Lymphocyte-rich	Lymphocytes outnumber tumor cells	None
Neutrophil-rich	Tumor produces granulocyte–colony-stimulating factor; neutrophilic infiltrate in the tumor	None
Chromophobe	Chromophobic to eosinophilic cytoplasm with abrupt nuclear atypia	Alternative lengthening of telomeres
Clear cell	>80% tumor shows glycogen-rich clear cells ± fat accumulation	None
Cirrhotomimetic	Multiple tumor nodules in a cirrhotic liver	None
Fibronodular	Multiple distinct nodules in a single tumor; "popcorn" appearance in contrast imaging	None

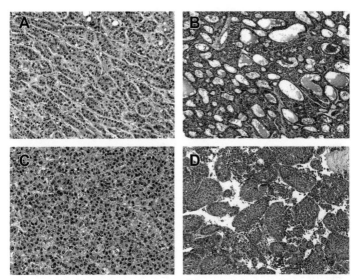

Fig. 1. HCC architectural growth patterns: (*A*) The tumor cells grow in trabecular pattern variable thickness and the trabeculae are lined by prominent sinusoidal endothelial cells. (*B*) The tumor cells grow in a pseudoglandular/acinar pattern with glandular or acinar structure. (*C*) The tumor cells grow in a solid/compact pattern without trabecular or pseudoglandular growth. (*D*) The tumor cells grow in a macrotrabecular pattern with thick trabeculae more than 10 cell layers (hematoxylin and eosin stain, original magnification ×100).

attempts to target this fusion with specific kinase inhibitors have not been promising so far.[53]

Scirrhous Hepatocellular Carcinoma

Scirrhous (SC)-HCC is characterized by nests or single tumor cells surrounded by a markedly fibrous stroma (**Fig. 2**B), which should constitute greater than 50% in the tumor.[10] The incidence of SC-HCC is estimated to be approximately 4.0%. The presence of dense fibrosis may lead to an erroneous impression of cholangiocarcinoma on imaging and gross examination.[45,54] The morphologic features are similar to a well to moderately differentiated HCC. Clear cell change and hyaline bodies have also been reported. Commonly used hepatocellular markers like HepPar-1 and pCEA are negative in more than 50% of SC-HCC, whereas markers commonly used to identify adenocarcinoma, like CK7, CK19, and EPCAM are positive in nearly two-thirds of cases.[26,55] Due to the dense fibrosis and overlapping morphologic and immunohistochemical features, SC-HCC is a mimic of fibrolamellar HCC. Although patient demographics are likely to be different in the 2 groups, molecular testing for *DNAJB1-PRKACA* fusion can be applied in cases that are difficult to classify based in morphology and immunohistochemical profile.[47,48,50] Although a few studies show a poorer prognosis in SC-HCC,[56] most studies have shown no differences in demographics, presence of chronic liver disease, presence of cirrhosis, serum AFP levels, or prognosis in SC-HCC compared with conventional HCC.[54,57,58]

Steatohepatitic Hepatocellular Carcinoma

Some of the HCCs have extensive ballooning, inflammation, Mallory-Denk bodies, and pericellular fibrosis (**Fig. 2**C), whereas others show predominantly steatosis. However,

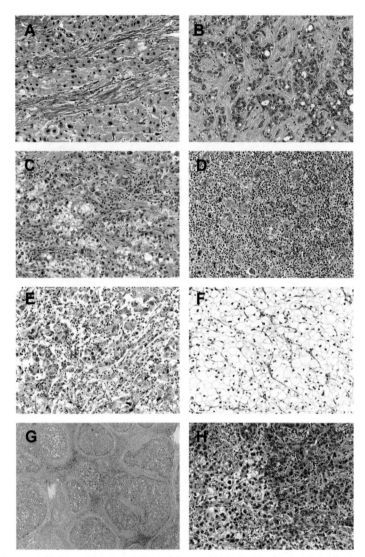

Fig. 2. Hepatocellular carcinoma major subtypes: (*A*) FL-HCC: The tumor cells show abundant eosinophilic cytoplasm, conspicuous macronucleoli, occasional pale bodies and bands of lamellar fibrosis (hematoxylin and eosin stain, Original magnification × 200). (*B*) SC-HCC: The tumor nests and single tumor cells are present in a dense desmoplastic background (hematoxylin and eosin stain, Original magnification × 200). (*C*) SH-HCC: The tumor shows macrovesicular steatosis, ballooning, Mallory-Denk bodies, inflammation and pericellular fibrosis (hematoxylin and eosin stain, Original magnification × 200). (*D*) LR-HCC: The tumor shows tumor cells in a background of dense lymphocytic infiltrate (hematoxylin and eosin stain, Original magnification × 200). (*E*) NR-HCC: The tumor shows abundant neutrophil infiltrate (hematoxylin and eosin stain, Original magnification × 200). (*F*) CC-HCC: The tumor cells have glycogen-rich clear cytoplasm (hematoxylin and eosin stain, Original magnification × 200). (*G*) FN-HCC: The tumor shows a fibronodular appearance characterized by extensive fibrosis dividing the tumor cells into multiple, well-circumscribed tumor nodules in a single tumor lesion (hematoxylin and eosin stain, Original magnification x 40). (*H*) Combined hepatocellular-cholangiocarcinoma: The tumor shows both HCC and cholangiocarcinoma components (hematoxylin and eosin stain, Original magnification × 200).

to make a diagnosis of steatohepatitic (SH)-HCC subtype, evidence of injury in the form of inflammation and ballooning with pericellular fibrosis is necessary. Presence of only steatosis is not enough.[45] Although many patients have metabolic syndrome–associated risk factors and the background non-neoplastic liver may show steatohepatitis, some patients may have none. It may be more common in NASH rather than alcoholic liver disease. Although data are still limited on this histologic subtype, studies have suggested that there is no difference in overall survival, disease-free survival, development of metastatic disease, or local recurrence compared with conventional HCC.[59,60] However, one study showed that patients with SH-HCC appear to have better disease-free survival.[61] The immunohistochemical profile of this subtype is similar to conventional HCC; however, it shows increased staining with inflammatory markers such as C-reactive protein (CRP) due to activation of *IL6/JAK/STAT* pathway.[62] These neoplasms are less likely to show beta-catenin mutations as compared with conventional HCC.[62,63] The differential diagnoses include steatohepatitis, in which case attention of architectural and cytologic atypia becomes necessary (IHC can be used for confirmation), and FNH with steatohepatitis-like change, in which case attention of features of FNH including thick-walled vessels, ductular reaction and thick fibrous bands are helpful to distinguish FNH from HCC.[64,65]

Macrotrabecular Hepatocellular Carcinoma

Macrotrabecular (MT)-HCC was recently described and has gained attention due to association with unique molecular signatures and prognostic implications.[62,66,67] MT-HCC is defined as hepatic trabeculae of $\geq$6 cell plate thickness and needs to constitute greater than 50% of the HCC by the World Health Organization (WHO) (see **Fig. 1**D).[10] However, HCCs with $\geq$30% MT component showed similar clinicopathologic correlates compared with HCCs with greater than 50% MT component.[66] This subtype HCC arises more commonly in noncirrhotic livers, especially in a setting of viral hepatitis B (HBV).[66,68] These tumors are often associated with higher AFP levels, larger size, more frequent vascular invasion, higher stage and grade, higher recurrence rate, and worse recurrence-free survival and overall survival.[66,67] Unique gene signatures associated with tumor angiogenesis such as angiopoietin 2, vascular endothelial growth factor A, and endothelial-specific molecule 1 (*ESM1*) have been reported in this subtype of HCC.[67,69]

Lymphocyte-Rich Hepatocellular Carcinoma

Lymphocyte-rich (LR)-HCC, also termed as lymphoepitheliomalike HCC, is characterized by presence of sheets or nests of poorly differentiated carcinoma cells admixed with dense lymphocytic infiltrate (**Fig. 2**D). Although a cutoff of greater than 100 tumor-infiltrating lymphocytes per 10 high-power fields has been proposed,[70] WHO did not establish such clear metrics for diagnosis, instead of proposing a definition of LR-HCC when lymphocytes outnumber tumor cells in most fields.[10] Although lymphoepitheliomalike cholangiocarcinoma is better described with strong association with Epstein-Barr virus (EBV), the association of EBV and LR-HCC is rare.[71,72] LR-HCC is estimated to represent fewer than 1% of HCCs, and have an overall favorable outcome compared with conventional HCC.[71] A recent study demonstrated that LR-HCCs often show focal amplification of chromosome *11q13.3*, that is strongly associated with the immune checkpoint signature.[73] Furthermore, LR-HCCs demonstrated high level of PD-L1 expression in intratumoral inflammatory cells.[39] These findings indicate LR-HCC might bear sensitivity to immune checkpoint inhibitor therapy.

Neutrophil-Rich Hepatocellular Carcinoma

Some HCCs elaborate granulocyte-colony stimulating factor (G-CSF), which attracts numerous and diffuse infiltrate of neutrophils within the tumor (**Fig. 2E**). Such tumors are rare and have been described in various organs (lung, tubular gut, thyroid, and pancreas) in additional to liver.[74–76] The patients may present with paraneoplastic syndrome such as leukocytosis, fever, coagulopathy and paraneoplastic symptoms.[77] Serum levels of G-CSF, CRP, and interlukin-6 (IL-6) may be elevated. Histology shows poorly differentiated HCC with focal or extensive sarcomatous differentiation and abundant neutrophilic infiltrate.[78,79] Although there are limited data regarding this rare subtype of HCC, the overall prognosis seems to be poor as compared with conventional HCC.[10]

Clear Cell Hepatocellular Carcinoma

Although clear cells are seen in many HCCs and in any of subtypes, the tumor needs to have greater than 80% clear cells to be designated as clear cell (CC)-HCC (**Fig. 2F**).[10] The cytoplasmic clearing in these neoplasms is due to accumulation of glycogen, whereas minor admixture of steatosis is also acceptable. CC-HCCs are usually well to moderately differentiated and show robust staining with hepatocellular markers. Based on available data, these tend to have better or at last similar prognosis as compared with conventional HCC.[80–82] In cases in which the lesions are seen in non-cirrhotic livers or in small biopsy specimens, metastases from other clear cell neoplasms, such as renal and gynecologic origins, should be considered and ruled out.[83]

Chromophobe Hepatocellular Carcinoma

Chromophobe (C)-HCC is composed of tumor cells with bland nuclear features and chromophobic to eosinophilic cytoplasm, and abrupt small clusters of tumor cells with marked nuclear anaplasia.[45,89] This subtype is associated with disruption of normal telomere-maintenance network resulting in alternative lengthening of telomeres, which can be detected by telomere fluorescence in situ hybridization.[89] Although the details are not known, it seems the prognosis of C-HCC is similar to conventional HCC.[10]

Cirrhotomimetic Hepatocellular Carcinoma

Cirrhotomimetic (CM)-HCC, also termed as diffuse cirrhosislike HCC, requires macroscopic correlation as the characteristic features are best appreciated on gross examination. The tumor forms multiple small nodules (usually >20) that are intimately admixed with the background nodules of a cirrhotic liver.[84,85] It is often diagnosed on the explant specimen at the time of transplantation or autopsy specimen, as it is often undetected radiographically or clinically. CM-HCC may occasionally be diagnosed by the discovery of HCC in a liver biopsy performed for medical reasons in absence of HCC by imaging. Most patients have no, or minimal, elevation in AFP and the individual tumor nodules show well or moderately differentiated HCC.[85] Although it is possible that the nodules may represent extensive intrahepatic metastasis, studies have demonstrated that the HCC nodules in this entity are synchronous multiclonal HCCs.[86,87] Based on limited data, these tumors often more likely have lower rates of complete pathologic necrosis after transcatheter arterial chemoembolization and poorer overall survival after transplant compared with conventional HCCs.[88]

Fibronodular Hepatocellular Carcinoma

In contrast to CM-HCC, fibronodular (FN)-HCC, a newly described subtype of HCC, is characterized by extensive fibrosis dividing a single tumor into multiple distinct nodules (**Fig. 2**G). Different from SC-HCC, FN-HCC does not show significant fibrosis between individual tumor nests or single tumor cells. FN-HCC exhibits a distinct "popcorn" appearance on contrast imaging and has a nodular appearance on cut surface. The tumors have shown association with noncirrhotic liver, earlier Barcelona Clinic Liver Cancer (BCLC) stage, lower rate of disease progression and longer time to progression as compared with SC-HCC and conventional HCC.[90]

Combined Hepatocellular-Cholangiocarcinoma

Combined hepatocellular-cholangiocarcinoma (cHCC-CCA) is a rare primary liver carcinoma. The diagnosis of cHCC-CCA requires unequivocal presence of both hepatocytic and cholangiocytic differentiation within the same tumor (**Fig. 2**H), whereas collision of HCC and iCCA arising separately in the same liver should not be included in this entity.[91,92] Based on the International Consensus Group on the nomenclature of cHCC-CCA, the diagnosis of cHCC-CCA can be made when there are both HCC and CCA components present, either intermixed or juxtaposed. The consensus group also included "intermediate cell carcinoma" as a form of cHCC-CCA, in which the tumor cells do not show classic HCC or iCCA morphologic features, but immunophenotypically display variably mixed hepatocytic and cholangiocytic markers at the cellular level.[92] Also, the 2019 WHO classification separated the cholangiolocellular carcinoma from previous cHCC-CCA with stem cell features when there is no associated HCC component, and now categorized it under iCCA.[91] Of note, the diagnosis of cHCC-CCA should be based on hematoxylin and eosin stain. IHC can be used to confirm morphologic components, but should not define the diagnosis on IHC alone.[92,93] Terms have been used such as mixed hepatobiliary carcinoma, biphenotypic (hepatobiliary) primary liver carcinoma, combined liver cell and bile duct carcinoma, HCC with dual phenotype, HCC with stem/progenitor cell should be abandoned and not be recommended to use.[92,93] Although molecular studies have shown that these carcinomas have stem cell features, it is known that these features are not unique to these combined carcinomas. The demographic and clinical features of cHCC-CC are highly variable.[94] Patients with cHCC-CCA often have worse prognosis compared with HCC and is more comparable to iCCA.[95] The prognosis of patients with cHCC-CCA undergoing liver transplantation and the roles of potential target therapies is still unclear.[96]

MORPHO-MOLECULAR CLASSIFICATION OF HEPATOCELLULAR CARCINOMA

The molecular classification of HCC has evolved dramatically over the past decade. The Cancer Genome Atlas Research Network results showed that *TERT* promoter, *TP53* and *CTNNB1* were seen in more than 70% of HCCs.[97] This work was further advanced by the French classification group, which not only provided molecular classification groups but also introduced several morphologic categories based on histologic and molecular correlation.[62] The HCCs were classified into 6 groups based on proliferative activity (G1-G3: high, G4-G6: low) and the molecular alterations were strongly associated morphologic patterns and subtypes.[62,68] The *CTNNB1*-mutated HCC shows a well-differentiated morphology with microtrabeculae, cholestasis, without much inflammation and with nuclear expression of beta-catenin and strong and diffuse GS positivity. The non-*CTNNB1*, non-*TP53* (low proliferation) category composed of smaller tumors with less aggressive biology and was enriched in steatohepatitic morphology and showed higher levels of staining with CRP as a result of alteration in the *JAK/STAT* pathway. The *TP53* mutated HCC are associated with a poorly differentiated/sarcomatous morphology and aggressive biologic behavior. In addition, the newly described macrotrabecular subtype is also strongly associated with *TP53* mutations and *FGF19* amplification with additional signature mutations in genes involved in angiogenesis (*ANGPT2* and *VEGFA*). The same study also confirmed the association of scirrhous subtype with stem cell markers and association with *TSC1/TSC2* mutations and upregulation of *PIK3/AKT* pathway.[62] Similarly, a prior study had shown macrotrabecular/compact histology to be associated with *YAP* and *EpCAM/KRT19* mutations, whereas *BMP4* mutations associated with pseudogland formations.[98] Further study shows that *TERT* promoter mutations represent an early event in carcinogenesis with likely role in tumor initiation and malignant transformation of precancerous lesions, while *TP53* mutations are seen in advanced neoplasms (especially the G3 macrotrabecular group).[99] A number of potentially targetable mutations in advanced HCC, specifically in the *AKT/mTOR, MET* pathways and ligand amplification genes such as *VEGFA* and *FGF19* have been identified.[99] Although multiple molecular signatures are common in HCC, it is important to filter out the genomic signatures that will have most prognostic and therapeutic value. The 5-gene score was developed with this notion, to identify the predictive molecular signatures. The 5-gene panel (*TAF9, RAMP3, HN1, KRT19,* and *RAN*) showed promise in identifying the G3 MT-HCCs and those with poor prognosis in the non-G3 category.[100] In fact, *KRT19* relates to CK19 expression by IHC, which has been shown to be related to a worse prognosis.[42,44,100]

SUMMARY

Comprehensive molecular profiling of HCC has ushered a new era in the pathology of hepatocellular neoplasms. morpho-molecular correlation studies have enabled identification of histologic features associated with specific molecular alterations. The role of pathology has shifted from mere diagnosis to prediction of prognosis and response to targeted therapy. In addition to guiding the surgeon's hand, pathology is now also guiding oncologists in treating patients in this era of precision medicine. The role of pathology will continue to evolve as we learn more about the complex underpinnings and continue to find more morphologic correlates of molecular alterations of HCC to offer better personalized care to patients.

DISCLOSURE

The authors have nothing to disclose.

REFERENCES

1. Marrero JA, Kulik LM, Sirlin CB, et al. Diagnosis, staging, and management of hepatocellular carcinoma: 2018 practice guidance by the American association for the study of liver diseases. Hepatology 2018;68(2):723–50.
2. Wu X, Li J, Gassa A, et al. Circulating tumor DNA as an emerging liquid biopsy biomarker for early diagnosis and therapeutic monitoring in hepatocellular carcinoma. Int J Biol Sci 2020;16(9):1551–62.
3. Ye Q, Ling S, Zheng S, et al. Liquid biopsy in hepatocellular carcinoma: circulating tumor cells and circulating tumor DNA. Mol Cancer 2019;18(1):114.
4. Mocan T, Simao AL, Castro RE, et al. Liquid biopsies in hepatocellular carcinoma: are we winning? J Clin Med 2020;9(5):1541.

5. Park YN, Yang CP, Fernandez GJ, et al. Neoangiogenesis and sinusoidal "capillarization" in dysplastic nodules of the liver. Am J Surg Pathol 1998;22(6): 656–62.

6. Hytiroglou P, Park YN, Krinsky G, et al. Hepatic precancerous lesions and small hepatocellular carcinoma. Gastroenterol Clin North Am 2007;36(4):867–87, vii.

7. Park YN. Update on precursor and early lesions of hepatocellular carcinomas. Arch Pathol Lab Med 2011;135(6):704–15.

8. Niu ZS, Niu XJ, Wang WH, et al. Latest developments in precancerous lesions of hepatocellular carcinoma. World J Gastroenterol 2016;22(12):3305–14.

9. International Consensus Group for Hepatocellular Neoplasia. Pathologic diagnosis of early hepatocellular carcinoma: a report of the international consensus group for hepatocellular neoplasia. Hepatology 2009;49(2):658–64.

10. Torbenson MS, Ng I, Park YN, et al. Hepatocellular carcinoma. 5th edition. Lyon (France): IARC; 2019.

11. Marginean EC, Gown AM, Jain D. Diagnostic approach to hepatic mass lesions and role of immunohistochemistry. Surg Pathol Clin 2013;6(2):333–65.

12. Roncalli M, Terracciano L, Di Tommaso L, et al. Liver precancerous lesions and hepatocellular carcinoma: the histology report. Dig Liver Dis 2011;43(Suppl 4): S361–72.

13. Park YN, Kojiro M, Di Tommaso L, et al. Ductular reaction is helpful in defining early stromal invasion, small hepatocellular carcinomas, and dysplastic nodules. Cancer 2007;109(5):915–23.

14. Choi WT, Ramachandran R, Kakar S. Immunohistochemical approach for the diagnosis of a liver mass on small biopsy specimens. Hum Pathol 2017;63:1–13.

15. Di Tommaso L, Franchi G, Park YN, et al. Diagnostic value of HSP70, glypican 3, and glutamine synthetase in hepatocellular nodules in cirrhosis. Hepatology 2007;45(3):725–34.

16. Di Tommaso L, Destro A, Seok JY, et al. The application of markers (HSP70 GPC3 and GS) in liver biopsies is useful for detection of hepatocellular carcinoma. J Hepatol 2009;50(4):746–54.

17. Tremosini S, Forner A, Boix L, et al. Prospective validation of an immunohistochemical panel (glypican 3, heat shock protein 70 and glutamine synthetase) in liver biopsies for diagnosis of very early hepatocellular carcinoma. Gut 2012;61(10):1481–7.

18. Chuma M, Sakamoto M, Yamazaki K, et al. Expression profiling in multistage hepatocarcinogenesis: identification of HSP70 as a molecular marker of early hepatocellular carcinoma. Hepatology 2003;37(1):198–207.

19. Di Tommaso L, Destro A, Fabbris V, et al. Diagnostic accuracy of clathrin heavy chain staining in a marker panel for the diagnosis of small hepatocellular carcinoma. Hepatology 2011;53(5):1549–57.

20. Yan BC, Gong C, Song J, et al. Arginase-1: a new immunohistochemical marker of hepatocytes and hepatocellular neoplasms. Am J Surg Pathol 2010;34(8): 1147–54.

21. Chandan VS, Shah SS, Torbenson MS, et al. Arginase-1 is frequently positive in hepatoid adenocarcinomas. Hum Pathol 2016;55:11–6.

22. Fujiwara M, Kwok S, Yano H, et al. Arginase-1 is a more sensitive marker of hepatic differentiation than HepPar-1 and glypican-3 in fine-needle aspiration biopsies. Cancer Cytopathol 2012;120(4):230–7.

23. Clark I, Shah SS, Moreira R, et al. A subset of well-differentiated hepatocellular carcinomas are Arginase-1 negative. Hum Pathol 2017;69:90–5.

24. Obiorah IE, Chahine J, Park BU, et al. Well differentiated arginase-1 negative hepatocellular carcinoma. Transl Gastroenterol Hepatol 2019;4:66.

25. Nguyen T, Phillips D, Jain D, et al. Comparison of 5 immunohistochemical markers of hepatocellular differentiation for the diagnosis of hepatocellular carcinoma. Arch Pathol Lab Med 2015;139(8):1028–34.

26. Krings G, Ramachandran R, Jain D, et al. Immunohistochemical pitfalls and the importance of glypican 3 and arginase in the diagnosis of scirrhous hepatocellular carcinoma. Mod Pathol 2013;26(6):782–91.

27. Fan Z, de Rijn MV, Montgomery K, et al. Hep Par 1 antibody stain for of hepatocellular carcinoma: the differential diagnosis 676 tumors tested using tissue microarrays and conventional tissue sections. Mod Pathol 2003;16(2):137–44.

28. Giedl J, Buttner-Herold M, Wach S, et al. Hepatocyte differentiation markers in adenocarcinoma of the prostate: hepatocyte paraffin 1 but not arginase-1 is specifically expressed in a subset of prostatic adenocarcinoma. Hum Pathol 2016;55:101–7.

29. Morrison C, Marsh W, Frankel WL. A comparison of CD10 to pCEA, MOC-31, and hepatocyte for the distinction of malignant tumors in the liver. Mod Pathol 2002;15(12):1279–87.

30. Kakar S, Gown AM, Goodman ZD, et al. Best practices in diagnostic immunohistochemistry: hepatocellular carcinoma versus metastatic neoplasms. Arch Pathol Lab Med 2007;131(11):1648–54.

31. Chu PGG, Ishizawa S, Wu E, et al. Hepatocyte antigen as a marker of hepatocellular carcinoma - an immunohistochemical comparison to carcinoembryonic antigen, CD10, and alpha-fetoprotein. Am J Surg Pathol 2002;26(8):978–88.

32. Ferrone CR, Ting DT, Shahid M, et al. The ability to diagnose intrahepatic cholangiocarcinoma definitively using novel branched DNA-enhanced albumin RNA in situ hybridization technology. Ann Surg Oncol 2016;23(1):290–6.

33. Shahid M, Mubeen A, Tse J, et al. Branched chain in situ hybridization for albumin as a marker of hepatocellular differentiation: evaluation of manual and automated in situ hybridization platforms. Am J Surg Pathol 2015;39(1):25–34.

34. Lin F, Shi JH, Wang HLL, et al. Detection of albumin expression by RNA in situ hybridization is a sensitive and specific method for identification of hepatocellular carcinomas and intrahepatic cholangiocarcinomas. Am J Clin Pathol 2018; 150(1):58–64.

35. Nasir A, Lehrke HD, Mounajjed T, et al. Albumin in situ hybridization can Be positive in adenocarcinomas and other tumors from diverse sites. Am J Clin Pathol 2019;152(2):190–9.

36. Goumard C, Desbois-Mouthon C, Wendum D, et al. Low levels of microsatellite instability at simple repeated sequences commonly occur in human hepatocellular carcinoma. Cancer Genomics Proteomics 2017;14(5):329–39.

37. Harding JJ, Nandakumar S, Armenia J, et al. Prospective genotyping of hepatocellular carcinoma: clinical implications of next-generation sequencing for matching patients to targeted and immune therapies. Clin Cancer Res 2019; 25(7):2116–26.

38. Llovet JM, Montal R, Sia D, et al. Molecular therapies and precision medicine for hepatocellular carcinoma. Nat Rev Clin Oncol 2018;15(10):599–616.

39. Calderaro J, Rousseau B, Amaddeo G, et al. Programmed death ligand 1 expression in hepatocellular carcinoma: relationship with clinical and pathological features. Hepatology 2016;64(6):2038–46.

40. Chen G, Chen YC, Reis B, et al. Combining expression of GPC3 in tumors and CD16 on NK cells from peripheral blood to identify patients responding to codrituzumab. Oncotarget 2018;9(12):10436–44.

41. Ortiz MV, Roberts SS, Glade Bender J, et al. Immunotherapeutic targeting of GPC3 in pediatric solid embryonal tumors. Front Oncol 2019;9:108.

42. Uenishi T, Kubo S, Yamamoto T, et al. Cytokeratin 19 expression in hepatocellular carcinoma predicts early postoperative recurrence. Cancer Sci 2003;94(10): 851–7.

43. Feng J, Zhu R, Chang C, et al. CK19 and glypican 3 expression profiling in the prognostic indication for patients with HCC after surgical resection. PLoS One 2016;11(3):e0151501.

44. Miltiadous O, Sia D, Hoshida Y, et al. Progenitor cell markers predict outcome of patients with hepatocellular carcinoma beyond Milan criteria undergoing liver transplantation. J Hepatol 2015;63(6):1368–77.

45. Torbenson MS. Morphologic subtypes of hepatocellular carcinoma. Gastroenterol Clin North Am 2017;46(2):365–91.

46. Ward SC, Huang JT, Tickoo SK, et al. Fibrolamellar carcinoma of the liver exhibits immunohistochemical evidence of both hepatocyte and bile duct differentiation. Mod Pathol 2010;23(9):1180–90.

47. Ross HM, Daniel HD, Vivekanandan P, et al. Fibrolamellar carcinomas are positive for CD68. Mod Pathol 2011;24(3):390–5.

48. Abdul-Al HM, Wang G, Makhlouf HR, et al. Fibrolamellar hepatocellular carcinoma: an immunohistochemical comparison with conventional hepatocellular carcinoma. Int J Surg Pathol 2010;18(5):313–8.

49. Honeyman JN, Simon EP, Robine N, et al. Detection of a recurrent DNAJB1-PRKACA chimeric transcript in fibrolamellar hepatocellular carcinoma. Science 2014;343(6174):1010–4.

50. Graham RP, Jin L, Knutson DL, et al. DNAJB1-PRKACA is specific for fibrolamellar carcinoma. Mod Pathol 2015;28(6):822–9.

51. Vyas M, Hechtman JF, Zhang Y, et al. DNAJB1-PRKACA fusions occur in oncocytic pancreatic and biliary neoplasms and are not specific for fibrolamellar hepatocellular carcinoma. Mod Pathol 2020;33(4):648–56.

52. Singhi AD, Wood LD, Parks E, et al. Recurrent rearrangements in PRKACA and PRKACB in intraductal oncocytic papillary neoplasms of the pancreas and bile duct. Gastroenterology 2020;158(3):573–82.e2.

53. Abou-Alfa GK, Mayer R, Venook AP, et al. Phase II multicenter, open-label study of oral ENMD-2076 for the treatment of patients with advanced fibrolamellar carcinoma. Oncologist 2020. [Epub ahead of print].

54. Kurogi M, Nakashima O, Miyaaki H, et al. Clinicopathological study of scirrhous hepatocellular carcinoma. J Gastroenterol Hepatol 2006;21(9):1470–7.

55. Matsuura S, Aishima S, Taguchi K, et al. 'Scirrhous' type hepatocellular carcinomas: a special reference to expression of cytokeratin 7 and hepatocyte paraffin 1. Histopathology 2005;47(4):382–90.

56. Lee JH, Choi MS, Gwak GY, et al. Clinicopathologic characteristics and long-term prognosis of scirrhous hepatocellular carcinoma. Dig Dis Sci 2012;57(6): 1698–707.

57. Jernigan PL, Wima K, Hanseman DJ, et al. Natural history and treatment trends in hepatocellular carcinoma subtypes: insights from a national cancer registry. J Surg Oncol 2015;112(8):872–6.

58. Kim SH, Lim HK, Lee WJ, et al. Scirrhous hepatocellular carcinoma: comparison with usual hepatocellular carcinoma based on CT-pathologic features and long-term results after curative resection. Eur J Radiol 2009;69(1):123–30.

59. Lee JS, Yoo JE, Kim H, et al. Tumor stroma with senescence-associated secretory phenotype in steatohepatitic hepatocellular carcinoma. PLoS One 2017; 12(3):e0171922.

60. Salomao M, Remotti H, Vaughan R, et al. The steatohepatitic variant of hepatocellular carcinoma and its association with underlying steatohepatitis. Hum Pathol 2012;43(5):737–46.

61. Shibahara J, Ando S, Sakamoto Y, et al. Hepatocellular carcinoma with steatohepatitic features: a clinicopathological study of Japanese patients. Histopathology 2014;64(7):951–62.

62. Calderaro J, Couchy G, Imbeaud S, et al. Histological subtypes of hepatocellular carcinoma are related to gene mutations and molecular tumour classification. J Hepatol 2017;67(4):727–38.

63. Ando S, Shibahara J, Hayashi A, et al. beta-catenin alteration is rare in hepatocellular carcinoma with steatohepatitic features: immunohistochemical and mutational study. Virchows Arch 2015;467(5):535–42.

64. Deniz K, Moreira RK, Yeh MM, et al. Steatohepatitis-like changes in focal nodular hyperplasia, A finding to distinguish from steatohepatitic variant of hepatocellular carcinoma. Am J Surg Pathol 2017;41(2):277–81.

65. Jain D. The steatohepatitic variant of hepatocellular carcinoma and its association with underlying steatohepatitis. Hum Pathol 2012;43(5):769 [author reply: 769–0].

66. Jeon Y, Benedict M, Taddei T, et al. Macrotrabecular hepatocellular carcinoma: an aggressive subtype of hepatocellular carcinoma. Am J Surg Pathol 2019; 43(7):943–8.

67. Ziol M, Pote N, Amaddeo G, et al. Macrotrabecular-massive hepatocellular carcinoma: a distinctive histological subtype with clinical relevance. Hepatology 2018;68(1):103–12.

68. Rebouissou S, Nault JC. Advances in molecular classification and precision oncology in hepatocellular carcinoma. J Hepatol 2020;72(2):215–29.

69. Calderaro J, Meunier L, Nguyen CT, et al. ESM1 as a marker of macrotrabecular-massive hepatocellular carcinoma. Clin Cancer Res 2019;25(19):5859–65.

70. Wada Y, Nakashima O, Kutami R, et al. Clinicopathological study on hepatocellular carcinoma with lymphocytic infiltration. Hepatology 1998;27(2):407–14.

71. Chan AW, Tong JH, Pan Y, et al. Lymphoepithelioma-like hepatocellular carcinoma: an uncommon variant of hepatocellular carcinoma with favorable outcome. Am J Surg Pathol 2015;39(3):304–12.

72. Labgaa I, Stueck A, Ward SC. Lymphoepithelioma-like carcinoma in liver. Am J Pathol 2017;187(7):1438–44.

73. Chan AW, Zhang Z, Chong CC, et al. Genomic landscape of lymphoepithelioma-like hepatocellular carcinoma. J Pathol 2019;249(2):166–72.

74. Shimakawa T, Asaka S, Usuda A, et al. Granulocyte-colony stimulating factor (G-CSF)-producing esophageal squamous cell carcinoma: a case report. Int Surg 2014;99(3):280–5.

75. Sato T, Omura M, Saito J, et al. Neutrophilia associated with anaplastic carcinoma of the thyroid: production of macrophage colony-stimulating factor (M-CSF) and interleukin-6. Thyroid 2000;10(12):1113–8.

76. Vinzens S, Zindel J, Zweifel M, et al. Granulocyte colony-stimulating factor producing anaplastic carcinoma of the pancreas: case report and review of the literature. Anticancer Res 2017;37(1):223–8.

77. Araki K, Kishihara F, Takahashi K, et al. Hepatocellular carcinoma producing a granulocyte colony-stimulating factor: report of a resected case with a literature review. Liver Int 2007;27(5):716–21.

78. Kohno M, Shirabe K, Mano Y, et al. Granulocyte colony-stimulating-factor-producing hepatocellular carcinoma with extensive sarcomatous changes: report of a case. Surg Today 2013;43(4):439–45.

79. Amano H, Itamoto T, Emoto K, et al. Granulocyte colony-stimulating factor-producing combined hepatocellular/cholangiocellular carcinoma with sarcomatous change. J Gastroenterol 2005;40(12):1158–9.

80. Liu Z, Ma W, Li H, et al. Clinicopathological and prognostic features of primary clear cell carcinoma of the liver. Hepatol Res 2008;38(3):291–9.

81. Ji SP, Li Q, Dong H. Therapy and prognostic features of primary clear cell carcinoma of the liver. World J Gastroenterol 2010;16(6):764–9.

82. Yang SH, Watanabe J, Nakashima O, et al. Clinicopathologic study on clear cell hepatocellular carcinoma. Pathol Int 1996;46(7):503–9.

83. Murakata LA, Ishak KG, Nzeako UC. Clear cell carcinoma of the liver: a comparative immunohistochemical study with renal clear cell carcinoma. Mod Pathol 2000;13(8):874–81.

84. Okuda K, Peters RL, Simson IW. Gross anatomic features of hepatocellular carcinoma from three disparate geographic areas. Proposal of new classification. Cancer 1984;54(10):2165–73.

85. Jakate S, Yabes A, Giusto D, et al. Diffuse cirrhosis-like hepatocellular carcinoma: a clinically and radiographically undetected variant mimicking cirrhosis. Am J Surg Pathol 2010;34(7):935–41.

86. Ng IOL, Guan XY, Poon RTP, et al. Determination of the molecular relationship between multiple tumour nodules in hepatocellular carcinoma differentiates multicentric origin from intrahepatic metastasis. J Pathol 2003;199(3):345–53.

87. Morimoto O, Nagano H, Sakon M, et al. Diagnosis of intrahepatic metastasis and multicentric carcinogenesis by microsatellite loss of heterozygosity in patients with multiple and recurrent hepatocellular carcinomas. J Hepatol 2003;39(2): 215–21.

88. Habibollahi P, Shamchi SP, Tondon R, et al. Combination of neoadjuvant transcatheter arterial chemoembolization and orthotopic liver transplantation for the treatment of cirrhotomimetic hepatocellular carcinoma. J Vasc Interv Radiol 2018;29(2):237–43.

89. Wood LD, Heaphy CM, Daniel HD, et al. Chromophobe hepatocellular carcinoma with abrupt anaplasia: a proposal for a new subtype of hepatocellular carcinoma with unique morphological and molecular features. Mod Pathol 2013; 26(12):1586–93.

90. Tefera J, Revzin M, Chapiro J, et al. Fibronodular hepatocellular carcinoma-a new variant of liver cancer: clinical, pathological and radiological correlation. J Clin Pathol 2020. https://doi.org/10.1136/jclinpath-2020-206574.

91. Sempoux C, Kakar S, Kondo F, et al. Combined hepatocellular-cholangiocarcinoma and undifferentiated primary liver carcinoma. 5th edition. Lyon (France): IARC; 2019.

92. Brunt E, Aishima S, Clavien PA, et al. cHCC-CCA: consensus terminology for primary liver carcinomas with both hepatocytic and cholangiocytic differentiation. Hepatology 2018;68(1):113–26.

93. Sciarra A, Park YN, Sempoux C. Updates in the diagnosis of combined hepato-cellular-cholangiocarcinoma. Hum Pathol 2020;96:48–55.

94. Jarnagin WR, Weber S, Tickoo SK, et al. Combined hepatocellular and cholan-giocarcinoma: demographic, clinical, and prognostic factors. Cancer 2002; 94(7):2040–6.

95. Lin G, Toh CH, Wu RC, et al. Combined hepatocellular cholangiocarcinoma: prognostic factors investigated by computed tomography/magnetic resonance imaging. Int J Clin Pract 2008;62(8):1199–205.

96. Komuta M, Yeh MM. A review on the update of combined hepatocellular cholan-giocarcinoma. Semin Liver Dis 2020;40(2):124–30.

97. Cancer Genome Atlas Research Network. Comprehensive and integrative genomic characterization of hepatocellular carcinoma. Cell 2017;169(7): 1327–41.e3.

98. Tan PS, Nakagawa S, Goossens N, et al. Clinicopathological indices to predict hepatocellular carcinoma molecular classification. Liver Int 2016;36(1):108–18.

99. Nault JC, Martin Y, Caruso S, et al. Clinical impact of genomic diversity from early to advanced hepatocellular carcinoma. Hepatology 2020;71(1):164–82.

100. Nault JC, De Reynies A, Villanueva A, et al. A hepatocellular carcinoma 5-gene score associated with survival of patients after liver resection. Gastroenterology 2013;145(1):176–87.

Surveillance for Hepatocellular Carcinoma

Jorge A. Marrero, MD, MS

KEYWORDS

• Surveillance • Alpha-fetoprotein • Ultrasound • Cirrhosis

KEY POINTS

- Patients with cirrhosis are at the highest risk for hepatocellular carcinoma and should undergo surveillance.
- Surveillance improves overall survival in patients with cirrhosis.
- Alpha-fetoprotein and ultrasound is the best strategy for the early detection of hepatocellular carcinoma.

INTRODUCTION

The decision to screen a population at risk for a specific cancer is based on well-established criteria.[1] Although the overall goal of surveillance for cancer is the reduction of overall cancer-specific mortality, the objective of surveillance is the application of a reliable and reproducible test in a large number of at-risk individuals to determine whether or not they are likely to develop the cancer for which they are being screened. Screening is the one-time application of an examination that allows detection of a disease at a curable stable and, thereby, reducing mortality, whereas surveillance refers to the continuous monitoring for disease occurrence in a population at risk with the same goals as those of screening. Surveillance is the best strategy that applies to the early detection of hepatocellular carcinoma (HCC).

The World Health Organization developed criteria to assess whether surveillance should be performed for a specific disease.[2] The criteria are as follows: (1) the disease in question should be an important health issue and a significant health burden, (2) there should be an identifiable target population, (3) treatment of disease before onset of symptoms (ie, early stage) should offer advantages compared with the treatment of symptomatic disease, (4) the surveillance examination should be affordable and provide benefits to justify its cost, (5) the surveillance examination should be acceptable to both patients and health care professionals, and (6) surveillance examinations should have an acceptable level of accuracy, and surveillance should result in

UT Southwestern Medical Center, Professional Office Building 1, Suite 520L, 5959 Harry Hines Boulevard, Dallas, TX 75390-8887, USA
E-mail address: jorge.marrero@utsouthwestern.edu

Clin Liver Dis 24 (2020) 611–621
https://doi.org/10.1016/j.cld.2020.07.013
1089-3261/20/© 2020 Elsevier Inc. All rights reserved.

reductions in mortality from the disease. HCC meets all criteria for surveillance and it is recommended to be performed in patients at risk to improve outcomes.[3] We review several of the important aspects for the surveillance of HCC.

AT-RISK POPULATION

Cirrhosis is found in more than 90% of individuals diagnosed with HCC.[4] Thus, any cause of chronic liver disease and ultimately cirrhosis should be considered as the main risk factor for HCC. The major causes of cirrhosis, and hence HCC, are chronic hepatitis B (HBV) infection, chronic hepatitis C (HCV), alcohol liver disease, and nonalcoholic fatty liver disease (NAFLD), but less prevalent conditions such as hereditary hemochromatosis, primary biliary cholangitis, and Wilson disease have also been associated with HCC development.

The decision to enter a patient into a surveillance program is determined by the level of risk for HCC while also taking into account the patient's age, overall health, functional status, and willingness and ability to comply with surveillance requirements. The level of HCC risk, in turn, is indicated by the estimated incidence of HCC. However, there are no experimental data to indicate the threshold incidence of HCC to trigger surveillance. Instead, decision analysis has been used to provide some guidelines as to the incidence of HCC at which surveillance may become effective. In general, an intervention is considered effective if it provides an increase in longevity of approximately 100 days, that is, approximately 3 months.[5] Interventions that can be achieved at a cost of less than approximately USD 50,000/y of life gained are considered cost-effective.[6] Several published decision analysis/cost-effectiveness models for HCC surveillance have reported that surveillance is cost-effective, although in some cases only marginally so, and most find that the effectiveness of surveillance depends on the incidence of HCC. For example, in a theoretic cohort of patients with Child-Pugh A cirrhosis, Sarasin and colleagues[7] reported that surveillance increased longevity by approximately 3 months if the incidence of HCC was 1.5%/year; if the incidence was lower, surveillance did not prolong survival. Conversely, Lin and colleagues[8] found that surveillance with alfa-fetoprotein (AFP) and ultrasound was cost-effective regardless of HCC incidence. Thus, although there is some disagreement between published models, surveillance should be offered for patients with cirrhosis of varying etiologies when the risk of HCC is 1.5%/year or greater. The preceding cost-effectiveness analyses, which were restricted to cirrhotic populations, cannot be applied to hepatitis B carriers without cirrhosis. A cost-effectiveness analysis of surveillance for hepatitis B carriers using ultrasound and AFP levels suggested that surveillance became cost-effective once the incidence of HCC exceeded 0.2%/year.[4] **Table 1** shows the populations at risk for HCC that should undergo surveillance. We will review the most common causes of cirrhosis.

Hepatitis B Virus

The evidence linking HBV with HCC is unquestioned.[9] Active viral replication is associated with higher risk of HCC and longstanding active infection with inflammation resulting in cirrhosis is the major event resulting in increased risk.[10,11] The incidence of HCC in inactive HBV carriers without liver cirrhosis is less than 0.3% per year. The role of specific HBV genotypes or mutations in hepatocarcinogenesis is not well established, especially outside Asia. HBV DNA integrates into the host cellular genome in most cases of chronic hepatitis B and induces genetic damage. DNA integration in nontumoral cells in patients with HCC suggests that genomic integration and damage precede the development of tumor. Thus, infection with HBV may be

Table 1 Patients at the highest risk for HCC	
Population Group	**Incidence of HCC**
Asian male hepatitis B carriers older than 40	0.4%–0.6% per y
Asian female hepatitis B carriers older than 50	0.3%–0.6% per y
Hepatitis B carrier with family history of HCC	Incidence higher than without family history
HBV cirrhosis	3%–8% per y
HCV cirrhosis	1%–3% per y
Hepatitis C cirrhosis	1%–3% per y
NAFLD cirrhosis	1%–3% per y
Alcohol-related cirrhosis	1%–3% per y
Genetic hemochromatosis and cirrhosis	1%–2% per y
Alpha-1 antitrypsin deficiency and cirrhosis	~1% per y
Primary biliary cholangitis cirrhosis	2%–5% per y
Autoimmune hepatitis cirrhosis	2%–3% per y

Abbreviations: HBV, hepatitis B; HCC, hepatocellular carcinoma; HCV, hepatitis C; NAFLD, nonalcoholic fatty liver disease.

correlated with the emergence of HCC even in the absence of liver cirrhosis. However, most studies show that the risk of HCC increases markedly in those with cirrhosis.[12] The HCC incidence among patients without cirrhosis ranged from 0.1 to 0.8 per 100 person-years, whereas the incidence in cirrhosis ranged from 2.2 to 4.3 per 100 person-years. There is strong evidence from prospective cohort studies that persistent HBV e antigen (HBeAg) and high levels of HBV serum DNA increase the risk of HCC. There is a multiplicative effect of heavy smoking and alcohol drinking in those with HBV infection, increasing the risk of HCC ninefold. The implementation of vaccination against HBV, as well as antiviral treatment of HBV infection has resulted in a significant decrease of HCC incidence.[13] Family history of HCC in patients with chronic HBV are at a significantly higher risk for developing HCC, and should undergo surveillance.[14]

Hepatitis C Virus

HCV is the most common cause of HCC in Western countries and fueled the increase in HCC in the United States. The prevalence of HCV in HCC cohorts varies according to the prevalence of HCV within each geographic area. HCC risk sharply increases after cirrhosis develops, with annual incidence ranging between 2% and 8%.[15] In addition, in patients with cirrhosis, the risk of HCC decreases but is not completely eliminated even after a sustained response to antiviral therapy.

Currently, well-tolerated combinations of direct-acting antivirals (DAAs) have replaced interferon-based therapy. The rates of sustained virological response (SVR) with combinations of DAAs exceed 95%.[16] Importantly, DAA therapy may lead to decreases in portal hypertension and change the natural history of patients with cirrhosis.[17] Successful DAA therapy is associated with a 71% reduction in HCC risk.[18] However, patients with cirrhosis continue to have a significantly elevated risk of HCC despite achieving SVR, with HCC being reported even 10 years after SVR. It is of critical importance to continue HCC surveillance in those with cirrhosis who have achieved SVR. DAA therapies have led to a significant reduction in HCC incidence from 3.6% per year to 1.8% per year,.[19]

An important question is whether those without cirrhosis should undergo surveillance. Those without cirrhosis have a lower HCC incidence of 1% per year and, therefore, would not warrant surveillance.[20] Another large study showed that those without cirrhosis but with a fibrosis-4 (Fib-4) score >3.25 had an incidence rate for HCC of 0.9% per 100 person-years (confidence interval [CI] 0.54–1.43).[19] Therefore, at this time, those without cirrhosis should not undergo surveillance for HCC because the incidence rate is too low for a survival benefit.

Nonalcoholic Fatty Liver Disease

It has been estimated that the worldwide prevalence of NAFLD is approximately 25%, and it is likely to continue to increase.[21] An association between NAFLD and HCC is well established.[22] In a study comparing the incidence of HCC among patients with HCV infection and NAFLD, 315 patients with cirrhosis secondary to HCV and 195 with cirrhosis due to NAFLD were followed for a median of 3.2 years.[23] The cumulative incidence of HCC was 2.6% in the NAFLD group compared with 4% in the HCV group (P = .09). The annual HCC incidence rate among patients with cirrhosis from NAFLD is approximately 1.8% per 100,000.[24]

The population attributable fraction (PAF) is the quantifiable contribution of a risk factor to a disease such as HCC. It is important for pursuing prevention of disease or interventions that may reduce disease burdens. A population-based study of 6991 patients with HCC older than 68 years evaluated the PAF.[25] The study showed that eliminating diabetes and obesity has the potential for a 40% reduction in the incidence of HCC and the impact would be higher than eliminating other factors including HCV. Therefore, the presence of the metabolic syndrome could be an important area for the prevention of HCC and a target for future interventions.

HCC does occur in patients without cirrhosis. HCC has been observed in patients with NAFLD without cirrhosis but incidence rates at lower than 1% a year.[26] Additional high-quality prospective studies are needed to confirm these observations, but at this time surveillance is not recommended in patients without cirrhosis. A recent review recommended surveillance for HCC among those with NAFLD with advanced fibrosis based on the difficulty of the available tools to distinguish cirrhosis from those with advanced fibrosis.[27]

Other Etiologies of Liver Disease

Alcohol-related cirrhosis is also associated with the development of HCC. The proportion of HCC attributed to alcoholic liver disease has been constant between 20% to 25%.[28] The risk of HCC among patients with alcoholic cirrhosis ranges from 1.3% to 3.0% annually.[29] The PAF for alcoholic liver disease is estimated to be between 13% and 23%, but this effect is modified by race and gender. Importantly, the effect of alcohol as an independent risk factor for HCC is potentiated by the presence of concurrent factors, especially viral hepatitis. Therefore, cirrhosis related to alcoholic liver disease remains an important risk factor for developing HCC.

Other causes of cirrhosis can also increase the risk of HCC. In a population-based cohort of patients with hereditary hemochromatosis and 5973 of their first-degree relatives, the authors found 62 patients developed HCC with a standardized incidence ratio of 21 (95% CI: 16–22).[30] Men were at higher risk than women, and there was no increased risk for development of nonhepatic malignancies. Cirrhosis from primary biliary cholangitis is also an important risk factor. In a study of 273 patients with cirrhosis from primary biliary cholangitis followed for 3 years, the incidence rate was 5.9%.[31] In a systematic review, a total of 6528 patients with autoimmune hepatitis with a median follow-up of 8 years were evaluated for HCC incidence.[32] The pooled incidence rate in the study was 3.1 per 1000 person-years, indicating that autoimmune hepatitis-related cirrhosis is a risk factor for HCC. In a prospective study of patients with cirrhosis due to alpha-1 antitrypsin deficiency, the annual incidence rate of HCC was 0.9% after a median follow-up time of 5.2 years.[33]

Liver Function and Hepatocellular Carcinoma Surveillance

Given the goal of HCC surveillance is to improve survival, this should be performed in patients who are eligible for HCC-related treatments. Therefore, prior studies have suggested HCC surveillance should be performed in patients with Child A or B cirrhosis but is not beneficial in Child C patients outside of liver transplant eligibility.[3,4] Moreover, if a patient's age, medical comorbidities, and poor performance status (ie, wheelchair bound) are clinically significant, then it is unlikely that these patients would have a survival benefit from surveillance for HCC, and palliative treatment should be considered. There are no studies that have indicated the best surveillance strategy for those on the liver transplant waiting list, although clearly surveillance for HCC is indicated given the increased priority these patients have for liver transplantation and the potential for curative therapy with this modality.

RISK STRATIFICATION FOR HEPATOCELLULAR CARCINOMA

The incidence rates for HCC among cirrhosis ranges from 1% to 3% per year, which means that the patients with cirrhosis are a group at a very high risk for developing HCC. However, the risk of developing HCC is not homogeneous among the patients with cirrhosis. For example, men have more than a 2:1 risk of developing HCC compared with women. The ability to stratify the risk of HCC is urgently needed to maximize the surveillance tests to those at the high risk. Unfortunately, prior predictive algorithms based on typical clinical risk factors such as age, gender, and degree of liver dysfunction have suboptimal performance when externally validated.[34] Recently, a tissue-based gene expression profile that predicts clinical progression in persons with HCV-induced cirrhosis and the development of HCC in individuals with cirrhosis has been developed. For the 186-gene expression panel that predicts clinical progression, classification in the high-risk group was associated with significantly increased risks of hepatic decompensation (hazard ratio [HR] 7.36, $P<.001$), overall death (HR 3.57, $P = .002$), liver-related death (HR 6.49, $P<.001$) and all liver-related adverse events (HR 4.98, $P<.001$).[35] For prediction of HCC development, the 186-gene panel was reduced to a 32-gene signature implemented on the Nanostring platform. In an independent cohort of 263 surgically treated patients with early-stage HCC, the probability of developing HCC was nearly fourfold higher in patients with a high-risk prediction score (41%/year) compared with those with a low-risk prediction score (11%/year).[36] Using these data, a recent Markov model was performed with an initial strategy of stratifying the risk HCC into a high-risk, intermediate-risk, or low-risk group using the molecular signature.[37] Once stratified into a risk group, a surveillance modality was for each group. Compared with biannual ultrasound and AFP, risk-stratified approach was more cost-effective. The surveillance of the high-risk group with MRI or abbreviated MRI was cost-effective with no surveillance of the low-risk group. Although this study needs prospective validation, it shows that surveillance strategies tailored to HCC risk are cost-effective and may improve overall utilization of surveillance. This panel looks promising to better define which of those with cirrhosis are at risk for development of HCC; however, it needs validation in serum as well as in different racial/ethnic groups and in different etiologies of liver disease before widespread use. It is likely that the ability to stratify the risk of HCC among patients with cirrhosis will ultimately be a combination of demographic, clinical, and genetic data.

SURVEILLANCE TESTS

At this time, HCC surveillance should be performed for all individuals with cirrhosis.[3] The modalities recommended for surveillance are liver ultrasound with or without AFP every 6 months. Ultrasound, with or without AFP, is recommended for surveillance because most of the studies showed a benefit of the combination of ultrasound and AFP in improving overall survival with a pooled sensitivity of 65% and specificity of 90%.[38]

Recently, guidelines have been developed for how surveillance ultrasound examinations should be performed, interpreted, and reported.[39] An ultrasound examination is considered negative if there are no focal abnormalities or if only definitely benign lesions such as cysts are identified. An examination is considered nondiagnostic if there are lesions measuring smaller than 10 mm that are not definitely benign. An examination is considered positive if there are lesions measuring $\geq$10 mm. A 10-mm threshold is used because lesions smaller than 10 mm are rarely malignant. Even if malignant, such nodules are difficult to diagnose reliably because of their small size and, so long as the patient is in regular surveillance, they may be followed safely. By comparison, lesion(s) $\geq$10 mm have a substantial likelihood of being malignant,[40] they are easier to diagnose reliably, and there is greater risk of harm from delaying the diagnosis.

AFP is considered positive if its value is >20 ng/mL, and negative if lower. Based on receiver operating curve analysis, this threshold provides a sensitivity of approximately 60% and a specificity of approximately 90%.[41] Assuming a 5% prevalence of HCC (approximately that expected in the HCC surveillance population), this is expected to provide 25% positive predictive value for HCC. Moreover, the addition of AFP is expected to increase the sensitivity of surveillance ultrasound, although the magnitude of the incremental gain is not yet known. More recent data suggest longitudinal changes in AFP may increase sensitivity and specificity than AFP interpreted at a single threshold of 20 ng/mL.[42] Other suggested strategies to increase AFP accuracy have included use of different cutoffs by cirrhosis etiology and AFP-adjusted algorithms but needs further validation.

In addition to AFP, a number of other biomarkers have been evaluated for surveillance. These include the *Lens culinaris* lectin binding sub-fraction of the AFP, or AFP-L3%, which measures a sub-fraction of AFP shown to be more specific although generally less sensitive than the AFP,[43] and des gamma carboxy prothrombin (DCP), also called protein induced by vitamin K absence/antagonist-II (PIVKA-II), a variant of prothrombin that is also specifically produced at high levels by a proportion of HCC.[44] These biomarkers are approved by the Food and Drug Administration for risk stratification but not HCC surveillance in the United States. In the past few years, a diagnostic model has been proposed that incorporates the levels of each of the 3 biomarkers AFP, AFP-L3%, and DCP, along with patient gender and age, into the Gender, Age, AFP-L3%, AFP, and DCP (GALAD) model.[45] GALAD has been shown to be promising in phase II (case-control) biomarker studies but still requires phase III and phase IV studies to evaluate its performance in large cohort studies.

There is also active development of novel cancer biomarker assays, including assays for cancer-specific DNA mutations, differentially methylated regions of DNA, microRNAs, long non-coding RNAs, native and posttranslationally modified proteins, and biochemical metabolites. Recent results suggest that there is differential expression of many biomolecules in exosomes released from tumor cells compared with those from normal cells.[46]

Despite their high diagnostic performance, cross-sectional multiphase contrast-enhanced computed tomography (CT) or MRI are not recommended for HCC surveillance given the paucity of data on its efficacy and cost-effectiveness. However, a recent cohort study of 407 patients with cirrhosis compared ultrasound with MRI (liver-specific contrast) for the surveillance of HCC.[47] A total of 43 patients developed HCC, with 1 detected by ultrasound only, 26 by MRI alone, 11 by both, and 5 missed by both modalities. MRI had a lower false-positive rate compared with ultrasound (3.0% vs 5.6%, $P = .004$). This is a provocative study that requires further validation as the primary surveillance test. Future studies should evaluate whether surveillance MRI may be better suited in those in whom the performance of ultrasound will be suboptimal due to body habitus or other criteria. To maximize the value of cross-sectional MRI while minimizing contrast exposure, scanning time, and cost, abbreviated MRI (AMRI) examination protocols have been developed and are being tested.[48] The abbreviated protocols typically include T1-weighted imaging obtained in the hepatobiliary phase post gadoxetate disodium injection, often supplemented with T2-weighted imaging and diffusion-weighted imaging. These protocols achieve sensitivities of 80% to 90% and specificities of 91% to 98% in small cohort studies. Ongoing studies may clarify the most appropriate niche for cost-effective and safe use of CT and MRI, AMRI protocols, perhaps particularly in those settings in which ultrasound performs the least reliably, such as in individuals with truncal obesity or marked parenchymal heterogeneity due to cirrhosis.

The surveillance strategy of biannual ultrasound versus MRI in patients with cirrhosis was shown to be cost-effective.[49] The study showed that MRI leads to increase in life-years and quality adjusted life years despite an increase in costs of >$5000; however, the importance of this study is that the annual HCC incidence was the most influential factor on determining the cost-effectiveness of this strategy. When the HCC incidence rate was greater than 1.81%, the strategy of using MRI was cost-effective; however, the surveillance strategy with MRI was not cost-effective at lower incidence rates, again further evidence that risk stratification is urgently needed. As reviewed previously, the HCC incidence rates in NAFLD, alcohol, and treated HCV cirrhosis, the most common chronic liver disease, have lower incidence rates than what this study shows to be cost-effective and therefore, this strategy of obtaining MRI every 6 months is not be feasible at this time. This study confirms the need and the importance for stratifying the risk of HCC among patients with cirrhosis to use MRI for those at the highest risk.

SURVEILLANCE UTILIZATION AND HARMS

An important limitation of the effectiveness of HCC surveillance in patients with cirrhosis has been the low utilization of this strategy in patients with cirrhosis.[50] In this systematic review, 29 studies with a total of 118,799 patients were evaluated and found to have a pooled estimate for surveillance utilization of 24.0% (95% CI 18.4–30.1). In subgroup analyses, the highest surveillance receipt was reported in studies with patients enrolled from subspecialty gastroenterology/hepatology clinics and lowest in studies characterizing surveillance in population-based cohorts. Commonly reported correlates of surveillance included higher receipt among patients followed by subspecialists and lower receipt among those with alcohol-related or nonalcoholic steatohepatitis–related cirrhosis. Modeling studies have shown that

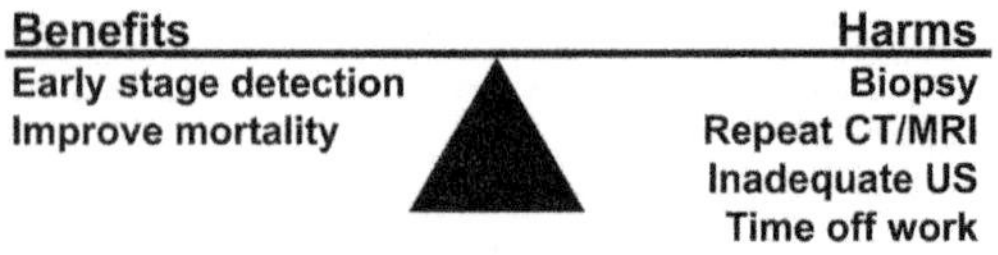

Benefits		Harms
Early stage detection		Biopsy
Improve mortality		Repeat CT/MRI
		Inadequate US
		Time off work

Fig. 1. The balance of benefits and harms of surveillance for HCC. US, ultrasound of the liver.

the minimal utilization of surveillance in patients with cirrhosis should be 34% of the population to improve outcomes.[51] The overall utilization of surveillance remains too low and is an important reason for the overall poor outcomes seen with this HCC.

Interventions to improve utilization of surveillance have been performed with outreach invitations, patient/provider educations, mailed/call reminders, and nurse navigators have resulted in an increase of surveillance utilization between 9% and 64%.[50] Unfortunately, these interventions proven to increase surveillance utilization have not been implemented in medical centers, so there is an opportunity to potentially improve outcomes if these interventions are applied. HCC surveillance utilization needs to markedly increase to improve overall impact of early detection for these patients.

The harms of surveillance are being recognized as an important aspect of early detection of cancer, and a balance between the benefits (early detection of the tumor) and harms is the best desired effect as shown in **Fig. 1**. The harms of surveillance were evaluated in a cohort of patients with cirrhosis undergoing surveillance, and it showed that the harms of surveillance (mostly related to false-positives and indeterminate tests) were more often associated with ultrasound when compared with AFP.[52] The harms were mostly physical related to follow-up imaging tests (CT, MRI, or angiogram) or performing a liver biopsy. There are also indirect harms related to potential loss of income by taking the time off to perform these tests or time off from family duties that also needs to be taken into account. Moreover, it has been estimated that 20% of ultrasounds are classified as inadequate for surveillance, and alternative surveillance modalities may be needed in those with inadequate surveillance ultrasound such as in obesity, alcohol, and NAFLD-related cirrhosis.[53] A recent model showed that accounting for both harms and benefits of ultrasound and AFP surveillance for HCC results in the best cost-effective strategy at this time.[54] Therefore, when assessing the surveillance strategy for the early detection of HCC, a balance between the benefits and harms is critically important, and overall AFP plus ultrasound is the best strategy.

SUMMARY

Patients with cirrhosis should undergo surveillance with AFP in combination with ultrasound. Harms and benefits of surveillance should be taken into account when deciding whether to start surveillance for a patient. Better tools for risk stratification and new surveillance strategies are being developed that may further improve the benefits of surveillance for HCC.

DISCLOSURE

Consultant Glycotest.

REFERENCES

1. Smith RA. Screening fundamentals. J Natl Cancer Inst Monogr 1997;(22):15–9.
2. Meissner HI, Smith RA, Rimer BK, et al. Promoting cancer screening: learning from experience. Cancer 2004;101:1107–17.

3. Heimbach JK, Kulik LM, Finn RS, et al. AASLD guidelines for the treatment of hepatocellular carcinoma. Hepatology 2017;67(1):358–80.

4. Marrero JA, Kulik L, Sirlin C, et al. Diagnosis, staging and management of hepatocellular carcinoma: 2018 practice guidance by the american association for the study of liver disease. Hepatology 2018;68(2):723–50.

5. Naimark D, Naglie G, Detsky AS. The meaning of life expectancy: what is a clinically significant gain? J Gen Intern Med 1994;9(12):702–7.

6. Laupacis A, Feeny D, Detsky AS, et al. How attractive does a new technology have to be to warrant adoption and utilization? Tentative guidelines for using clinical and economic evaluations. CMAJ 1992;146(4):473–81.

7. Sarasin FP, Giostra E, Hadengue A. Cost-effectiveness of screening for detection of small hepatocellular carcinoma in western patients with Child-Pugh class A cirrhosis. Am J Med 1996;101(4):422–34.

8. Lin OS, Keeffe EB, Sanders GD, et al. Cost-effectiveness of screening for hepatocellular carcinoma in patients with cirrhosis due to chronic hepatitis C. Aliment Pharmacol Ther 2004;19(11):1159–72.

9. Bréchot C. Pathogenesis of hepatitis B virus—related hepatocellular carcinoma: old and new paradigms. Gastroenterology 2004;127(5):S56–61.

10. Chen C, Yang HI, Su J, et al. Risk of hepatocellular carcinoma across a biological gradient of serum hepatitis B virus DNA level. JAMA 2006;295(1):65–73.

11. Yang HI, Lu S-N, Liaw YF, et al. Hepatitis B e antigen and the risk of hepatocellular carcinoma. N Engl J Med 2002;347(3):168–74.

12. Fattovich G, Stroffolini T, Zagni I, et al. Hepatocellular carcinoma in cirrhosis: incidence and risk factors. Gastroenterology 2004;127(5 Suppl 1):S35–50.

13. Lok AS. Does antiviral therapy for hepatitis B and C prevent hepatocellular carcinoma? J Gastroenterol Hepatol 2011;26(2):221–7.

14. Loomba R, Liu J, Yang HI, et al. Synergistic effects of family history of hepatocellular carcinoma and hepatitis B virus infection on risk for incident hepatocellular carcinoma. Clin Gastroenterol Hepatol 2013;11(12):1636–45.e3.

15. Goodgame B. The risk of end stage liver disease and hepatocellular carcinoma among persons infected with hepatitis C virus: publication bias? Am J Gastroenterol 2003;98(11):2535–42.

16. Falade-Nwulia O, Suarez-Cuervo C, Nelson DR, et al. Oral direct-acting agent therapy for hepatitis C virus infection. Ann Intern Med 2017;166(9):637.

17. Mandorfer M, Kozbial K, Schwabl P, et al. Sustained virologic response to interferon-free therapies ameliorates HCV-induced portal hypertension. J Hepatol 2016;65(4):692–9.

18. Ioannou GN, Green PK, Berry K. HCV eradication induced by direct-acting antiviral agents reduces the risk of hepatocellular carcinoma. J Hepatol 2017. https://doi.org/10.1016/j.jhep.2017.08.030. S0168-8278(17):32273-0.

19. Kanwal F, Kramer JR, Asch SM, et al. Risk of hepatocellular cancer in HCV patients treated with direct-acting antiviral agents. Gastroenterology 2017;153(4):996–1005.

20. Ioannou GN, Beste LA, Green PK, et al. Increased risk for hepatocellular carcinoma persists up to 10 years after HCV eradiction in patients with baseline cirrhosis or high fib-4 scores. Gastroenterology 2019;157(5):1264–78.

21. Younossi ZM, Koenig AB, Abdelatif D, et al. Global epidemiology of nonalcoholic fatty liver disease-Meta-analytic assessment of prevalence, incidence, and outcomes. Hepatology 2016;64(1):73–84.

22. Ascha MS, Hanouneh IA, Lopez R, et al. The incidence and risk factors of hepatocellular carcinoma in patients with nonalcoholic steatohepatitis. Hepatology 2010;51(6):1972–8.

23. Kawamura Y, Arase Y, Ikeda K, et al. Large-scale long-term follow-up study of Japanese patients with non-alcoholic Fatty liver disease for the onset of hepatocellular carcinoma. Am J Gastroenterol 2012;107(2):253–61.

24. Bertot LC, Adams LA. Trends in hepatocellular carcinoma due to non-alcoholic fatty liver disease. Expert Rev Gastroenterol Hepatol 2019;13(2):179–87.

25. Welzel TM, Graubard BI, Quraishi S, et al. Population-attributable fractions of risk factors for hepatocellular carcinoma in the United States. Am J Gastroenterol 2013;108(8):1314–21.

26. Perumpail RB, Wong RJ, Ahmed A, et al. Hepatocellular carcinoma in the setting of non-cirrhotic nonalcoholic fatty liver disease and the metabolic syndrome: US experience. Dig Dis Sci 2015;60:3142–8.

27. Loomba R, Lim JK, Patton H, et al. AGA clinical practice update on screening and surveillance for hepatocellular carcinoma in patients with nonalcoholic fatty liver disease: expert review. Gastroenterology 2020;158(6):1822–30.

28. Massarweh NN, El-Serag HB. Epidemiology of hepatocellular carcinoma and intrahepatic cholangiocarcinoma. Cancer Control 2017;24(3). 1073274817729245.

29. Ganne-Carrie N, Chaffaut C, Bourcier V, et al. Estimate of hepatocellular carcinoma incidence in patients with alcoholic cirrhosis. J Hepatol 2018;69(6):1274–83.

30. Elmberg M, Hultcrantz R, Ekbom A, et al. Cancer risk in patients with hereditary hemochromatosis and in their first-degree relatives. Gastroenterology 2003;125(6):1733–41.

31. Rong G, Wang H, Bowlus CL, et al. Incidence and risk factors for hepatocellular carcinoma in primary biliary cirrhosis. Clin Rev Allergy Immunol 2015;48(2–3):132–41.

32. Tansel A, Katz LH, El-Serag HB, et al. Incidence and determinants of hepatocellular carcinoma in autoimmune hepatitis: a systematic review and meta-analysis. Clin Gastroenterol Hepatol 2017;15(8):1207–17.e4.

33. Antoury C. Alpha-1 antitrypsin deficiency and the risk of hepatocellular carcinoma in end-stage liver disease. World J Hepatol 2015;7(10):1427.

34. Singal AG, Nehra M, Adams-Huet B, et al. Detection of hepatocellular carcinoma at advanced stages among patients in the HALT-C trial: where did surveillance fail? Am J Gastroenterol 2013;108:425–32.

35. Hoshida Y, Villanueva A, Kobahashi M, et al. Gene expression in fixed tissues and outcome in hepatocellular carcinoma. N Engl J Med 2008;359:1995–2004.

36. Hoshida Y, Villanueva A, Sangiovanni A, et al. Prognostic gene expression signature for patients with hepatitis C related early stage cirrhosis. Gastroenterology 2013;144(5):1024–30.

37. Goossens N, Singal AG, King LY, et al. Cost-effectiveness of risk score stratified hepatocellular carcinoma screening in patients with cirrhosis. Clin Transl Gastroenterol 2017;(6):e101.

38. Singal AG, Anjana A, Tiro J. Early detection, curative treatment, and survival rates for hepatocellular carcinoma surveillance in patients with cirrhosis: a meta-analysis. PLoS Med 2014;11(4):e1001624.

39. Fetzer DT, Rodgers SK, Harris AC, et al. Screening and surveillance of hepatocellular carcinoma: an introduction to ultrasound liver imaging reporting and data system. Radiol Clin North Am 2017;55(6):1197–209.

40. Willatt JM, Hussain HK, Adusumilli S, et al. MR imaging of hepatocellular carcinoma in the cirrhotic liver: challenges and controversies. Radiology 2008; 247(2):311–30.
41. Gupta S. Test characteristics of α-fetoprotein for detecting hepatocellular carcinoma in patients with hepatitis C. Ann Intern Med 2003;139(1):46.
42. Tayob N, Lok ASF, Do K-A, et al. Improved detection of hepatocellular carcinoma by using a longitudinal alpha-fetoprotein screening algorithm. Clin Gastroenterol Hepatol 2016;14(3):469–75.e2.
43. Leerapun A, Suravarapu SV, Bida JP, et al. The utility of Lens culinaris agglutinin-reactive alpha-fetoprotein in the diagnosis of hepatocellular carcinoma: evaluation in a United States referral population. Clin Gastroenterol Hepatol 2007;5(3): 394–402.
44. Marrero JA, Wang Y. Alpha-fetoprotein, des-gamma carboxyprothrombin, and lectin-bound alpha-fetoprotein in early hepatocellular carcinoma. Gastroenterology 2009;137(1):110–8.
45. Johnson PJ, Pirrie SJ, Cox TF, et al. The detection of hepatocellular carcinoma using a prospectively developed and validated model based on serological biomarkers. Cancer Epidemiol Biomarkers Prev 2013;23(1):144–53.
46. Taouli B, Hoshida Y, Kakite S, et al. Imaging-based surrogate markers of transcriptome subclasses and signatures in hepatocellular carcinoma: preliminary results. Eur Radiol 2017;27(11):4472–81.
47. Kim SY, An J, Lim Y-S, et al. MRI with liver-specific contrast for surveillance of patients with cirrhosis at high risk of hepatocellular carcinoma. JAMA Oncol 2017; 3(4):456.
48. Marks RM, Ryan A, Heba ER, et al. Diagnostic per-patient accuracy of an abbreviated hepatobiliary phase gadoxetic acid–enhanced MRI for hepatocellular carcinoma surveillance. AJR Am J Roentgenol 2015;204(3):527–35.
49. Kim HL, An J, Park JA, et al. Magnetic resonance imaging is cost-effective for hepatocellular carcinoma surveillance in high-risk patients with cirrhosis. Hepatology 2019;69(4):1599–613.
50. Wolf E, Rich NE, Marrero JA, et al. Utilization of hepatocellular carcinoma surveillance in patients with cirrhosis: a systematic review and meta-analysis. Hepatology 2020. https://doi.org/10.1002/hep.31309. Online ahead of print.
51. Mourad A, Deuffic-Burban S, Ganne-Carrie N, et al. Hepatocellular carcinoma screening in patients with compensated hepatitis C-related cirrhosis aware of their HCV status improves survival: a modeling approach. Hepatology 2014; 59(4):1471–81.
52. Atiq O, Tiro J, Yopp AC, et al. An assessment of benefits and harms of hepatocellular carcinoma surveillance in patients with cirrhosis. Hepatology 2016; 65(4):1196–205.
53. Simmons O, Fetzer DT, Yokoo T, et al. Predictors of adequate ultrasound quality for hepatocellular carcinoma surveillance in patients with cirrhosis. Aliment Pharmacol Ther 2016;45(1):169–77.
54. Parikh ND, Singal AG, Hutton DW, et al. Cost-effectiveness of hepatocellular carcinoma surveillance: as assessment of benefits and harms. Am J Gastroenterol 2020. https://doi.org/10.14309/ajg.0000000000000715. Online ahead of print.

Imaging Diagnosis of Hepatocellular Carcinoma

The Liver Imaging Reporting and Data System, Why and How?

Guilherme Moura Cunha, MD[a],*, Kathryn J. Fowler, MD[a],
Farid Abushamat, MD[b], Claude B. Sirlin, MD[a],
Yuko Kono, MD, PhD[b],*

KEYWORDS

• Liver • Hepatocellular carcinoma • Imaging diagnosis

KEY POINTS

- Imaging modalities carry high specificity for the diagnosis of hepatocellular carcinoma (HCC) when stringent criteria are applied in at-risk patients, thus enabling many HCCs to be diagnosed without biopsy.
- The Liver Imaging Reporting and Data System (LI-RADS) aims to standardize the lexicon, technique, interpretation, and reporting of liver imaging in patients at risk for HCC.
- For diagnosis, 2 LI-RADS algorithms are available covering cross-sectional imaging techniques (CT/MRI LI-RADS) and contrast-enhanced ultrasound (CEUS LI-RADS).
- Although both algorithms provide high positive predictive value (PPV) and high specificity in the diagnosis of HCC, the algorithms are not identical, reflecting intrinsic differences between imaging modalities.
- Users should be aware of and consider the unique advantages and disadvantages of CEUS, CT, and MRI when deciding which imaging method to use.

INTRODUCTION

Approximately 90% of hepatocellular carcinomas (HCCs) develop in people with risk factors such as cirrhosis or noncirrhotic chronic hepatitis B infection.[1] In patients with chronic hepatitis B infection without cirrhosis, the 5-year cumulative risk of HCC is up to 3%, whereas in patients with liver cirrhosis the 5-year cumulative risk can reach up to 30%.[2–6] Tumors detected at early stages are amenable to curative therapies such

[a] Liver Imaging Group, Department of Radiology, University of California, 9500 Gilman Drive, San Diego, CA 92093, USA; [b] Division of Gastroenterology & Hepatology, University of California, 9500 Gilman Drive, San Diego, CA 92093, USA
* Corresponding authors.
E-mail addresses: gcunha@health.ucsd.edu (G.M.C.); ykono@health.ucsd.edu (Y.K.)

Clin Liver Dis 24 (2020) 623–636
https://doi.org/10.1016/j.cld.2020.07.002
1089-3261/20/© 2020 Elsevier Inc. All rights reserved.
liver.theclinics.com

as surgical resection, thermal ablation, and liver transplantation, resulting in 5-year survival rates of 80%.[7] Patients with advanced-stage disease have fewer options and poor prognosis. Imaging plays a crucial role in the management of HCC. Given the benefit of early detection, high-risk individuals are recommended to undergo HCC surveillance, typically with ultrasound with or without serum alpha fetoprotein measurement.[8] When a nodule is detected on screening, patients should undergo diagnostic imaging with either contrast-enhanced computed tomography (CT), contrast-enhanced MRI or contrast-enhanced ultrasound (CEUS). All 3 imaging modalities carry high specificity for the diagnosis of HCC when stringent criteria are applied in at-risk patients, thus enabling many HCCs to be diagnosed without biopsy (ie, by imaging alone).

Different imaging diagnostic systems for HCC have been proposed worldwide. The Liver Imaging Reporting and Data System (LI-RADS), the most comprehensive of these, aims to standardize the lexicon, technique, interpretation, and reporting of liver imaging in at-risk patients. LI-RADS is updated by an international and multispecialty consortium informed by evidence and expertise. LI-RADS comprises 4 different imaging modalities, covering 3 imaging contexts (screening/surveillance, diagnosis, and treatment response) with algorithms for each:

1. US LI-RADS for screening ultrasound
2. CEUS LI-RADS for diagnosis
3. CT/MRI LI-RADS for diagnosis and staging
4. TR LI-RADS for locoregional treatment response assessment (a systemic treatment response algorithm has not yet been developed)

Currently, LI-RADS does not apply to nuclear imaging modalities (ie, positron emission tomography), as the benefits of these techniques for HCC diagnosis, particularly in early disease, are unclear.[9]

In 2018, LI-RADS ultrasound and CT/MRI algorithms were incorporated by the American Association for the Study of Liver Diseases (AASLD) into the 2018 practice guidance for HCC, promoting a unified approach for diagnostic, staging, and management recommendations.[10] The AASLD has not yet adopted the CEUS algorithm for diagnosis of HCC or the LI-RADS TR algorithm for treatment response, but the authors anticipate it might do so in the future as evidence continues to accrue and these algorithms mature.

This article focuses on similarities and differences between the CT/MRI diagnostic algorithm (CT/MRI LI-RADS) and the CEUS diagnostic algorithm (CEUS LI-RADS). Both algorithms rely on the dynamic postcontrast imaging features of HCC, leverage the high pretest probability of HCC in at-risk patients, and provide high positive predictive value (PPV) and high specificity in the noninvasive diagnosis of HCC. However, reflecting intrinsic differences between the applied modalities and corresponding contrast agents, the algorithms are not identical. Users should be aware of and consider the unique advantages and disadvantages of CEUS, CT, and MRI when deciding which imaging method to use.

KEY CONCEPTS
Imaging Algorithms Must Be Applied Only in the Appropriate Population

In order to achieve the desired high PPV, LI-RADS should be applied only in a population with high pretest probability of HCC. This at-risk population (ie, LI-RADS population) includes patients with cirrhosis, chronic hepatitis B viral infection, or current/prior HCC. LI-RADS should not be applied to children (<18 years old) or patients with vascular etiologies of cirrhosis (eg, Budd-Chiari syndrome or cardiac congestion) or congenital hepatic fibrosis.[11] In these circumstances, the pre-test probability for HCC is not as well established and likely lower. For instance, in patients with Budd-Chiari and congenital hepatic fibrosis, the presence of benign hypervascular nodules that resemble HCC at imaging may reduce the specificity of the diagnosis. Ultimately, in the LI-RADS population, PPV for HCC diagnosis is expected to be greater than 95%. CT/MRI and CEUS LI-RADS apply to the same population.

Although it is plausible that the LI-RADS criteria could provide high PPV in populations with less elevated risk, such as patients with longstanding NAFLD (non-alcoholic fatty liver disease) or patients with stage 2 or 3 fibrosis caused by viral hepatitis,[12] there is currently insufficient literature on the diagnostic performance of LI-RADS to recommend widespread application in such populations. From the radiologist's perspective, the diagnosis of cirrhosis for defining an at-risk patient is based on information provided by the referring physician. A complete discussion of how clinicians make the diagnosis of cirrhosis is beyond the scope of this article, but this determination is usually based on clinical context, histology findings (when available), and clinical indicators of advanced liver disease. Quantitative imaging methods such as transient elastography (TE), ultrasound shear wave elastography (SWE), and magnetic resonance elastography (MRE) can assist in the diagnosis of cirrhosis[13,14] by informing the decision to perform liver biopsy, but these technologies usually do not have sufficient PPV to diagnose cirrhosis reliably in the absence of confirmatory biopsy or other findings.

Imaging Studies Must Meet Technical Standards to Yield Desired Results

Although detailed technical descriptions are reserved for the radiology audience, clinicians should be aware of basic technical differences between CT/MRI and CEUS that are relevant for daily clinical practice. CEUS is an advanced form of ultrasound that uses intravenous blood pool microbubble contrast agents for the dynamic characterization of hepatic observations with high temporal resolution. CEUS requires an ultrasound scanner with contrast-specific imaging capability to visualize signals specific to microbubbles, a feature available on most modern commercially available machines. Of note, the addition of contrast to a standard ultrasound examination requires some preparation, including the placement of an intravenous catheter, which is not otherwise needed for ultrasound. Additionally, the coding and billing of standard ultrasound and CEUS differ, requiring separate orders and insurance authorization in the United States. Because the contrast used in CEUS does not impose any nephrotoxic risk, there is no need for renal function testing prior to administration. It is important to note that perfluorobutane, a contrast agent that has prolonged liver uptake because of greater stability and Kupffer cell phagocytosis, has not yet been adopted by CEUS LI-RADS and is not yet approved for use in the United States. Further details on CEUS LI-RADS technical standards, including imaging protocols and techniques, are described elsewhere.[15,16]

CT/MRI examinations also must be performed according to technical standards. Administration of intravenous contrast and acquisition of a multiphase liver protocol (eg, before contrast, late hepatic arterial phase, portal venous phase, and delayed phase images) is mandatory to allow for diagnosis of HCC.[1,17–19] For CT, multidetector CT (≥8 detectors) is a requisite, whereas for MRI, 1.5 or 3 T magnets are required, according to LI-RADS. For additional description of the technical standards, the interested reader is referred to https://www.acr.org/Clinical-Resources/Reporting-and-Data-Systems/LI-RADS.[20]

Differences Between Contrast Agents Used in Contrast-Enhanced Ultrasound and Computed Tomography/MRI

CEUS contrast agents are considered blood pool (intravascular) agents that do not diffuse out into tissues. CT/MRI contrast agents transition from the intravascular space to the interstitial and/or intracellular space of tissues. MRI contrast agents are divided in 2 major classes based on the ability to be taken up by hepatocytes (extracellular contrast agents [ECAs] and hepatobiliary agents [HBAs]). This difference in the distribution of the contrast agents results in specific imaging features. Most importantly, the feature washout is characterized differently on CEUS than on CT/MRI. The characterization of washout appearance helps in the imaging differentiation between HCC and non-HCC malignancies. The high temporal resolution of CEUS allows for differentiation between early versus late washout, an important distinction to achieve a specific diagnosis. With CEUS, washout is classified into 2 subtypes based on onset and degree. One subtype (early or marked washout) is suggestive of cholangiocarcinoma and other non-HCC malignancies (LR-M), while the other subtype (late and mild washout) indicates HCC (LR-5). Conversely, on CT and MRI with ECA, washout is classified based on morphology. One subtype (peripheral washout) is suggestive of cholangiocarcinoma and other non-HCC malignancies, while the other subtype (nonperipheral) is suggestive of HCC in particular (**Fig. 1** shows an example of LR-5 observation on CEUS and contrast-enhanced CT). On MRI with HBA, washout is characterized based on morphology and onset. Similar to CT and MRI with ECA, peripheral versus nonperipheral washout distinguishes LR-M versus LR-5 observations, but for nonperipheral washout to be considered a feature of HCC, the onset needs to be in the PVP. On CT/MRI, the degree of washout is not taken into account.

Beyond the differences in imaging appearance between CEUS and CT/MRI contrast agents, there are practical considerations also. Microbubble contrast agents used in CEUS have virtually no adverse reactions. Therefore, they can be used for lesion characterization in patients with contraindications to gadolinium-based and iodine-based contrast agents such as allergies or renal dysfunction. Additionally, CEUS is real-time imaging, which eliminates the risk of arterial phase mistiming and may be useful to characterize arterial phase hyperenhancement (APHE) deemed equivocal on CT or MRI. CEUS is also useful in differentiating true nodules from pseudolesions such as arterio-portal (AP) shunts encountered on CT and MRI. For these reasons, CEUS is often used as a problem-solving tool for indeterminate lesions on CT or MRI. On the other hand, CEUS requires separate injections for each lesion evaluated, and so is less well suited to patients with multifocal disease or those who require staging of intrahepatic tumor burden and/or extrahepatic spread. CT and MRI allow for assessment of the whole liver and adjacent anatomic structures and are preferred for assessing tumor extent (ie, staging).[10] Finally, CEUS is not currently recognized by the organ procurement and transplantation network (OPTN) and so cannot be used for establishing automatic transplant eligibility, which will be discussed further.

Diagnostic Algorithms Provide Hierarchical Features for Assigning Categories

In LI-RADS, to assign a diagnostic category that reflects the risk of benignity, malignancy or HCC, radiologists appraise combinations of imaging features in accordance to the diagnostic algorithms. On CT/MRI, LI-RADS major imaging criteria for the diagnosis of HCC are size, in combination with nonrim arterial phase hyperenhancement (APHE), enhancing capsule appearance, washout appearance, and threshold growth. For CEUS LI-RADS, major imaging features are size, APHE, and washout (onset and degree). In addition, both CT/MRI and CEUS algorithms list ancillary imaging features

A

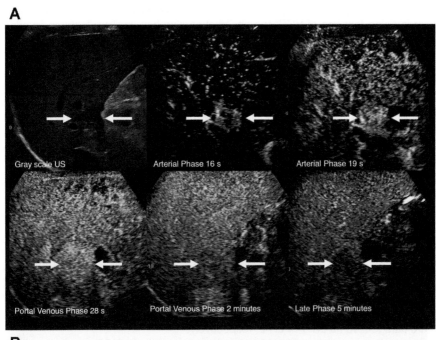

B

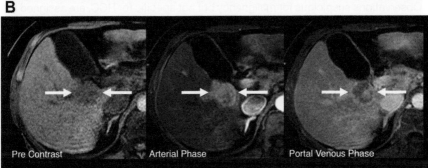

Fig. 1. 62-year-old woman with cirrhosis secondary to chronic hepatitis C viral infection and alcohol abuse. (*A*) Precontrast ultrasound and CEUS images show a 3.0 cm hypoechoic nodule in segment 5. The combination of size ≥10 mm and major features (*arrows*: non rim APHE, late and mild washout at 5 minutes) indicates a CEUS LR-5 lesion (definite HCC). (*B*) Same observation on pre- and postcontrast MRI. The presence of nonrim APHE, washout appearance, capsule appearance (*arrows*), and ≥20 mm are major features of definite HCC (LR-5).

that can be used to increase confidence or adjust the final diagnostic category. These ancillary features (AFs) may favor benignity, malignancy in general, or HCC in particular. For the latter, although AFs can be used to upgrade observations to a higher probability of HCC (ie, LR-4 vs LR-3), they are not specific enough to allow for observations to be upgraded from probably HCC (LR-4) to definite HCC (LR-5) based on their presence. Finally, if the user is still unsure between 2 categories, a tie-breaking rule is applied, whereby the category with lower certainty between the two should be chosen. All these steps are intended to assure the highest possible specificity for HCC in both algorithms. **Fig. 2** shows an LR-5 observation with CT/MRI LI-RADS major imaging features of HCC; the observation also has ancillary features favoring HCC, but these do not contribute to the category assignment in this case.

Diagnostic Algorithms Provide Probabilistic Categories for Diagnosing Hepatocellular Carcinoma

The CT/MRI and CEUS algorithms define 8 diagnostic categories to reflect the relative probability of HCC. Although not identical, each algorithm is applied at the individual observation level and starts with a stepwise decision tree designed to narrow in on nodules of hepatocellular origin that may represent HCC.[11,16] In brief, this stepwise process comprises the following

1. Determine if the imaging study is adequate for categorizing a particular observation that is devoid of significant artifact or technical failure. An observation is categorized as LR-NC (not categorizable) if image omissions or degradation precludes the assessment of its imaging features such that it is not possible to determine if it is more likely benign (ie, should be categorized LR-1 or LR-2) or more likely malignant (ie, should be categorized LR-4, LR-5, or LR-M).
2. The presence of tumor in vein (TIV) should be ruled out. If a positive finding of tumor in vein is detected, an LR-TIV category should be assigned and whenever possible its most likely etiology (due to HCC or non-HCC malignancy) specified.
3. Benign lesions should be recognized. Definitely or probably benign observations are categorized as LR-1 or LR-2, respectively.
4. Observations suspicious for malignancy but not specific for HCC, are assigned LR-M.

If an observation(s) does not fit into one of these categories, it should be assessed using the diagnostic table. The diagnostic table uses the major imaging features of

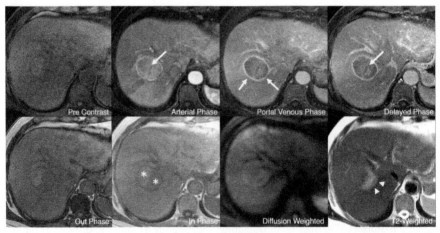

Fig. 2. 67-year-old man, chronic hepatitis C viral infection, pre- and postcontrast MRI. The combination of size ≥20 mm and major features (*arrows*: APHE, washout appearance, and capsule appearance) indicates an LR-5 mass (definite HCC). Incidentally, the mass also shows ancillary features favoring malignancy (*arrowheads*: mild-moderate T2 hyperintensity) and HCC in particular (*asterisks*: mosaic appearance), but these ancillary features do not contribute to the category assignment in this case. The mass would be LR-5 even if all these ancillary features were absent.

HCC to assign categories ranging from intermediate probability to definite HCC (LR-3, LR-4, LR-5). The diagnostic table differs between CT/MRI LI-RADS and CEUS LI-RADS accounting for the different imaging features observed in each modality. Importantly, no single major imaging feature in the diagnostic table is specific enough to categorize an observation as LR-5 (definite HCC)I rather the combination of features stratifies the risk between intermediate, probable or definite. **Fig. 3** shows CT/MRI and CEUS LI-RADS diagnostic algorithms and corresponding tables.

On both CEUS and CT/MRI, the categories LR-3 to LR-5 have increasing probability for being malignant and HCC. Hence, LR-3 observations may be benign or malignant. The LR-4 category implies an observation is highly suspicious for HCC, but there is not 100% certainty. These are often distinctive nodules or masses with imaging features of HCC but lacking a combination of findings that confers high specificity to the diagnosis. LR-5 observations meet criteria for definite HCC, and patients should be assessed for treatment options, usually without need for histologic confirmation.

The CT/MRI criteria for definite HCC are identical between LI-RADS and AASLD, and except for minor differences, are consistent with the European Association of Study of the Liver (EASL) and the Organ Procurement and Transplantation Network (OPTN).[1,17,18] Several publications have shown that CEUS provides high PPV and specificity for the diagnosis of HCC.[21–23] The advances in knowledge led to the endorsement of CEUS for the diagnosis of HCC by the American College of Radiology (ACR), EASL, European guidelines, and various individual countries,[1,19,20,24] although it has not been adopted by AASLD at the time of publication of this article.[10] Current OPTN policies have no mention on the use of CEUS for HCC diagnosis.

The diagnostic performance of the outermost categories (definitely benign [LR-1] and definitely HCC [LR-5]) is extremely high, with reported percentage of HCC in the LR-1 category of 0% and 94% in the LR-5.[21,25] In CT/MRI LI-RADS, the LR-5 category provides high specificity and PPV for the diagnosis of HCC.[26–28] **Table 1** shows

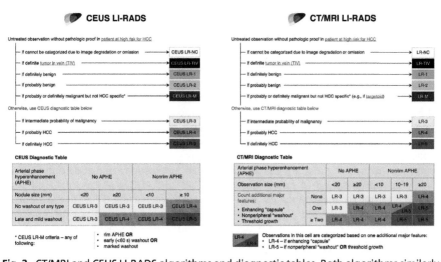

Fig. 3. CT/MRI and CEUS LI-RADS algorithms and diagnostic tables. Both algorithms similarly, although not identically, start with a stepwise decision tree until determining the probability of HCC. Greater differences are noted in the diagnostic table because of differences in imaging features for the diagnosis of HCC. (*From* https://www.acr.org/Clinical-Resources/Reporting-and-Data-Systems/LI-RADS Accessed Dec 10, 2019; with permission.)

Table 1
Performance of the LR-5 category for the diagnosis of hepatocellular carcinoma in studies using computed tomography/MRI Liver Imaging Reporting and Data System v2018 and contrast-enhanced ultrasound Liver Imaging Reporting and Data System v2017

LI-RADS Algorithm	Specificity	Sensitivity	PPV	NPV	Modality/Contrast
CT/MRI	.	.	88%	.	CT
CT/MRI	90%	78%–80%	94%–96%	58%–69%	MRI/ECA
CT/MRI	89%–98%	67%–81%	92%–99%	50%–79%	MRI/EOB
CEUS	96%–97%	57%–73%	94%–99%	70%	CEUS

Data from Refs.[21,23,28,29]

the reported performance of the CT/MRI and CEUS LR-5 for the diagnosis of HCC. Percentages of HCCs described in prior studies using CT or MRI in the remaining categories are: 0% to 14.8% for LR-2, 16.7% to 40.5% for LR-3, and 47.6% to 74% for LR-4.[23,27,29] Some studies have demonstrated a slightly higher sensitivity of MRI compared with CT, especially for observations less than 20 mm, with HBA-enhanced MRI having the highest sensitivity.[30] Nevertheless, LI-RADS provides 1 single diagnostic algorithm (CT/MRI LI-RADS) and does not recommend 1 cross-sectional method over another, recognizing that the choice of imaging techniques and contrast agents may depend on clinical and institutional factors and the radiologist's expertise. For CEUS LI-RADS, in 2 large studies with more than 1000 observations each, the rates of HCC in the LR-1, LR-2, LR-3, LR-4, and LR-5 categories were 0%, 0%, 11.5% to 47%, 72.3% to 86.0%, and 93.3% to 98.5%, respectively.[21,22]

Not all Malignancies Are Hepatocellular Carcinoma–the Role of LR-M

The LR-M category (probably or definitely malignant, not specific for HCC) describes an observation that is highly suspicious for malignancy but cannot be definitively categorized as HCC. The LR-M category was designed to preserve the specificity of the LI-RADS algorithm for diagnosis of HCC while not losing sensitivity for the diagnosis of malignancy.[31] Accordingly, the LR-M category has high sensitivity for liver malignancies overall, although the performance parameters for this category may vary because of different study designs and populations, and percentages of combined tumors (cHCC-CCA) that impose a diagnostic challenge on imaging.[32–34] The imaging features of LR-M differ between CEUS and CT/MRI. CT/MRI imaging features of LR-M dominantly are described with targetoid morphology or nontargetoid masses that do not meet LR-5 criteria but have infiltrative appearance, marked diffusion restriction, or necrosis. Targetoid appearance includes rim enhancement in the arterial phase (rim APHE), peripheral washout, and progressive central enhancement on delayed phases.[11] Of note, any of these features may be seen in isolation and are sufficient for assigning LR-M categorization. CEUS LI-RADS features of LR-M also include a targetoid appearance (ie, rim APHE). However, unlike CT/MRI, the assessment of washout is based on the time of onset and degree and not morphology. The presence of early (within 60 seconds) and marked washout (observations becoming very dark) are features of LR-M on CEUS.[16] **Fig. 4** shows an example of LR-M observation on CEUS and CT. Conversely, the combination of nonrim APHE with late (onset after 60 seconds) and mild washout permits diagnosis of HCC with almost 99% PPV in the at-risk population.[21]

Almost any liver malignancy can show features of LR-M, although the most common entities in the population of patients at risk for HCC are intrahepatic

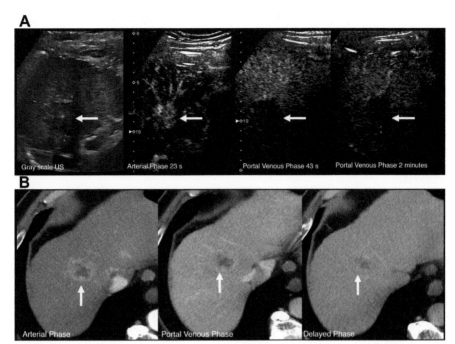

Fig. 4. 62-year-old man with cirrhosis secondary to chronic hepatitis C viral infection and alcohol abuse. (*A*) Gray scale ultrasound and CEUS showing a 32 mm hypoechoic nodule in the right liver lobe. The nodule shows nonrim APHE and early (<1 min) and marked washout. Both early and marked washout is a major feature for CEUS LR-M and typical washout pattern for nonhepatocellular malignancy. (*B*) Pre- and post-contrast CT images show major features for LR-M (*arrows*). Rim APHE and progressive central enhancement with peripheral washout. Histology results showed an intrahepatic cholangiocarcinoma. Different washout pattern is seen between the pure intravascular microbubble contrast agent for CEUS and small molecular contrast agent for CT (and MRI).

cholangiocarcinoma (ICC), combined tumors (cHCC-CCA), and atypical HCC. A common misconception is that LR-M means non-HCC malignancy. Rather, LR-M may still be HCC. The true percentage of LR-M lesions that are subsequently proven to be HCC on biopsy is not fully understood. In a meta-analysis, CT/MRI LR-M observations revealed 36% were HCC (95% confidence interval [CI]: 26%–48%), and 93% overall were malignant (95% CI 87%–97%).[25] An analysis of 288 CEUS LR-M lesions showed 59.7% (172/288) were HCCs; 33% (95/288) were non-HCC malignancies, and 7.3% (21/288) were benign.[22] Hence, LR-M observations should undergo multidisciplinary discussion of diagnostic and treatment options.

The differentiation between HCC from other malignancies in patients with cirrhosis has critical management and prognostic implications. Patients with HCC within stage T2 are eligible for curative treatment through transplantation, but transplantation is often contraindicated in patients with non-HCC malignancies because of the poor long-term survival and high recurrence rates.[35] LI-RADS aims to achieve a very high specificity/PPV for HCC to avoid transplantation misallocation. It is important to note, however, that because of the stringent nature of the LI-RADS criteria, not all HCCs are categorized as LR-5, and some may be categorized as LR-3, LR-4 ,or LR-M.[28] Rarely, other malignancies may potentially be categorized as LR-5; cHCC-

CCA may have imaging features from both lineages, and up to 54% of these lesions may be categorized LR-5.[32]

Emerging data suggest that imaging features and the final LI-RADS category may correlate with biologic behavior and provide prognostic information, regardless of the pathologic diagnosis. Choi and colleagues[33] described that among HCCs, tumors exhibiting imaging features of LR-M had worse overall survival and recurrence-free survival than tumors categorized as LR-4 or LR-5. In a study by Jeon and colleagues[34] cHCC-CCA categorized as LR-M on imaging showed higher recurrence rates than cHCC-CCA categorized as LR-4 or LR-5. Although these retrospective studies suggest that imaging information might have prognostic value, prospective trials are needed to determine how this information should be used in guiding management decisions.

MANAGEMENT TAILORED TO CATEGORY

The management of observations detected on imaging in patients at risk for HCC usually follows guidelines proposed by individual medical societies. These guidelines are often broad to accommodate institutional practices, clinical scenarios, and treatment options inherent to certain geographic regions or populations. In 2018, CT/MRI LI-RADS was incorporated into the AASLD practice guidelines for HCC, leading to a unified management algorithm.[17] Nevertheless, it is important to note that these are informative recommendations, and the AASLD/LI-RADS algorithm does not dictate management. Management decisions should incorporate other clinically available information and institutional practices, ideally supported by multidisciplinary discussions. **Fig. 5** illustrates AASLD-LI-RADS unified management algorithm (CT/MRI) and CEUS LI-RADS management recommendations, which are not currently endorsed by AASLD.

Observations categorized as LR-5 are considered definite HCC, and therefore, staging and treatment planning are recommended without the need of additional imaging or invasive tests. Eventually, biopsy can be pursued in certain scenarios, such as the need for molecular profiling to determine systemic therapy options or in clinical trials.

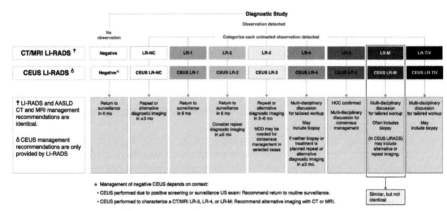

Fig. 5. CT/MRI AASLD-LI-RADS and CEUS LIRADS management recommendations condensed. Both algorithms are similar with minor differences noticed for negative studies and in the LR-M category. (*Adapted from* https://www.acr.org/Clinical-Resources/Reporting-and-Data-Systems/LI-RADS. Accessed Dec 10, 2019; with permission.)

CT/MRI LR-5 observations count toward T staging to determine patient eligibility for transplantation. In the United States, OPTN is the organization that regulates organ allocation for transplantation. The criteria for definite HCC are similar between LI-RADS and OPTN, with the exception of observations 10 to 19 mm in size, with APHE and washout appearance. According to LI-RADS, these observations meet criteria for LR-5, whereas they are not considered definite HCC by OPTN (OPTN Class 5), and hence, do not count toward T staging.[36] Additionally, OPTN does not routinely recognize CEUS LR-5 for transplantation eligibility.

Management of observations with high probability of malignancy but not definite HCCs (LR-4 and LR-M observations) should be individualized based on specific patient factors and multidisciplinary discussions. Biopsy may be recommended for LR-4 observations when it is critical to obtain a definitive HCC diagnosis for transplant eligibility or resection. LR-M observations are commonly biopsied to dictate appropriate therapy for the underlying malignancy. For observations categorized as LR-NC, both algorithms recommend repeat or alternative imaging within 3 months. LR-1 and LR-2 observations should return to routine surveillance at 6-month intervals, while LR-3 observations should undergo short follow-up imaging in 3 to 6 months.[17]

Selection of Modality: Contrast-Enhanced Ultrasound or Computed Tomography/MRI

Institutional, societal, or geographic practices and recommendations affect the choice of imaging modality. Currently, US guidelines only recognize CEUS as a problem-solving tool and recommend CT/MRI for characterizing liver lesions.[17]

At this time, AASLD and OPTN have not adopted CEUS as a tool for the definitive diagnosis of HCC. EASL and the Asian Pacific Association for the Study of the Liver Disease (APASL) recommend CEUS,[1,19] contrast-enhanced CT, or MRI for characterizing nodules detected during surveillance. CEUS for noncardiac applications was introduced in the United States much later than in Asian and European countries because of its late approval by the US Food and Drug Administration (FDA) in April 2016. As a result, the availability and recognition of CEUS in the United States remain low.

In addition to societal and local practices, modality selection should also take into account the advantages and limitations of each individual method. For example, CEUS can immediately characterize an observation after it is located on surveillance ultrasound, a potential cost- and time-effective approach that minimizes loss to follow-up. Its use over more expensive cross-sectional modalities could also be favored in patients with risk factors other than cirrhosis, as less heterogeneous background liver parenchyma could yield higher diagnostic accuracy to this imaging modality. Recent studies have shown that CEUS may provide improved visibility and higher effectiveness for imaging-guided ablation therapies for primary liver tumors.[37] Conversely, in the setting of tumor resection or transplantation, CT/MRI would likely be preferred to concurrently diagnose and stage the malignancy. Additional research is required to assess the preferred use of HBA to provide balance between sensitivity and specificity ECA in specific clinical scenarios as recommended by some medical societies.[19]

SUMMARY

LI-RADS provides a standardized and rigorous imaging system that aims to improve clinical practice for the care of patients with or at risk for HCC. Although CT/MRI and

CEUS LI-RADS diagnose HCC in at-risk patients with comparably high specificity and PPV, clinicians should be aware of the inherent advantages and limitations of the individual modalities to maximize the utility of the algorithms. Familiarity with the similarities and differences between CT/MRI LI-RADS and CEUS LI-RADS will allow for efficient and appropriate clinical decisions based on individualized patient factors.

In conclusion, the adoption of LI-RADS improves the communication among health care professionals and researchers participating in the care of patients with or at risk for HCC. Its probabilistic rather than binary approach provides clear, granular information to guide personalized management strategies. Additionally, the standardization of many aspects of HCC imaging not only results in increased accuracy of the current methods, but also facilitates the use of clinical data for further refinements and improvements, as well as the development of new clinical practices.

DISCLOSURE

All authors involved in this work have no conflicts of interest or industry support to disclose with regard to the current article.

REFERENCES

1. European Association For The Study Of The Liver. EASL clinical practice guidelines: management of hepatocellular carcinoma. J Hepatol 2018;69(1):182–236.
2. Fattovich G, Stroffolini T, Zagni I, et al. Hepatocellular carcinoma in cirrhosis: incidence and risk factors. Gastroenterology 2004;127(5):S35–50.
3. Di Costanzo GG, Rodríguez M, Velázquez RF. Prospective analysis of risk factors for hepatocellular carcinoma on patients with cirrhosis. Hepatology 2003;38(4): 1061.
4. Calvaruso V, Cabibbo G, Cacciola I, et al. Incidence of hepatocellular carcinoma in patients with HCV-associated cirrhosis treated with direct-acting antiviral agents. Gastroenterology 2018;155(2):411–21.
5. Fattovich G, Bortolotti F, Donato F. Natural history of chronic hepatitis B: special emphasis on disease progression and prognostic factors. J Hepatol 2008; 48(2):335–52.
6. Raffetti E, Fattovich G, Donato F. Incidence of hepatocellular carcinoma in untreated subjects with chronic hepatitis B: a systematic review and meta-analysis. Liver Int 2016;36(9):1239–51.
7. Bruix J, Reig M, Sherman M. Evidence-based diagnosis, staging, and treatment of patients with hepatocellular carcinoma. Gastroenterology 2016;150(4):835–53.
8. Tzartzeva K, Obi J, Rich NE, et al. Surveillance imaging and alpha fetoprotein for early detection of hepatocellular carcinoma in patients with cirrhosis: a meta-analysis. Gastroenterology 2018;154(6):1706–18.
9. Castilla-Lièvre MA, Franco D, Gervais P, et al. Diagnostic value of combining 11 C-choline and 18 F-FDG PET/CT in hepatocellular carcinoma. Eur J Nucl Med Mol Imaging 2016;43(5):852–9.
10. Heimbach JK, Kulik LM, Finn RS, et al. AASLD guidelines for the treatment of hepatocellular carcinoma. Hepatology 2018;67(1):358–80.
11. Chernyak V, Fowler KJ, Kamaya A, et al. Liver Imaging Reporting and Data System (LI-RADS) version 2018: imaging of hepatocellular carcinoma in at-risk patients. Radiology 2018;289(3):816–30.
12. Fraum TJ, Cannella R, Ludwig DR, et al. Assessment of primary liver carcinomas other than hepatocellular carcinoma (HCC) with LI-RADS v2018: comparison of

the LI-RADS target population to patients without LI-RADS-defined HCC risk factors. Eur Radiol 2020;30(2):996–1007.

13. Singh S, Venkatesh SK, Loomba R, et al. Magnetic resonance elastography for staging liver fibrosis in non-alcoholic fatty liver disease: a diagnostic accuracy systematic review and individual participant data pooled analysis. Eur Radiol 2016;26(5):1431–40.

14. Herrmann E, de Lédinghen V, Cassinotto C, et al. Assessment of biopsy-proven liver fibrosis by two-dimensional shear wave elastography: an individual patient data-based meta-analysis. Hepatology 2018;67(1):260–72.

15. Lyshchik A, Kono Y, Dietrich CF, et al. Contrast-enhanced ultrasound of the liver: technical and lexicon recommendations from the ACR CEUS LI-RADS working group. Abdom Radiol (NY) 2018;43(4):861–79.

16. Wilson SR, Lyshchik A, Piscaglia F, et al. Ceus LI-RADS: algorithm, implementation, and key differences from CT/MRI. Abdom Radiol (NY) 2018;43(1):127–42.

17. Marrero JA, Kulik LM, Sirlin CB, et al. Diagnosis, staging, and management of hepatocellular carcinoma: 2018 practice guidance by the American Association for the Study of Liver Diseases. Hepatology 2018;68(2):723–50.

18. Available at: https://optn.transplant.hrsa.gov/governance/policies/. Accessed December 10, 2019.

19. Omata M, Cheng AL, Kokudo N, et al. Asia–Pacific clinical practice guidelines on the management of hepatocellular carcinoma: a 2017 update. Hepatol Int 2017; 11(4):317–70.

20. Available at: https://www.acr.org/Clinical-Resources/Reporting-and-Data-Systems/LI-RADS. Accessed December 10, 2019.

21. Terzi E, Iavarone M, Pompili M, et al. Contrast ultrasound LI-RADS LR-5 identifies hepatocellular carcinoma in cirrhosis in a multicenter restropective study of 1,006 nodules. J Hepatol 2018;68(3):485–92.

22. Li J, Ling W, Chen S, et al. The interreader agreement and validation of contrast-enhanced ultrasound liver imaging reporting and data system. Eur J Radiol 2019; 120:108685.

23. Huang JY, Li JW, Lu Q, et al. Diagnostic accuracy of CEUS LI-RADS for the characterization of liver nodules 20 mm or smaller in patients at risk for hepatocellular carcinoma. Radiology 2020;294(2):329–39.

24. Vogel A, Cervantes A, Chau I, et al. Hepatocellular carcinoma: ESMO clinical practice guidelines for diagnosis, treatment and follow-up. Ann Oncol 2019; 30(5):871–3.

25. van der Pol CB, Lim CS, Sirlin CB, et al. Accuracy of the liver imaging reporting and data system in computed tomography and magnetic resonance image analysis of hepatocellular carcinoma or overall malignancy—a systematic review. Gastroenterology 2019;156(4):976–86.

26. Ronot M, Fouque O, Esvan M, et al. Comparison of the accuracy of AASLD and LI-RADS criteria for the non-invasive diagnosis of HCC smaller than 3 cm. J Hepatol 2018;68(4):715–23.

27. Kim YY, An C, Kim S, et al. Diagnostic accuracy of prospective application of the liver imaging reporting and data system (LI-RADS) in gadoxetate-enhanced MRI. Eur Radiol 2018;28(5):2038–46.

28. Kim YY, Kim MJ, Kim EH, et al. Hepatocellular carcinoma versus other hepatic malignancy in cirrhosis: performance of LI-RADS version 2018. Radiology 2019;291(1):72–80.

29. Ren AH, Zhao PF, Yang DW, et al. Diagnostic performance of MR for hepatocellular carcinoma based on LI-RADS v2018, compared with v2017. J Magn Reson Imaging 2019;50(3):746–55.

30. Semaan S, Violi NV, Lewis S, et al. Hepatocellular carcinoma detection in liver cirrhosis: diagnostic performance of contrast-enhanced CT vs. MRI with extracellular contrast vs. gadoxetic acid. Eur Radiol 2020;30(2):1020–30.

31. Fowler KJ, Potretzke TA, Hope TA, et al. LI-RADS M (LR-M): definite or probable malignancy, not specific for hepatocellular carcinoma. Abdom Radiol (NY) 2018; 43(1):149–57.

32. Potretzke TA, Tan BR, Doyle MB, et al. Imaging features of biphenotypic primary liver carcinoma (hepatocholangiocarcinoma) and the potential to mimic hepatocellular carcinoma: LI-RADS analysis of CT and MRI features in 61 cases. AJR Am J Roentgenol 2016;207(1):25–31.

33. Choi SH, Lee SS, Park SH, et al. LI-RADS classification and prognosis of primary liver cancers at gadoxetic acid–enhanced MRI. Radiology 2019;290(2):388–97.

34. Jeon SK, Joo I, Lee DH, et al. Combined hepatocellular cholangiocarcinoma: LI-RADS v2017 categorisation for differential diagnosis and prognostication on gadoxetic acid-enhanced MR imaging. Eur Radiol 2019;29(1):373–82.

35. Lee DD, Croome KP, Musto KR, et al. Liver transplantation for intrahepatic cholangiocarcinoma. Liver Transpl 2018;24(5):634–44.

36. Wald C, Russo MW, Heimbach JK, et al. New OPTN/UNOS policy for liver transplant allocation: standardization of liver imaging, diagnosis, classification, and reporting of hepatocellular carcinoma. Radiology 2013;266(2):376–82.

37. Francica G, Meloni MF, Riccardi L, et al. Ablation treatment of primary and secondary liver tumors under contrast-enhanced ultrasound guidance in field practice of interventional ultrasound centers. A multicenter study. Eur J Radiol 2018; 105:96–101.

Surgical Resection
Old Dog, Any New Tricks?

Yoshikuni Kawaguchi, MD, PhD[a,b], Heather A. Lillemoe, MD[a],
Jean-Nicolas Vauthey, MD[a],*

KEYWORDS

- Hepatocellular carcinoma • Surgery • Liver resection • Laparoscopic liver resection
- Future liver remnant • Portal vein embolization • Major resection • Immunotherapy

KEY POINTS

- Treatment guidelines of hepatocellular carcinoma (HCC) vary between Western and Eastern countries, taking into account local factors (eg, the availability of donors for liver transplant).
- The minimal requirement of future liver remnant/standardized liver volume is 40% in patients with cirrhosis, whereas it is 20% to 25% for patients with normal liver.
- A new 3-level complexity classification effectively stratifies 11 common liver resection procedures with respect to surgical and postoperative outcomes and may be useful as a training pathway.
- For patients with small HCCs (ie, <3 cm), both resection and ablation can be recommended from the results of 5 randomized controlled trials.
- New medical therapies, including multikinase inhibitors and immunotherapies, are promising, and perioperative use of these therapies may further improve outcomes in patients undergoing HCC resection.

INTRODUCTION

Liver cancer is the sixth most common cancer and, in 2018, was the fourth leading cause of cancer-related death worldwide.[1] The rates of incidence and mortality are approximately 2 to 3 times higher for men than for women. Hepatocellular carcinoma (HCC) is the most common primary liver cancer and accounts for 75% to 85% of diagnoses, followed by intrahepatic cholangiocarcinoma (10%–15%), and other rare liver histologies. The improvement and safety of surgical techniques for liver resection and transplant, and advancements in ablation, transarterial chemoembolization

[a] Department of Surgical Oncology, The University of Texas MD Anderson Cancer Center, 1515 Holcombe Boulevard, Unit 1484, Houston, TX 77030, USA; [b] Hepato-Biliary-Pancreatic Surgery Division, Department of Surgery, Graduate School of Medicine, The University of Tokyo, 7-3-1 Hongo, Bunkyo-ku, Tokyo 113-8655, Japan
* Corresponding author. Hepato-Biliary-Pancreatic Surgery Division, Department of Surgery, Graduate School of Medicine, The University of Tokyo, 7-3-1 Hongo, Bunkyo-ku, Tokyo 113-8655.
E-mail address: jvauthey@mdanderson.org

Clin Liver Dis 24 (2020) 637–655
https://doi.org/10.1016/j.cld.2020.07.004
1089-3261/20/© 2020 Elsevier Inc. All rights reserved.

(TACE), and systemic therapies have expanded the treatment options for patients with HCC. Liver transplant is the ideal treatment option for patients with HCC and poorly compensated liver disease because it removes both HCC and damaged liver and reduces the risk for early recurrence. However, shortages in donor liver and long waiting times to transplant are significant barriers to this treatment approach. As such, liver resection remains an effective treatment option for patients with HCC. The use of a multidisciplinary approach and the knowledge of each therapeutic option is critical in the management of patients with HCC. This article reviews the current evidence surrounding resection of HCC, including alternative and multimodal treatment approaches to the management of this disease.

TREATMENT GUIDELINES FOR HEPATOCELLULAR CARCINOMA: DIFFERENCES BETWEEN WEST AND EAST

The Barcelona Clinic Liver Cancer (BCLC) staging classification is widely used in Western countries. The classification recommends surgery only for patients with single HCCs in very early stage 0 disease[2] (solitary HCC <2 cm and Child-Pugh grade A) and in early stage A (single and Child-Pugh grade A–B) (**Fig. 1A**). It recommends ablation or liver transplant for patients with early stage A (largest HCC ≤3 cm and number of s ≤3).[3–5] Compared with Western countries, the selection criteria for liver resection are generally more lenient and indications for transplant are stricter in Eastern countries.[6,7] The Japanese clinical practice guidelines for HCC (fourth Japan Society of Hepatology [JSH] HCC guidelines) recommend both liver resection and radiofrequency ablation for patients who have less than or equal to 3 HCCs and Child-Pugh grade A to B, and recommend liver transplant for patients who have HCCs within Milan criteria and Child-Pugh grade C (**Fig. 1B**).[6] Importantly, these treatment guidelines are influenced by the availability of donors for liver transplant. Clearly, the treatment guidelines vary between Western and Eastern countries, taking into account local factors.

Liver Resection of Hepatocellular Carcinoma

Minimal future liver remnant requirements

Liver resection remains the treatment of choice for HCC. Two major preoperative considerations for HCC resection are the patient's liver function and the predicted future liver remnant (FLR). The intrinsic liver function of patients with HCC is often impaired because this patient population generally has chronic liver disease, including viral hepatitis, alcoholic hepatitis, and nonalcoholic steatohepatitis. As such, studies report that more FLR is needed for patients undergoing resection for HCC than for patients undergoing resection of secondary liver cancer (ie, metastatic disease).[8] The minimal requirement of FLR/standardized liver volume (standardized liver volume = $-794 + 1267.28 \times$ body surface area)[9] is 30% in patients with hepatic injury and fibrosis and 40% in patients with cirrhosis,[10] whereas it is 20% to 25% for patients with normal liver.[11,12]

New 3-level complexity classification

The assessment of FLR is important to avoid postoperative hepatic insufficiency. As a useful indicator for hepatic insufficiency, liver resection has historically been categorized in the binary fashion of major versus minor, from the number of resected segments. Major liver resection is generally defined as the resection of 3 or more contiguous Couinaud segments,[13–16] and is associated with higher rates of postoperative hepatic insufficiency than minor liver resection for both open and laparoscopic approaches.[17–21] However, the minor/major classification system does not necessarily stratify procedures effectively with respect to surgical and postoperative

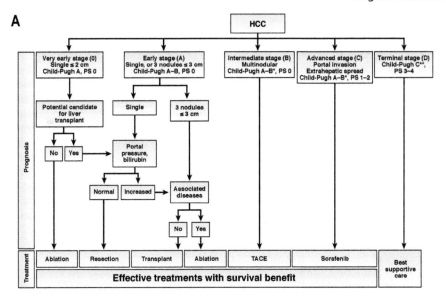

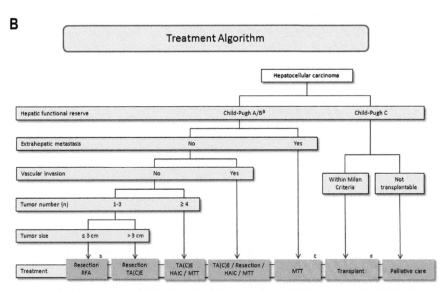

Fig. 1. Clinical practice guidelines in Western countries and Japan. (*A*) Staging and treatment according to the BCLC system.[96] (*B*) Clinical practice guidelines for hepatocellular carcinoma: The Japan Society of Hepatology 2017 (fourth JSH-HCC guidelines) 2019 update.[6] *Note that Child-Pugh classification is not sensitive to accurately identify those patients with advanced liver failure that would deserve liver transplant consideration. **Patients with end stage cirrhosis due to heavily impaired liver function (Child-Pugh C or earlier stage with predictors of poor prognosis, high Model for End-Stage Liver Disease score) should be considered for liver transplantation. In them, HCC may become a contraindication if exceeding the enlistment criteria. [a] Assessment based on liver damage is recommended in the case of hepatectomy. [b] For solitary hepatocellular carcinoma, resection is recommended as first-line therapy, and ablation as second-line therapy. [c] Patients with Child-Pugh A only. [d] Patients aged less than or equal to 65 years. HAIC, hepatic arterial infusion chemotherapy; MTT, molecular-targeted therapy; RFA, radiofrequency ablation; TACE, transcatheter arterial

outcomes.[17,19,22,23] Our group has recently reported a 3-level complexity classification and categorized 11 common liver resection procedures as being of low, intermediate, or high complexity (grade) (**Fig. 2**).[19–21] Our data showed that the new 3-level classification system effectively stratified 11 liver resection procedures with respect to surgical and postoperative outcomes in Western and Eastern cohorts for both open and laparoscopic liver resections.[19–21,24] **Fig. 3** shows details related to duration of operation, estimated blood loss, and comprehensive complication index[25] for the procedures individually and stratified by grade using the 3-level classification scale. There was a clear, incremental increase in each of these factors as surgical complexity progressively increased from grade I to grade III. This scale predicts surgical complexity and postoperative morbidity better than the minor/major classification for both open and laparoscopic approaches.[20,21] Therefore, our 3-level classification may be useful as a training pathway for performing liver resections, and for tailoring management after liver resection (**Fig. 4**).

Anatomic resection versus nonanatomic resection

Anatomic resection of Couinaud segment for small HCC was reported in 1981 by Makuuchi and colleagues.[26] HCC frequently invades to the intrahepatic vascular structures and spreads through the portal vein. As such, the complete removal of tumor-bearing portal territory was reported to be theoretically superior to nonanatomic resection. The technique proposed by Makuuchi and colleagues[26] is detailed as follows: (1) under the guidance of intraoperative ultrasonography, the portal vein of interest is identified and punctured using a 22-gauge needle; (2) blue dye is injected into the portal vein; (3) the territory of the dyed surface is marked using electrocautery; and (4) liver resection is performed using ultrasonography guidance and intersegmental hepatic veins are exposed. This technique was recently refined using fluorescence imaging.[27–29] By using transportal injection or systemic intravenous injection of indocyanine green, the portal vein territory was more clearly visualized on the liver surface compared with the traditional method (**Fig. 5**). Many retrospective studies reported that anatomic resection was associated with better survival and lower recurrence than nonanatomic resection.[30–33] In contrast, other studies showed that survival did not differ significantly between patients undergoing anatomic resection and those undergoing nonanatomic resection.[34,35] Therefore, this clinical question remains unanswered and needs to be further elucidated.

Portal vein embolization

FLR is one of the most important factors when determining the technical resectability of HCC. To induce the hypertrophy of FLR and avoid the risk of postoperative hepatic insufficiency,[36] portal vein embolization (PVE) has been used.[8] The use of PVE was reported by Makuuchi and colleagues,[37] Matsuoka and colleagues,[38] and Kinoshita and colleagues[39] in the 1980s. PVE has now been adopted as a safe procedure frequently used to increase the volume of FLR for patients undergoing liver resection.[40–44]

----

chemoembolization. PS, posterosuperior. (*From* [A] Bruix J, Reig M, Sherman M. Evidence-Based Diagnosis, Staging, and Treatment of Patients With Hepatocellular Carcinoma. *Gastroenterology.* 2016;150(4):835-853; with permission; and [B] Kokudo N, Takemura N, Hasegawa K, et al. Clinical practice guidelines for hepatocellular carcinoma: The Japan Society of Hepatology 2017 (4th JSH-HCC guidelines) 2019 update. *Hepatology research: the official journal of the Japan Society of Hepatology.* 2019, with permission.)

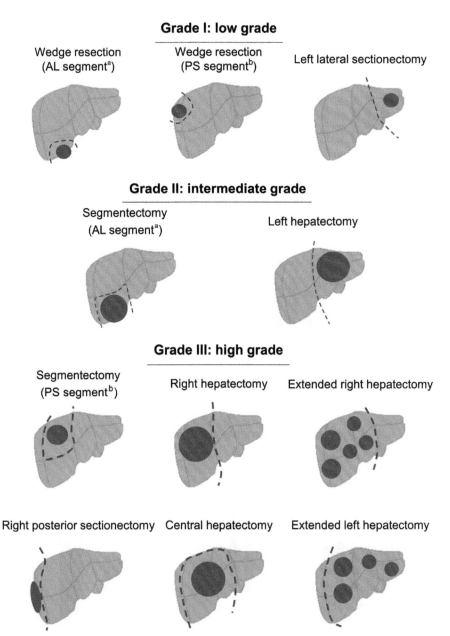

Fig. 2. New 3-level complexity classification. [a] Anterolateral (AL) segments are defined as Couinaud segments 2, 3, 4b, 5, and 6, and [b] PS segments are defined as Couinaud segments 1, 4a, 7, and 8.

Liver resection for HCC following PVE is feasible and safe, with reported morbidity rates of 19% to 55% and mortalities of 0% to 12% (**Table 1**).[41,45–52] The 5-year overall survival ranged from 44% to 72% in patients who underwent combined PVE and HCC resection. Studies also report that sequential TACE and PVE before liver resection is a feasible and useful treatment option.[53–56] This tactic prevents tumor progression and

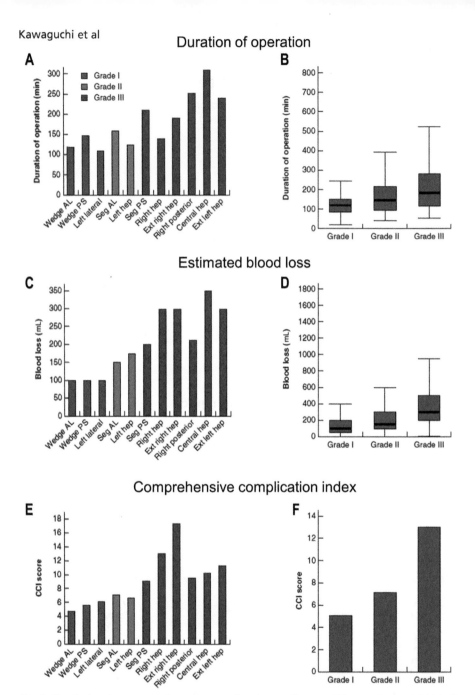

Fig. 3. Surgical and postoperative outcomes for 11 open liver resection procedures (*A, C, E*) and 3 grades (*B, D, F*) in our 3-level classification. (*A, B*) Duration of operation, (*C, D*) estimated blood loss, and (*E, F*) comprehensive complication index (CCI).[25] Central hep, central hepatectomy; Ext left hep, extended left hepatectomy; Ext right hep, extended right hepatectomy; Left hep, left hepatectomy; Left lateral, left lateral sectionectomy; Right hep, right hepatectomy; Right posterior, right posterior sectionectomy; Seg-AL, anterolateral segmentectomy; Seg-PS, PS segmentectomy; Wedge-AL, wedge resection of anterolateral segment; Wedge-PS, wedge resection of PS segment. (*Adapted from* Kawaguchi Y, Hasegawa K, Tzeng CD, et al. Performance of a modified three-level classification in stratifying open liver resection procedures in terms of complexity and postoperative morbidity. *The British journal of surgery.* 2020 Feb;107(3):258-267; with permission.)

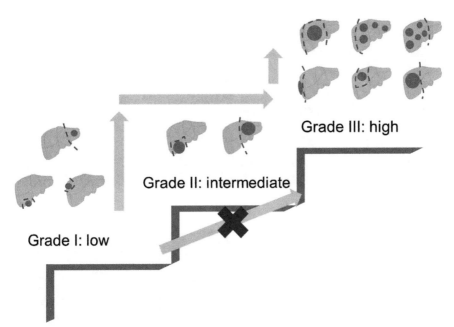

Fig. 4. Proposed training pathway based on 3-level complexity classification.

may increase hypertrophy in the FLR because arterial flow is also occluded. Ogata and colleagues[54] showed that the hypertrophy of the FLR was greater in patients who underwent TACE plus PVE than in patients who underwent PVE alone.

Laparoscopic liver resection

Laparoscopic liver resection (LLR) has been increasingly used worldwide.[57] In their systemic review, Nguyen and colleagues[58] reported on the safety of LLR with low rates of morbidity and mortality for both major and minor resections, as well as appropriate oncologic results compared with open liver resection (OLR). These results are most likely caused by patient selection and the advantages of the laparoscopic approach, including a magnified view[59,60] and the hemostatic effect caused by pneumoperitoneum.[61,62] Three retrospective studies including more than 200 patients showed that the 5-year overall survival (OS) was not significantly different between patients undergoing LLR for HCC and those undergoing OLR for HCC.[63–65] However, no randomized controlled trials (RCTs) comparing long-term outcomes in patients undergoing LLR versus OLR for HCC have been reported. For patients with colorectal liver metastases, a recent RCT (Oslo-CoMet study) showed that median OS in patients undergoing LLR was similar to those undergoing OLR: 80 months versus 81 months.[66]

Liver Resection Versus Ablation

It remains unclear whether liver resection or ablation is the most effective treatment of small HCC lesions. To answer this clinical question, 5 RCTs have been reported (**Table 2**).[67–71] Two of these studies showed that liver resection was associated with better survival than radiofrequency ablation[68,70] and 3 showed that survival did not differ significantly between patients undergoing resection and those undergoing ablation.[67,69,71] The shortcomings of these RCTs include insufficient patient follow-up; unclear treatment allocation; and different inclusion criteria, including tumor number,

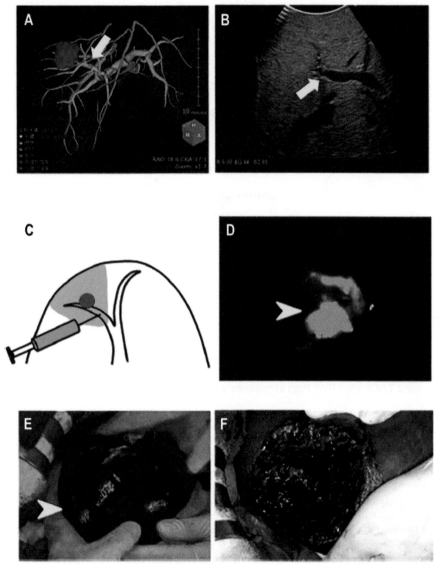

Fig. 5. Portal vein territory identification using fluorescence imaging. (*A*) P8 dorsal branch (*arrow*) was shown by three-dimensional simulation. (*B*) P8 dorsal branch (*arrow*) was visualized by intraoperative ultrasonography. (*C*) Schema of portal vein territory identification. (*D*) Fluorescence imaging clearly showed the territory of P8 dorsal branch (*arrowhead*). (*E*) Blue dye-stained regions (*arrowhead*) were unclear on gross examination of the liver. (*F*) Cut surface of the liver after anatomic resection of P8 dorsal branch territory. (*From* Kobayashi Y, Kawaguchi Y, Kobayashi K, et al. Portal vein territory identification using indocyanine green fluorescence imaging: Technical details and short-term outcomes. *Journal of surgical oncology.* 2017;116(7):921-931. with permission.)

Table 1
Outcomes of resection after preoperative portal vein embolization for hepatocellular carcinoma

Author, Year	Regions	N	Morbidity (%)	Mortality (%)	5-y DFS (%)	5-y OS (%)
PVE						
Azoulay et al,[41] 2000	Europe	10	55	0	21	44
Tanaka et al,[45] 2000	Asia	33	NA	2	33	50
Wakabayashi et al,[46] 2001	Asia	26	NA	12	40	46
Sugawara et al,[47] 2002	Asia	66	NA	0	38	59
Seo et al,[48] 2007	Asia	32	19	0	37	72
Palavecino et al,[49] 2009	United States	21	24	0	56	72
Siriwardana et al,[51] 2012	Asia	34	47	6	Approximately 40[a]	Approximately 60[a]
TACE + PVE						
Aoki et al,[53] 2004	Asia	24	24	0	47	56
Ogata et al,[54] 2006	Europe	18	39	NA	37	NA
Yoo et al,[55] 2011	Asia	68	NA	0	61	72
Ronot et al,[56] 2016	Europe	39	NA	8	NA	Approximately 30[a]

Abbreviations: DFS, disease-free survival; NA, not available; OS, overall survival.
[a] Estimated by the Kaplan-Meier curve.

tumor diameter, and Child-Pugh grade. Nonetheless, for patients with small HCCs (ie, <3 cm), the current evidence shows that both resection and ablation can be recommended.

Liver Resection Versus Transarterial Chemoembolization

There has been 1 RCT comparing the outcomes of patients undergoing resection for HCC with those undergoing TACE.[72] For patients outside of Milan criteria,[73] resection was associated with better survival than TACE (**Table 3**). The authors found 8 cohort studies comparing outcomes after resection with TACE using the propensity score adjustment.[72,74–81] Although the studies had different inclusion criteria, the data

Table 2
Liver resection versus ablation, randomized controlled trials

Author, Year	Regions	N	Tumor Number	Tumor Diameter (cm)	Child-Pugh Grade	Result
Chen et al,[67] 2006	Asia	180	1	≤ 5	A	Not significant
Huang et al,[68] 2010	Asia	230	Milan criteria[a]		A, B	Favor for resection
Feng et al,[69] 2012	Asia	168	≤ 2	≤ 4	A, B	Not significant
Liu et al,[70] 2016	Asia	200	Milan criteria[a]		A, B	Favor for resection
Izumi et al,[71] 2019	Asia	308	≤ 3	≤ 3	A, B	Not significant

[a] A solitary HCC nodule of 5 cm or less, or up to 3 nodules of 3 cm or less.[73]

show that resection is associated with better survival than TACE in selected patients who have multiple HCCs.

Liver Resection Versus Liver Transplant

Liver transplant is an established treatment option for patients who have early-stage HCC and poorly compensated cirrhosis and/or portal hypertension.[73,82] However, the preferred treatment of patients who have early-stage HCC and well-compensated cirrhosis is not established. Several retrospective studies have evaluated outcomes after liver resection for HCC in this setting, comparing them with those of transplant. However, most are limited by small sample sizes and low statistical power. No prospective studies have been performed on this topic given the inability to randomize patients to liver resection versus transplant. The authors found 2 studies including more than 200 patients (**Table 4**). They both suggest that transplant is associated with better survival than liver resection in patients within Milan criteria and Child-Pugh A or B.[83,84] Nonetheless, it should be noted that graft availability and waiting times for transplant differ between countries, which greatly influences the selection of liver resection versus transplant for patients with early-stage HCC.

New Medical Therapies and Liver Resection

In 2009, studies showed that sorafenib was an effective medical therapy for HCC.[85,86] The STORM trial compared patients who were assigned to receive either sorafenib or placebo after resection or ablation of HCC. The study did not show a significant survival benefit in those receiving sorafenib in the adjuvant setting.[87]

Recent studies have shown the effectiveness of new medical therapies for HCC as first and second lines (**Table 5**). These new therapies include multikinase inhibitors and immunotherapies. The REFLECT study showed that lenvatinib was noninferior to sorafenib for patients with untreated advanced HCC in first-line settings.[88] The CELESTIAL study, the REACH-II study, and the RESOURCE study respectively showed cabozantinib, ramucirumab, and regorafenib were associated with longer survival than placebo for the treatment of HCC in the second-line setting.[89–91] Recent results of immunotherapy trials are also promising in both first-line and second-line settings.[92–94] For first-line therapy in HCC, CheckMate-459 found that nivolumab was associated with better survival than sorafenib[92] and IMbrave150 showed that the

Table 3
Liver resection versus transarterial chemoembolization, randomized controlled trials and cohort studies using adjustment of propensity score

Author, Year	Regions	N	Tumor Number	Tumor Diameter (cm)	Child-Pugh Grade	OS
RCT
Yin et al,[72] 2014	Asia	173	Outside of Milan criteria[a]		A, B	Favor for resection
Cohort Studies Using Adjustment of Propensity Score
Hsu et al,[74] 2012	Asia	292	Outside of Milan criteria[a]		A, B	Favor for resection
Guo et al,[75] 2014	Asia	304	BCLC stage A[c]		A	Favor for resection
Zhu et al,[76] 2014	Asia	108	BCLC stage A[c]		A, B	Favor for resection
Yang et al,[77] 2014	Asia	118	1	≤3	A, B	Not significant
Shi et al,[78] 2014	Asia	1296	NA	NA	NA	Not significant
Liu et al,[79] 2014	Asia	216	Any with portal vein tumor thrombosis		A, B	Favor for resection
Lee et al,[80] 2015	Asia	118	1	≥ 5	A	Not significant
Zhong et al,[81] 2018	Asia	488	UICC stage (seventh) T3[b]		A, B	Favor for resection

[a] Milan criteria, a solitary HCC nodule of 5 cm or less, or up to 3 nodules of 3 cm or less.[73]
[b] Multiple lesions with any lesion larger than 5 cm (stage IIIa), or involving a major portal vein or hepatic veins (stage IIIb).
[c] A single tumor of any size or 2 to 3 tumors less than or equal to 3 cm.

Table 4
Liver resection versus transplant, retrospective studies including more than 200 patients

Author, Year	Regions	N	Tumor Number	Tumor Diameter (cm)	Child-Pugh Grade	5-y OS
Shah et al,[83] 2007	Europe	261	Milan criteria[a]		Child-Pugh A, B	Favor for transplant
Bellavance et al,[84] 2008	United States and Europe	379	Milan criteria[a]		Child-Pugh A, B	Favor for transplant

[a] Milan criteria, a solitary HCC nodule of 5 cm or less, or up to 3 nodules of 3 cm or less.[73]

Table 5
New medical therapy for hepatocellular carcinoma

Author, Year	Drug	Target	Study	Phase	Design	Median OS (mo) HR; 95% CI
First Line						
Kudo et al,[88] 2018	Lenvatinib	Multi-kinase	REFLECT	3	Vs sorafenib	13.6 vs 12.3 0.92; 0.79–1.06
Yau et al,[92] 2019	Nivolumab	PD-1	ChekMate-459	3	Vs Sorafenib	16.4 vs 14.7 0.85; 0.72–1.02
Cheng et al,[94] 2019	Atezolizumab + Bevacizumab	PD-L1 + VEGF	IMbrave150	3	Vs Sorafenib	6.8 vs 4.3 0.59; 0.47–0.76
Second Line						
Abou-Alfa et al,[89] 2018	Cabozantinib	Met/VEGFR-2	CELESTIAL	3	Vs Placebo	10.2 vs 8.0 0.76; 0.63–0.92
Zhu et al,[90] 2019	Ramucirumab	VEGFR-2	REACH-II	3	Vs Placebo	8.5 vs 7.3 0.71; 0.53–0.95
Bruix et al,[91] 2017	Regorafenib	Multi-kinase	RESORCE	3	Vs placebo	10.7 vs 7.8 0.63; 0.50–0.79
Finn et al,[93] 2019	Pembrolizumab	PD-1	KEYNOTE240	3	Vs Placebo	13.9 vs 10.6 0.78; 0.61–0.998

Abbreviations: CI, confidence interval; HR, hazard ratio; PD-1, programmed cell death protein 1; PD-L1, programmed death-ligand 1; VEGFR, vascular endothelial growth factor receptor.

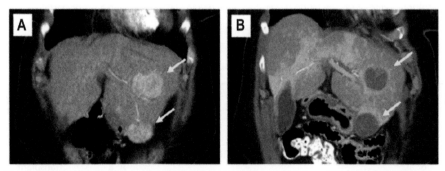

Fig. 6. Pretreatment and posttreatment computed tomography with arterial phase in patient with resectable hepatocellular carcinoma (*arrows*) treated with perioperative immunotherapy. (*A*) Pretreatment. (*B*) After 1 dose of nivolumab and ipilimumab followed by 1 dose of single-agent nivolumab. (*From* Kaseb AO, Vence L, Blando J, et al. Immunologic Correlates of Pathologic Complete Response to Preoperative Immunotherapy in Hepatocellular Carcinoma. *Cancer immunology research.* 2019;7(9):1390-1395; with permission.)

regimen of atezolizumab and bevacizumab was associated with better survival than sorafenib.[94] In the second-line setting, KEYNOTE240 showed that pembrolizumab provided better survival than placebo.[93]

Our group is conducting a randomized pilot study of perioperative immunotherapy for resectable HCC (ClinicalTrial.gov, NCT03222076). The clinical trial has 3 treatment arms: perioperative nivolumab alone in patients with resectable HCC (arm A), perioperative nivolumab plus ipilimumab in patients with resectable HCC (arm B), and perioperative nivolumab plus ipilimumab in patients with potentially resectable HCC (arm C). Our trial has accrued 9 patients, of whom 3 had complete response.[95] **Fig. 6** shows a representative case of a patient who showed complete response after treatment in arm B.[95] After 1 dose of nivolumab and ipilimumab followed by 1 dose of single-agent nivolumab, both lesions were downsized and had a cystlike appearance (see **Fig. 6**B). The patient underwent anatomic resection of segment 3. Histopathologic examination showed 2 hemorrhagic and necrotic liver lesions with no viable tumor cells.

SUMMARY

Liver resection remains an effective treatment option for HCC. The knowledge of liver function and minimal FLR requirement, combined with PVE when necessary, can help ensure the safety of liver resection for patients with HCC and underlying liver disease. The authors suggest a newly proposed 3-level classification system, which better categorizes procedures based on surgical complexity and perioperative morbidity. This classification can be used to guide the training for residents and fellows and improve postoperative management. LLR is one of the breakthroughs in liver resection for HCC in recent years and outcomes have been promising.

Note that guidelines for liver resection differ by country. In Western countries, liver resection is recommended for single lesions and ablation or liver transplant is recommended for small and multiple HCCs. In Eastern countries, liver resection is recommended for both single and multiple HCCs. Liver transplant is not generally performed for patients with well-compensated liver function because of donor shortages, especially in Eastern countries. The current evidence suggests that, for patients with small HCC lesions (<3 cm), OS is likely to be similar for patients undergoing liver resection versus ablation. For selected patients with multiple HCCs, liver resection may be associated with better OS than TACE. For the past 10 years, sorafenib has been the only effective medical therapy available for unresectable HCC. Recently, several promising new therapies, including multikinase inhibitors and immunotherapies, have been reported. Perioperative use of these new therapies may further improve outcomes in patients undergoing liver resection for HCC and potentially change the current treatment guidelines.

ACKNOWLEDGMENTS

The authors thank Ms Ruth Haynes for administrative support in the preparation of this article.

DISCLOSURE

The authors have nothing to disclose.

REFERENCES

1. Marengo A, Rosso C, Bugianesi E. Liver cancer: connections with obesity, fatty liver, and cirrhosis. Annu Rev Med 2016;67:103–17.

2. Takayama T, Makuuchi M, Hirohashi S, et al. Early hepatocellular carcinoma as an entity with a high rate of surgical cure. Hepatology 1998;28(5):1241–6.
3. Bruix J, Sherman M. Management of hepatocellular carcinoma: an update. Hepatology 2011;53(3):1020–2.
4. Llovet JM, Bruix J. Novel advancements in the management of hepatocellular carcinoma in 2008. J Hepatol 2008;48(Suppl 1):S20–37.
5. Duffy JP, Hiatt JR, Busuttil RW. Surgical resection of hepatocellular carcinoma. Cancer J 2008;14(2):100–10.
6. Kokudo N, Takemura N, Hasegawa K, et al. Clinical practice guidelines for hepatocellular carcinoma: the Japan Society of Hepatology 2017 (4th JSH-HCC guidelines) 2019 update. Hepatol Res 2019;49(10):1109–13.
7. Yau T, Tang VY, Yao TJ, et al. Development of Hong Kong Liver Cancer staging system with treatment stratification for patients with hepatocellular carcinoma. Gastroenterology 2014;146(7):1691–700.e3.
8. Kawaguchi Y, Lillemoe HA, Vauthey JN. Dealing with an insufficient future liver remnant: portal vein embolization and two-stage hepatectomy. J Surg Oncol 2019;119(5):594–603.
9. Vauthey JN, Abdalla EK, Doherty DA, et al. Body surface area and body weight predict total liver volume in Western adults. Liver Transplant 2002;8(3):233–40.
10. Shindoh J, Tzeng CW, Aloia TA, et al. Optimal future liver remnant in patients treated with extensive preoperative chemotherapy for colorectal liver metastases. Ann Surg Oncol 2013;20(8):2493–500.
11. Vauthey JN, Chaoui A, Do KA, et al. Standardized measurement of the future liver remnant prior to extended liver resection: methodology and clinical associations. Surgery 2000;127(5):512–9.
12. Kishi Y, Abdalla EK, Chun YS, et al. Three hundred and one consecutive extended right hepatectomies: evaluation of outcome based on systematic liver volumetry. Ann Surg 2009;250(4):540–8.
13. de Haas RJ, Wicherts DA, Andreani P, et al. Impact of expanding criteria for resectability of colorectal metastases on short- and long-term outcomes after hepatic resection. Ann Surg 2011;253(6):1069–79.
14. Wu C-Y, Chen Y-J, Ho HJ, et al. Association between nucleoside analogues and risk of hepatitis B virus–related hepatocellular carcinoma recurrence following liver resection. JAMA 2012;308(18):1906.
15. Han HS, Shehta A, Ahn S, et al. Laparoscopic versus open liver resection for hepatocellular carcinoma: case-matched study with propensity score matching. J Hepatol 2015;63(3):643–50.
16. Cloyd JM, Mizuno T, Kawaguchi Y, et al. Comprehensive complication index validates improved outcomes over time despite increased complexity in 3707 consecutive hepatectomies. Ann Surg 2018;271(4):724–31.
17. Jang JS, Cho JY, Ahn S, et al. Comparative performance of the complexity classification and the conventional major/minor classification for predicting the difficulty of liver resection for hepatocellular carcinoma. Ann Surg 2018;267(1):18–23.
18. Tanaka S, Kawaguchi Y, Kubo S, et al. Validation of index-based IWATE criteria as an improved difficulty scoring system for laparoscopic liver resection. Surgery 2019;165(4):731–40.
19. Kawaguchi Y, Fuks D, Kokudo N, et al. Difficulty of laparoscopic liver resection: proposal for a new classification. Ann Surg 2018;267(1):13–7.
20. Kawaguchi Y, Tanaka S, Fuks D, et al. Validation and performance of three-level procedure-based classification for laparoscopic liver resection. Surg Endosc 2019;34(5):2056–66.

21. Kawaguchi Y, Hasegawa K, Tzeng CD, et al. Performance of a modified three-level classification in stratifying open liver resection procedures in terms of complexity and postoperative morbidity. Br J Surg 2019;107(3):258–67.
22. Lee MK, Gao F, Strasberg SM. Completion of a liver surgery complexity score and classification based on an International Survey of Experts. J Am Coll Surgeons 2016;223(2):332–42.
23. Lee MKt, Gao F, Strasberg SM. Perceived complexity of various liver resections: results of a survey of experts with development of a complexity score and classification. J Am Coll Surgeons 2015;220(1):64–9.
24. Russolillo N, Aldrighetti L, Cillo U, et al. Risk-adjusted benchmarks in laparoscopic liver surgery in a national cohort. Br J Surg 2020;107(7):845–53.
25. Slankamenac K, Graf R, Barkun J, et al. The comprehensive complication index: a novel continuous scale to measure surgical morbidity. Ann Surg 2013;258(1):1–7.
26. Makuuchi M, Hasegawa H, Yamazaki S. Intraoperative ultrasonic examination for hepatectomy. Jpn J Clin Oncol 1981;11:367–90.
27. Kawaguchi Y, Ishizawa T, Miyata Y, et al. Portal uptake function in veno-occlusive regions evaluated by real-time fluorescent imaging using indocyanine green. J Hepatol 2013;58(2):247–53.
28. Kawaguchi Y, Nomura Y, Nagai M, et al. Liver transection using indocyanine green fluorescence imaging and hepatic vein clamping. Br J Surg 2017;104(7):898–906.
29. Kobayashi Y, Kawaguchi Y, Kobayashi K, et al. Portal vein territory identification using indocyanine green fluorescence imaging: technical details and short-term outcomes. J Surg Oncol 2017;116(7):921–31.
30. Hasegawa K, Kokudo N, Imamura H, et al. Prognostic impact of anatomic resection for hepatocellular carcinoma. Ann Surg 2005;242(2):252–9.
31. Eguchi S, Kanematsu T, Arii S, et al. Comparison of the outcomes between an anatomical subsegmentectomy and a non-anatomical minor hepatectomy for single hepatocellular carcinomas based on a Japanese nationwide survey. Surgery 2008;143(4):469–75.
32. Tanaka S, Mogushi K, Yasen M, et al. Surgical contribution to recurrence-free survival in patients with macrovascular-invasion-negative hepatocellular carcinoma. J Am Coll Surgeons 2009;208(3):368–74.
33. Cucchetti A, Qiao GL, Cescon M, et al. Anatomic versus nonanatomic resection in cirrhotic patients with early hepatocellular carcinoma. Surgery 2014;155(3):512–21.
34. Okamura Y, Ito T, Sugiura T, et al. Anatomic versus nonanatomic hepatectomy for a solitary hepatocellular carcinoma: a case-controlled study with propensity score matching. J Gastrointest Surg 2014;18(11):1994–2002.
35. Marubashi S, Gotoh K, Akita H, et al. Anatomical versus non-anatomical resection for hepatocellular carcinoma. Br J Surg 2015;102(7):776–84.
36. Mullen JT, Ribero D, Reddy SK, et al. Hepatic insufficiency and mortality in 1,059 noncirrhotic patients undergoing major hepatectomy. J Am Coll Surgeons 2007;204(5):854–62 [discussion: 862–4].
37. Makuuchi M, Takayasu K, Takuma T, et al. Preoperative transcatheter embolization of the portal venous branch for patients receiving extended lobectomy due to the bile duct carcinoma. J Jpn Soc Clin Surg 1984;45:14–21.
38. Matsuoka T, Nakatsuka H, Kobayashi N, et al. [Portal vein embolization for hepatoma with lipiodol-fibrin adhesive mixture]. Nihon Igaku Hoshasen Gakkai Zasshi 1984;44(11):1411–3.

39. Kinoshita H, Sakai K, Hirohashi K, et al. Preoperative portal vein embolization for hepatocellular carcinoma. World J Surg 1986;10(5):803–8.
40. de Baere T, Roche A, Elias D, et al. Preoperative portal vein embolization for extension of hepatectomy indications. Hepatology 1996;24(6):1386–91.
41. Azoulay D, Castaing D, Krissat J, et al. Percutaneous portal vein embolization increases the feasibility and safety of major liver resection for hepatocellular carcinoma in injured liver. Ann Surg 2000;232(5):665–72.
42. Abulkhir A, Limongelli P, Healey AJ, et al. Preoperative portal vein embolization for major liver resection: a meta-analysis. Ann Surg 2008;247(1):49–57.
43. Giraudo G, Greget M, Oussoultzoglou E, et al. Preoperative contralateral portal vein embolization before major hepatic resection is a safe and efficient procedure: a large single institution experience. Surgery 2008;143(4):476–82.
44. Mueller L, Hillert C, Moller L, et al. Major hepatectomy for colorectal metastases: is preoperative portal occlusion an oncological risk factor? Ann Surg Oncol 2008; 15(7):1908–17.
45. Tanaka H, Hirohashi K, Kubo S, et al. Preoperative portal vein embolization improves prognosis after right hepatectomy for hepatocellular carcinoma in patients with impaired hepatic function. Br J Surg 2000;87(7):879–82.
46. Wakabayashi H, Ishimura K, Okano K, et al. Is preoperative portal vein embolization effective in improving prognosis after major hepatic resection in patients with advanced-stage hepatocellular carcinoma? Cancer 2001;92(9):2384–90.
47. Sugawara Y, Yamamoto J, Higashi H, et al. Preoperative portal embolization in patients with hepatocellular carcinoma. World J Surg 2002;26(1):105–10.
48. Seo DD, Lee HC, Jang MK, et al. Preoperative portal vein embolization and surgical resection in patients with hepatocellular carcinoma and small future liver remnant volume: comparison with transarterial chemoembolization. Ann Surg Oncol 2007;14(12):3501–9.
49. Palavecino M, Chun YS, Madoff DC, et al. Major hepatic resection for hepatocellular carcinoma with or without portal vein embolization: perioperative outcome and survival. Surgery 2009;145(4):399–405.
50. Shindoh J, D Tzeng CW, Vauthey JN. Portal vein embolization for hepatocellular carcinoma. Liver Cancer 2012;1(3–4):159–67.
51. Siriwardana RC, Lo CM, Chan SC, et al. Role of portal vein embolization in hepatocellular carcinoma management and its effect on recurrence: a case-control study. World J Surg 2012;36(7):1640–6.
52. Aoki T, Kubota K. Preoperative portal vein embolization for hepatocellular carcinoma: consensus and controversy. World J Hepatol 2016;8(9):439–45.
53. Aoki T, Imamura H, Hasegawa K, et al. Sequential preoperative arterial and portal venous embolizations in patients with hepatocellular carcinoma. Arch Surg 2004; 139(7):766–74.
54. Ogata S, Belghiti J, Farges O, et al. Sequential arterial and portal vein embolizations before right hepatectomy in patients with cirrhosis and hepatocellular carcinoma. Br J Surg 2006;93(9):1091–8.
55. Yoo H, Kim JH, Ko GY, et al. Sequential transcatheter arterial chemoembolization and portal vein embolization versus portal vein embolization only before major hepatectomy for patients with hepatocellular carcinoma. Ann Surg Oncol 2011; 18(5):1251–7.
56. Ronot M, Cauchy F, Gregoli B, et al. Sequential transarterial chemoembolization and portal vein embolization before resection is a valid oncological strategy for unilobar hepatocellular carcinoma regardless of the tumor burden. HPB (Oxford) 2016;18(8):684–90.

57. Kawaguchi Y, Hasegawa K, Wakabayashi G, et al. Survey results on daily practice in open and laparoscopic liver resections from 27 centers participating in the second International Consensus Conference. J Hepatobiliary Pancreat Sci 2016; 23(5):283–8.

58. Nguyen KT, Gamblin TC, Geller DA. World review of laparoscopic liver resection-2,804 patients. Ann Surg 2009;250(5):831–41.

59. Hoznek A, Salomon L, Olsson LE, et al. Laparoscopic radical prostatectomy. The Creteil experience. Eur Urol 2001;40(1):38–45.

60. Kawaguchi Y, Velayutham V, Fuks D, et al. Operative techniques to avoid near misses during laparoscopic hepatectomy. Surgery 2017;161(2):341–6.

61. Eiriksson K, Fors D, Rubertsson S, et al. High intra-abdominal pressure during experimental laparoscopic liver resection reduces bleeding but increases the risk of gas embolism. Br J Surg 2011;98(6):845–52.

62. Kawaguchi Y, Nomi T, Fuks D, et al. Hemorrhage control for laparoscopic hepatectomy: technical details and predictive factors for intraoperative blood loss. Surg Endosc 2016;30(6):2543–51.

63. Li W, Zhou X, Huang Z, et al. Short-term and long-term outcomes of laparoscopic hepatectomy, microwave ablation, and open hepatectomy for small hepatocellular carcinoma: a 5-year experience in a single center. Hepatol Res 2017;47(7): 650–7.

64. Cheung TT, Dai WC, Tsang SH, et al. Pure laparoscopic hepatectomy versus open hepatectomy for hepatocellular carcinoma in 110 patients with liver cirrhosis: a propensity analysis at a single center. Ann Surg 2016;264(4):612–20.

65. Ker CG, Chen JS, Kuo KK, et al. Liver surgery for hepatocellular carcinoma: laparoscopic versus open approach. Int J Hepatol 2011;2011:596792.

66. Fretland ÅA, Aghayan D, Edwin B, et al. Long-term survival after laparoscopic versus open resection for colorectal liver metastases. J Clin Oncol 2019; 37(18_suppl):LBA3516.

67. Chen MS, Li JQ, Zheng Y, et al. A prospective randomized trial comparing percutaneous local ablative therapy and partial hepatectomy for small hepatocellular carcinoma. Ann Surg 2006;243(3):321–8.

68. Huang J, Yan L, Cheng Z, et al. A randomized trial comparing radiofrequency ablation and surgical resection for HCC conforming to the Milan criteria. Ann Surg 2010;252(6):903–12.

69. Feng K, Yan J, Li X, et al. A randomized controlled trial of radiofrequency ablation and surgical resection in the treatment of small hepatocellular carcinoma. J Hepatol 2012;57(4):794–802.

70. Liu H, Wang ZG, Fu SY, et al. Randomized clinical trial of chemoembolization plus radiofrequency ablation versus partial hepatectomy for hepatocellular carcinoma within the Milan criteria. Br J Surg 2016;103(4):348–56.

71. Izumi N, Hasegawa K, Nishioka Y, et al. A multicenter randomized controlled trial to evaluate the efficacy of surgery vs. radiofrequency ablation for small hepatocellular carcinoma (SURF trial). J Clin Oncol 2019;37(15_suppl):4002.

72. Yin L, Li H, Li AJ, et al. Partial hepatectomy vs. transcatheter arterial chemoembolization for resectable multiple hepatocellular carcinoma beyond Milan Criteria: a RCT. J Hepatol 2014;61(1):82–8.

73. Mazzaferro V, Regalia E, Doci R, et al. Liver transplantation for the treatment of small hepatocellular carcinomas in patients with cirrhosis. N Engl J Med 1996; 334(11):693–9.

74. Hsu CY, Hsia CY, Huang YH, et al. Comparison of surgical resection and trans-arterial chemoembolization for hepatocellular carcinoma beyond the Milan criteria: a propensity score analysis. Ann Surg Oncol 2012;19(3):842–9.

75. Guo Z, Zhong JH, Jiang JH, et al. Comparison of survival of patients with BCLC stage A hepatocellular carcinoma after hepatic resection or transarterial chemo-embolization: a propensity score-based analysis. Ann Surg Oncol 2014;21(9): 3069–76.

76. Zhu SL, Ke Y, Peng YC, et al. Comparison of long-term survival of patients with solitary large hepatocellular carcinoma of BCLC stage A after liver resection or transarterial chemoembolization: a propensity score analysis. PLoS One 2014; 9(12):e115834.

77. Yang HJ, Lee JH, Lee DH, et al. Small single-nodule hepatocellular carcinoma: comparison of transarterial chemoembolization, radiofrequency ablation, and he-patic resection by using inverse probability weighting. Radiology 2014;271(3): 909–18.

78. Shi HY, Wang SN, Wang SC, et al. Preoperative transarterial chemoembolization and resection for hepatocellular carcinoma: a nationwide Taiwan database anal-ysis of long-term outcome predictors. J Surg Oncol 2014;109(5):487–93.

79. Liu PH, Lee YH, Hsia CY, et al. Surgical resection versus transarterial chemoem-bolization for hepatocellular carcinoma with portal vein tumor thrombosis: a pro-pensity score analysis. Ann Surg Oncol 2014;21(6):1825–33.

80. Lee YB, Lee DH, Cho Y, et al. Comparison of transarterial chemoembolization and hepatic resection for large solitary hepatocellular carcinoma: a propensity score analysis. J Vasc Interv Radiol 2015;26(5):651–9.

81. Zhong C, Zhang YF, Huang JH, et al. Comparison of hepatic resection and trans-arterial chemoembolization for UICC stage T3 hepatocellular carcinoma: a pro-pensity score matching study. BMC Cancer 2018;18(1):643.

82. Llovet JM, Fuster J, Bruix J. Intention-to-treat analysis of surgical treatment for early hepatocellular carcinoma: resection versus transplantation. Hepatology 1999;30(6):1434–40.

83. Shah SA, Cleary SP, Tan JC, et al. An analysis of resection vs transplantation for early hepatocellular carcinoma: defining the optimal therapy at a single institu-tion. Ann Surg Oncol 2007;14(9):2608–14.

84. Bellavance EC, Lumpkins KM, Mentha G, et al. Surgical management of early-stage hepatocellular carcinoma: resection or transplantation? J Gastrointest Surg 2008;12(10):1699–708.

85. Cheng A-L, Kang Y-K, Chen Z, et al. Efficacy and safety of sorafenib in patients in the Asia-Pacific region with advanced hepatocellular carcinoma: a phase III rand-omised, double-blind, placebo-controlled trial. Lancet Oncol 2009;10(1):25–34.

86. Llovet JM, Ricci S, Mazzaferro V, et al. Sorafenib in advanced hepatocellular car-cinoma. N Engl J Med 2008;359(4):378–90.

87. Bruix J, Takayama T, Mazzaferro V, et al. Adjuvant sorafenib for hepatocellular carcinoma after resection or ablation (STORM): a phase 3, randomised, double-blind, placebo-controlled trial. Lancet Oncol 2015;16(13):1344–54.

88. Kudo M, Finn RS, Qin S, et al. Lenvatinib versus sorafenib in first-line treatment of patients with unresectable hepatocellular carcinoma: a randomised phase 3 non-inferiority trial. Lancet 2018;391(10126):1163–73.

89. Abou-Alfa GK, Meyer T, Cheng AL, et al. Cabozantinib in patients with advanced and progressing hepatocellular carcinoma. N Engl J Med 2018;379(1):54–63.

90. Zhu AX, Kang Y-K, Yen C-J, et al. Ramucirumab after sorafenib in patients with advanced hepatocellular carcinoma and increased α-fetoprotein concentrations

(REACH-2): a randomised, double-blind, placebo-controlled, phase 3 trial. Lancet Oncol 2019;20(2):282–96.

91. Bruix J, Qin S, Merle P, et al. Regorafenib for patients with hepatocellular carcinoma who progressed on sorafenib treatment (RESORCE): a randomised, double-blind, placebo-controlled, phase 3 trial. Lancet 2017;389(10064):56–66.

92. Yau T, Park JW, Finn RS, et al. LBA38_PRCheckMate 459: a randomized, multicenter phase III study of nivolumab (NIVO) vs sorafenib (SOR) as first-line (1L) treatment in patients (pts) with advanced hepatocellular carcinoma (aHCC). Ann Oncol 2019;30(Supplement_5).

93. Finn RS, Ryoo B-Y, Merle P, et al. Results of KEYNOTE-240: phase 3 study of pembrolizumab (Pembro) vs best supportive care (BSC) for second line therapy in advanced hepatocellular carcinoma (HCC). J Clin Oncol 2019;37(15_suppl): 4004.

94. Cheng A-L, Qin S, Ikeda M, et al. LBA3IMbrave150: efficacy and safety results from a ph III study evaluating atezolizumab (atezo) + bevacizumab (bev) vs sorafenib (Sor) as first treatment (tx) for patients (pts) with unresectable hepatocellular carcinoma (HCC). Ann Oncol 2019;30(Supplement_9).

95. Kaseb AO, Vence L, Blando J, et al. Immunologic correlates of pathologic complete response to preoperative immunotherapy in hepatocellular carcinoma. Cancer Immunol Res 2019;7(9):1390–5.

96. Bruix J, Reig M, Sherman M. Evidence-based diagnosis, staging, and treatment of patients with hepatocellular carcinoma. Gastroenterology 2016;150(4): 835–53.

The Impact of Allocation Changes on Patients with Hepatocellular Carcinoma

Lavanya Yohanathan, MD, Julie K. Heimbach, MD*

KEYWORDS

- Hepatocellular carcinoma • Organ allocation • Waitlist mortality
- Liver transplantation

KEY POINTS

- Liver allocation policy for hepatocellular carcinoma (HCC) has continued to evolve steadily over the past 20 years.
- HCC exception candidates have been overprioritized relative to nonexception waitlisted patients, and model for end-stage liver disease inflation.
- National Liver Review Board and Acuity Circle model represent a recent, significant change in the liver allocation system, and the net effect for patients with HCC is uncertain but potentially may ameliorate differences in access for HCC and nonexception patients awaiting LT.

INTRODUCTION

In the United States, mortality for HCC has increased faster than for any other tumor primarily due to cirrhosis from hepatitis C virus (HCV) as well as other causes such as alcohol, nonalcoholic fatty liver disease (NAFLD), and HBV.[1,2] Although recently the age-adjusted incidence rates seem to be plateauing, the combination of the high disease incidence with the demonstrated effectiveness of liver transplantation (LT) as a treatment of HCC treatment and an allocation policy that prioritized patients with HCC has led to HCC being the most common indication for LT in the United States.[3]

The observation that HCC is now a leading indication for LT is especially notable because the initial experience of LT for patients with HCC was associated with such poor outcome that in 1989 the Department of Health and Human Services listed HCC as a contraindication for LT.[4,5] The early dismal outcomes led to the conclusion that LT was not an acceptable treatment of HCC, although notably LT was used only as a therapy for last resort for those with very extensive tumors. However, patients undergoing LT for other indications noted to have incidental tumors in the explanted liver

Mayo Clinic College of Medicine, 200 First Street Southwest, Rochester, MN 55905, USA
* Corresponding author.
E-mail address: heimbach.julie@mayo.edu

Clin Liver Dis 24 (2020) 657–663
https://doi.org/10.1016/j.cld.2020.07.003
1089-3261/20/© 2020 Elsevier Inc. All rights reserved.

demonstrated low recurrence rates and good survival, suggesting that patients with limited tumor burden may benefit from LT. The landmark publication from Mazzafero and colleagues[6] in 1996 demonstrated 83% recurrence-free survival and 75% actuarial survival at 4 years for patients undergoing LT for HCC within the Milan criteria (1 tumor between 2–5 cm or 2–3 tumors between 1–3 cm), defining the importance of patient selection and also establishing LT for unresectable HCC as a standard of care.

However, a major remaining challenge is the availability of deceased-donor organs. Because of the extreme shortage, a system of allocation is required. Before 2002, the allocation of deceased donor livers was based on waiting time and medical status (measured by the Child-Turcotte-Pugh score as well as hospitalization/intensive care unit status) and did not offer any additional priority for patients with HCC.[7] Thus, access to transplantation for HCC was very limited as the patient's HCC would progress while their liver function remained relatively stable and priority for transplant remained low. With the adoption of the model for end-stage liver disease (MELD) allocation system, which included additional prioritization for patients with complications of cirrhosis such as HCC, access was markedly improved.

As depicted in **Fig. 1**, the system has undergone multiple revisions to the priority granted for HCC patients, as well as other system enhancements such as a standardized pathology form and standard imaging criteria. More recent changes are anticipated to have a more notable impact on patients with HCC, including the adoption of standard down-sizing criteria, the development of a national liver review board, and the revision of the distribution of allocated livers to a circle-based system, and will require close monitoring.

Evolution of Hepatocellular Carcinoma Liver Allocation Policy

The MELD-based system for allocation of deceased donor livers was adopted in the United States in 2002 and has been associated with a decrease in waitlist mortality and an increase in post-LT survival.[8,9] This system was updated to include sodium in 2016, which has led to a further decrease in waitlist mortality without any impact

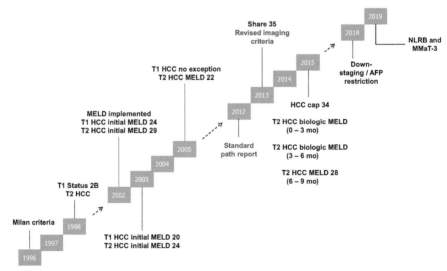

Fig. 1. OPTN/UNOS HCC policy timeline.

on post-LT survival.[10,11] Patients with HCC as well as other complications of cirrhosis and certain metabolic conditions have an increased mortality risk without access to timely LT, which is not predicted by their calculated MELD or MELD-Na score. Therefore, they are allowed to receive assigned MELD scores commonly referred to as MELD exception scores. Since inception, the MELD system has continued to evolve through multiple revisions as summarized in **Fig. 1**.

The process of awarding exception scores for HCC in the United States is automated for patients whose tumors are within designated criteria. Historically, assigned MELD score exceptions for HCC meeting standard criteria were set at a score intended to reflect a 15% risk of waitlist drop out over a 3-month period, and this score increased every 3 months by a value anticipated to reflect a 10% increased risk of mortality without transplantation. Patients who did not meet standard criteria for HCC could still receive an MELD exception score through a process of appeal to a regional review board system, similar to the process for patients with other indications for MELD score exception that are not covered by allocation policy. Although nearly 70% of MELD exception scores are granted for patients with HCC, there are 6 additional policy-based diagnoses for patients meeting specific criteria (hepatopulmonary syndrome, hilar cholangiocarcinoma, familial amyloidosis, primary hyperoxaluria, portopulmonary hypertension, and cystic fibrosis) who also receive policy-based MELD exception scores.

Problems with the Hepatocellular Carcinoma Exception System

Following the adoption of the exception point policy, challenges have arisen. It was immediately identified that the initial scores for patients with HCC were too high and they were reduced twice with T2 HCC starting score going from 28 down to 25, then to 22 and the priority for T1 being eliminated altogether.[12–14] Even with these downward adjustments, with ongoing monitoring it was still evident that patients with HCC were transplanted at a much higher rate than non-HCC patients and removed from the list at lower rates.[15–17]

Another issue that potentially may be related to the system of MELD score exceptions is MELD inflation. Until very recently, there has been a steady increase in the median MELD score at the time of transplant across all regions. In a compelling manuscript by Northup and colleagues,[16] the investigators link the steady increase in the MELD score needed to access transplant to the increased numbers of patients transplanted with exception scores. They proposed the increasing MELD score may be due to the fixed thresholds for exception patients, which included a large number of patients who are relatively stable, and required those with calculated score to increase higher than these thresholds in order to access LT.

Finally, it was noted that there was significant variability in the approval of MELD exception points by regional review boards for patients with HCC not meeting criteria. Some regions were approving patients who had been successfully downsized from UCSF criteria, whereas other regions did not require downstaging. Still others were not allowing any exceptions for patients beyond Milan criteria. There were also concerns about different rates of approval for nonstandard indications for exceptions across the different regions and additional concerns about inefficiencies and delays, as well as concerns about lack of expertise, particularly for pediatric waitlist candidates, and the potential for there to be a conflict of interest when reviewing cases within the same allocation region.

Policy Solutions: National Liver Review Board

The overprioritization for patients with HCC was addressed by the "cap and delay" policy revision, which was adopted in 2015.[18] This revision added a 6-month waiting period before patients could be transplanted based on their assigned HCC exception score; although the score granted after 6 months was MELD 28, the same exception score as they would have had after 6 months under the prior system, which avoided further disadvantaging of patients waiting in high-MELD regions, yet importantly, allowed for biological selection by delaying access to transplant.[19] A recent analysis of transplant rates for patients with HCC and those without HCC in the United States before and after the policy change determined that HCC candidates had a 37% lower risk of waitlist mortality/dropout prepolicy and a comparable risk of mortality/dropout postpolicy and concluded that the revised policy established equity between HCC and non-HCC waitlist candidates.[20]

Addressing the issues of MELD inflation and inconsistent approaches by regional review boards for patients with HCC and those without HCC required more significant change. First, in December 2017, a national downstaging policy was created, incorporating downstaging criteria initially proposed by UCSF to define the allowable tumor burden before downstaging treatment (1 lesion between 5–8 cm; 2–3 lesions with at least one greater than 3 cm although none greater than 5 cm and sum of all less than 8 cm; 4–5 lesions all less than 3 cm and sum <8 cm), as well as a cap on the maximum alpha-fetoprotein at 1000 ng/mL (influencing waitlist and post-LT outcomes).[21] This policy created a standardized approach applied across all regions for patients initially presenting with HCC beyond Milan criteria.

Following the adoption of a unified approach to downstaging, the National Liver Review Board (NLRB) was adopted in May 2019. The primary goal was to improve consistency and efficiency in the allocation of MELD exception points across the United States. However, because it was necessary to set scores using a national board even though there are regional differences in the scores needed to access transplantation, the scoring system was also revised to one that is based on the median MELD at transplant in the area of distribution where the patient is listed.

The newly adopted NLRB has 3 distinct boards:

- Adult HCC: staffed by reviewers with special interest in HCC in order to handle HCC exception requests that do not meet standard exception policy criteria
- Adult other: to address non-HCC adult exception requests
- Pediatric: staffed by reviewers with pediatric expertise

Each case will be reviewed by 5 randomly assigned reviewers from the appropriate board and requires a supermajority (4/5) for approval. Centers with an approved pediatric program may have a representative on the pediatric board, whereas adult centers may provide representation to both the HCC and the adult other boards. If the case is denied, the center may appeal in writing to the same group of 5 reviewers, providing any additional data/information to support their appeal. If the appeal is still not approved, the center may request a conference call with a separate group of preselected reviewers called the appeal review team (ART). The ART consists of NLRB reviewers who are expected to serve a 1-month term. If the case is still not approved, the transplant center may appeal to the OPTN Liver/Intestine committee, which is the same final step as under the previous regional review board system.

In addition to changing the structure to 3 separate boards focused on specific content areas, the review process for the 6 other policy-based diagnoses became an automated process done via computer, as it already had been for HCC, instead of requiring a manual review by the chair of the regional review board. In order to try to improve the consistency of the review boards, guidance documents addressing the most common nonpolicy-based scenarios were created for the board and centers to reference when considering or preparing nonpolicy-based exception requests, including for patients with HCC not meeting policy criteria. However, it is anticipated that the most significant change for patients with HCC is that with the adoption of the NLRB, the MELD scores assigned to exception points are now set at a fixed value (currently set at −3) relative to the median MELD score at transplantation (MMaT) for the area of organ distribution for the transplant center where the patient is listed, which until February of 2020 was the median for the donor service area. Transplants performed using nationally shared allografts, allografts from DCD donors, and allografts from living donors are excluded from the calculation of MMaT.

The purpose of this is 2-fold. First, given that the review board is now a national instead of regional system, it allows the initial awarded score for both policy and nonpolicy-based exceptions to be adjusted to the score needed to access transplantation where the patient is listed. It is also hoped that this fixed point system will reduce or at least prevent further escalation in the MMaT and will hopefully also further reduce the imbalance in transplant rate between patients with and without exceptions. The median MELD is recalculated for each center every 6 months based on the prior 12 months of data.

Acuity Circle Model

Geographic disparity in access to transplantation has been noted for decades and affects both patients with and without HCC. Following an OPTN Board directive in 2012, the Liver-Intestine Committee began in earnest to attempt to create a system that reduced variability in access to liver transplant. After a very arduous process, a circle-based model of distribution which creates a series of progressively larger circles around the donor hospital was adopted in February 2020. After offering the liver broadly for Status 1A/1B patients, the Acuity circle model then reverts to a 150 mile circle around the donor hospital for patients with an MELD score of 37 to 40. The system only requires sharing over larger circles if the liver is not accepted for a patient within the smaller circle and thus provides an attempted surrogate for population-based circles. The liver is then offered to patients with MELD 37 to 40 within 250 miles of the donor hospital, then 500 miles of the donor hospital. If no suitable patient is identified, the liver is then offered back to the smaller circle for MELD 34 to 36, then if not accepted, it is offered to the 250 nm and subsequently the 500 nm circles for MELD 34 to 36. This continues for MELD 29 to 33 and then for MELD 15 to 28 before being offered nationally. Because the donor service area is no longer the unit of distribution, the calculation of the median MELD at transplant is based on a 250 nm circle around the transplant hospital.

Going forward, it may be necessary to further adjust the size of the circles depending on the performance of the new system, and this adjustment may ideally be made according to population density rather than uniformly being applied across the United States. An additional issue created by the new system, which is specific to exception patients, including those with HCC, is that because organ distribution is based on a circle around the donor hospital, while the MMaT is based on a 250 nm circle around the recipient hospital, there will be situations where patients listed at different transplant centers with an exception score for HCC will have different exception scores for the same organ offer even though they both may be within 150 miles of the donor hospital and they both may have been waiting for the same amount of time. Patients from transplant center A will still be eligible for different organ offers from donor hospitals located, for example, north and west of transplant center A, which would not come within 150 nm of transplant center B, which is located east and south. However, it is unknown whether this system will ultimately provide equitable access given that centers and populations are not evenly distributed. A potential revision recently proposed is to generate equivalent MMaT scores for each donor match run by taking the highest, lowest, or average MMaT for all transplant centers contained within the distribution circle. Although this may be more complex from a programming standpoint, it would allow patients with the same exception score diagnosis to be ranked according to time at score for each organ offer. Consideration for adopting a national MMaT has also been proposed although this would underprioritize HCC in the higher MELD areas and overprioritize HCC (relative to patients without HCC) in the low-MELD areas.

SUMMARY

Liver transplantation for HCC within defined criteria is an optimal treatment modality, as it addresses both the tumor and also underlying cirrhosis. The cap-and-delay policy has reduced the disparity in access between patients with and without HCC, thus potentially increasing the waiting times for patients with HCC and thus making the role of bridging therapies and living donor liver transplantation more prominent. The creation of national downstaging policy has standardized the approach for patients presenting with HCC beyond Milan. The adoption of the NLRB is expected to increase efficiency and consistency, whereas the new scoring system may reduce MELD inflation and MELD scores overall. However, with the adoption of the Acuity circle model in February of 2020, the calculation of the MMaT moved from a DSA-based calculation to a circle around the transplant center model, creating some match runs where patients have different scores for the same diagnosis, even if they have the same waiting time at that exception score. Thus, it remains essential to have the continued engagement and collaboration of members in order to optimize the new policy through innovative solutions to issues that will continue to arise. A potential next step may include artificial intelligence and machine learning techniques as analysis tools to further optimize the system.

DISCLOSURE

The authors have nothing to disclose.

REFERENCES

1. White DL, Thrift AP, Kanwal F, et al. Incidence of hepatocellular carcinoma in all 50 United States, from 2000 through 2012. Gastroenterology 2017;152(4): 812–20.e5.
2. Singal AG, El-Serag HB. Hepatocellular carcinoma from epidemiology to prevention: translating knowledge into practice. Clin Gastroenterol Hepatol 2015;13(12): 2140–51.
3. Yang JD, Larson JJ, Watt KD, et al. Hepatocellular carcinoma is the most common indication for liver transplantation and placement on the waitlist in the United States. Clin Gastroenterol Hepatol 2017;15(5):767–75.e3.
4. Iwatsuki S, Starzl TE, Sheahan DG, et al. Hepatic resection versus transplantation for hepatocellular carcinoma. Ann Surg 1991;214(3):221–9.
5. Ringe B, Pichlmayr R, Wittekind C, et al. Surgical treatment of hepatocellular carcinoma: experience with liver resection and transplantation in 198 patients. World J Surg 1991;15(2):270–85.
6. Mazzaferro V, Regalia E, Doci R, et al. Liver transplantation for the treatment of small hepatocellular carcinomas in patients with cirrhosis. N Engl J Med 1996; 334(11):693–700.

7. Lucey MR, Brown KA, Everson GT, et al. Minimal criteria for placement of adults on the liver transplant waiting list: a report of a national conference organized by the American Society of Transplant Physicians and the American Association for the Study of Liver Diseases. Liver Transpl Surg 1997;3(6):628–37.

8. Wiesner R. MELD and PELD: application of survival models to liver allocation. Liver Transplant 2001;7(7):567–80.

9. Kamath PS, Kim WR. The model for end-stage liver disease (MELD). Hepatology 2007;45(3):797–805.

10. Biggins SW, Kim WR, Terrault NA, et al. Evidence-based incorporation of serum sodium concentration into MELD. Gastroenterology 2006;130(6):1652–60.

11. Nagai S, Chau LC, Schilke RE, et al. Effects of allocating livers for transplantation based on model for end-stage liver disease–sodium scores on patient outcomes. Gastroenterology 2018;155(5):1451–62.e3.

12. Wiesner RH, Freeman RB, Mulligan DC. Liver transplantation for hepatocellular cancer: the impact of the MELD allocation policy. Gastroenterology 2004; 127(5):S261–7.

13. Sharma P, Harper AM, Hernandez JL, et al. Reduced priority MELD score for hepatocellular carcinoma does not adversely impact candidate survival awaiting liver transplantation. Am J Transplant 2006;6(8):1957–62.

14. Massie AB, Caffo B, Gentry SE, et al. . MELD exceptions and rates of waiting list outcomes. Am J Transplant 2011;11(11):2362–71.

15. Washburn K, Edwards E, Harper A, et al. Hepatocellular carcinoma patients are advantaged in the current liver transplant allocation system. Am J Transplant 2010;10(7):1643–8.

16. Northup PG, Intagliata NM, Shah NL, et al. Excess mortality on the liver transplant waiting list: unintended policy consequences and model for end-stage liver disease (MELD) inflation. Hepatology 2015;61(1):285–91.

17. Mathur AK, Schaubel DE, Gong Q, et al. Racial and ethnic disparities in access to liver transplantation. Liver Transpl 2010;16(9):1033–40.

18. Heimbach JK, Hirose R, Stock PG, et al. Delayed hepatocellular carcinoma model for end-stage liver disease exception score improves disparity in access to liver transplant in the United States. Hepatology 2015;61(5):1643–50.

19. Halazun KJ, Patzer RE, Rana AA, et al. Standing the test of time: outcomes of a decade of prioritizing patients with hepatocellular carcinoma, results of the UNOS natural geographic experiment. Hepatology 2014;60(6):1957–62.

20. Ishaque T, Massie AB, Bowring MG, et al. Liver transplantation and waitlist mortality for HCC and non-HCC candidates following the 2015 HCC exception policy change. Am J Transplant 2019;19(2):564–72.

21. Ross K, Patzer RE, Goldberg DS, et al. Sociodemographic determinants of waitlist and posttransplant survival among end-stage liver disease patients. Am J Transplant 2017;17(11):2879–89.

Downstaging to Liver Transplant

Success Involves Choosing the Right Patient

Kali Zhou, MD, MAS[a], Neil Mehta, MD[b],*

KEYWORDS

- Hepatocellular carcinoma • Liver cancer • Downstaging • Liver transplantation
- Hepatocellular carcinoma therapy • Outcomes

KEY POINTS

- Downstaging of patients with hepatocellular carcinoma outside Milan criteria through local-regional therapy increasingly is used to expand access to lifesaving transplant.
- Those patients within modest expansion of tumor criteria successfully downstaged into Milan criteria have excellent post-transplant outcomes, on par with those starting within Milan criteria.
- Optimal selection of patients for the downstaging pathway includes an assessment of tumor burden, liver function, and surrogate markers for tumor biology, including α-fetoprotein.
- Response to therapy and no disease progression over at least 6 months prior to transplant are key to maintaining desired post-transplant outcomes.

DEFINITION AND RATIONALE FOR DOWNSTAGING (COMPARED WITH EXPANDED CRITERIA)

Liver transplantation (LT) remains the optimal treatment strategy for patients with early-stage hepatocellular carcinoma (HCC). LT restores normal hepatic function, replaces the diseased liver, and is thought to be the best oncologic resection. The incidence of HCC has continued to rise for more than 2 decades in the United States, largely due to the epidemic of ease and the aging population with cirrhosis due to chronic hepatitis C virus.[1,2] Consequently, the number of HCC waitlist registrations in the United States has risen considerably,[3] with HCC now accounting for approximately 30% of all LTs performed in the United States, compared with less than 5%

a Department of Medicine, Division of Gastrointestinal and Liver Diseases, University of Southern California, 1450 San Pablo Street, HC4 3000, Los Angeles, CA 90033, USA;
b Department of Medicine, Division of Gastroenterology and Hepatology, University of California, San Francisco, 513 Parnassus Avenue Box 0538, San Francisco, CA 94143, USA
* Corresponding author.
E-mail address: neil.mehta@ucsf.edu
Twitter: @kalizhouMD (K.Z.)

Clin Liver Dis 24 (2020) 665–679
https://doi.org/10.1016/j.cld.2020.07.005
1089-3261/20/© 2020 Elsevier Inc. All rights reserved.

liver.theclinics.com

before the implementation of the Model for End-Stage Liver Disease (MELD) system of organ allocation for HCC in 2002.[4–6] Expanding LT indications for HCC to meet this growing demand while ensuring acceptable post-LT outcomes has been challenging. For patients with HCC exceeding the Milan criteria[7] (1 lesion $\leq$5 cm or 2–3 lesions $\leq$3 cm), survival after LT incrementally decreases with increasing tumor size and number.[8–10] A modest expansion of tumor criteria, such as with the University of California, San Francisco (UCSF) criteria (1 lesion $\leq$6.5 cm or 2–3 lesions $\leq$4.5 cm with total tumor diameter $\leq$8 cm)[11,12] and the Up-to-7 criteria (sum of largest tumor diameter and tumor number up to 7),[8] achieves post-LT survival nearly that achieved with the Milan criteria. Examples of other expanded selection criteria include total tumor volume ($\leq$115 cm^3), the Kyoto criteria, extended Toronto criteria, and National Cancer Center, Korea, criteria, all of which attempt to include laboratory or imaging surrogates for tumor biology (ie, α-fetoprotein [AFP] and fludeoxyglucose F 18 positron emission tomography [PET] [FDG]-PET scans) rather than rely on tumor burden alone for initial patient selection.[13–16]

In recent years, there has been a shift away from expanded criteria, especially in areas with limited organ availability, given concerns that implementation could reduce access to LT for those with a better post-LT prognosis.[17,18] Additionally, there is increasing evidence that tumor burden is just one of several factors that predict post-LT outcome,[10,19] and increasing transplant wait times have necessitated use of local-regional therapy (LRT) as a bridge to LT. LRT frequently is used with the aim of controlling tumor growth and reducing the risk of waitlist dropout. One of the limitations of expansion of tumor size limits alone is that they do not account for the effects of LRT whereas selection criteria now commonly include surrogates of tumor biology, such as AFP and response to LRT.[9,16,20–22] High AFP and tumor progression despite LRT identify aggressive tumors with a greater risk for tumor recurrence after LT.[19,20,22–24]

Tumor downstaging combines expanded criteria and the effects of LRT (**Fig. 1**). Downstaging of HCC is defined as a reduction in tumor burden using LRT to meet

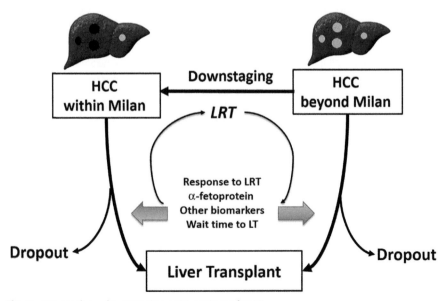

Fig. 1. Approach to downstaging HCC patients for LT.

acceptable criteria for LT (eg, Milan criteria). Tumor response should be based on multiphase contrast-enhanced computed tomography or magnetic resonance imaging measurement of the size of only viable tumors, and the measurements should not include the area of necrosis resulting from LRT.[24] The rationale of tumor downstaging is to select suitable LT candidates with initial tumors exceeding Milan criteria who have favorable tumor biology because objective response to downstaging treatment also may serve as a prognostic marker and a tool to select a subgroup of patients who likely will do well after LT.[24] According to an international consensus conference on LT for HCC, LT after successful downstaging should achieve a 5-year survival rate comparable to that of HCC patients initially meeting conventional LT criteria and not requiring tumor downstaging.[17]

HISTORY OF DOWNSTAGING AND INCORPORATION AS NATIONAL POLICY

Over the past 10 years to 15 years, several different downstaging studies have been published using Milan criteria as the endpoint but each allowing for various upper limits in initial tumor burden[25–31] with the goal of achieving comparable post-LT recurrence and survival after downstaging to those within Milan criteria at the outset. Two of these studies included a control group (within Milan criteria), had well-defined upper limits in the tumor size and number, and had adequate follow-up after LT. In the study from Bologna, Italy,[27] the upper limits included a single lesion less than or equal to 6 cm, 2 tumors each less than or equal to 5 cm, and 3 to 5 tumors each less than or equal to 4 cm with the sum of maximal diameters less than or equal to 12 cm. Under this downstaging protocol, identical 3-year, disease-free post-LT survival of 71% was observed in both the down-staging group (n = 32) and Milan criteria group (n = 88). In the second study, from UCSF,[26] the upper limits of tumor burden included a single lesion less than or equal to 8 cm, 2 to 3 lesions less than 5 cm, with total tumor diameter less than 8 cm, or 4 to 5 nodules all less than 3 cm also with total tumor diameter less than 8 cm. The application of downstaging also involved a minimum observation period of 3 months of disease stability from successful downstaging to LT. Patients were excluded from LT if they had macrovascular tumor invasion, extrahepatic tumor spread, or tumor progression to beyond inclusion criteria. In this study, nearly two-thirds (n = 77/118) had successful downstaging with 5-year post-transplant survival of 78%. There were no significant differences in intention-to-treat survival, post-transplant survival, or recurrence-free probabilities compared with the control group of 488 patients listed for LT with HCC initially meeting Milan criteria. A follow-up multi-center downstaging study from United Network for Organ Sharing (UNOS) Region 5,[32] showed similar results with a low likelihood of unfavorable explant features and excellent 5-year post-LT survival of 80% with recurrence rate of less than 15% in patients meeting these inclusion criteria who were successfully downstaged prior to LT. Therefore, UNOS/Organ Procurement and Transplantation Network adopted the UCSF/Region 5 down-staging protocol (**Box 1**) in 2017 (hereafter referred to as UNOS-DS) with patients successfully downstaged to within Milan criteria eligible to receive automatic MELD exception after the mandatory 6-month waiting period.[33]

FREQUENCY OF DOWNSTAGING SUCCESS

Although downstaging is a well-accepted mechanism in the United States for transplantation for patients beyond Milan criteria and newly accepted national policy, frequency of referral of candidates beyond Milan criteria into the downstaging pathway largely is unknown. Among those referred with applications for MELD exception between 2005 and 2011, 42% were within Milan criteria, 27% within UNOS-DS

Box 1
United Network for Organ Staging protocol

Inclusion criteria
  HCC exceeding UNOS T2 criteria (Milan criteria) but meeting 1 of the following:
  1. Single lesion 5.1–8 cm
  2. 2–3 lesions each ≤5 cm with the sum of the maximal tumor diameters ≤8 cm
  3. 4–5 lesions each ≤3 cm with the sum of the maximal tumor diameters ≤8 cm
  Plus the absence of vascular invasion or extrahepatic disease based on cross-sectional imaging

Criteria for successful downstaging
  1. Residual tumor size and diameter within Milan criteria (1 lesion ≤5 cm or 2–3 lesions ≤3 cm)
    a. Only viable tumor(s) are considered; tumor diameter measurements should not include the area of necrosis from tumor-directed therapy
    b. If there is more than 1 area of residual tumor enhancement, then the diameter of the entire lesion should be counted toward the overall tumor burden

Criteria for downstaging failure and exclusion from LT
  1. Progression of tumor(s) to beyond inclusion/eligibility criteria for downstaging (as defined previously)
  2. Tumor invasion of a major hepatic vessel based on cross-sectional imaging
  3. Lymph node involvement by tumor or extrahepatic spread of tumor
  4. Infiltrative tumor growth pattern
  5. Per current UNOS policy, if AFP ≥1000 ng/mL, then transplant cannot be undertaken unless AFP level decreases to <500 ng/mL with LRT

Additional guidelines
  Per current UNOS policy, patient must remain within Milan criteria for 6 months after successful downstaging before receiving MELD exception points

---

criteria, and 18% beyond UNOS-DS criteria.[34] A vast majority of applications were accepted—including 90% of those within and 71% beyond UNOS-DS criteria. Looking temporally at UNOS data, the proportion of HCC patients listed with MELD exception and tumor burden beyond Milan criteria at any point has increased slowly over time (*P* trend <0.001) (**Fig. 2**) and in 2018 accounted for approximately 13% of HCC patients listed for LT. Success of downstaging into Milan criteria in the literature has been variable due to heterogeneity in selection criteria, and ranged between 39% and 58% in a systematic review.[25] More recent US multicenter data demonstrated downstaging to be quite feasible, with less than 20% never able to be successfully downstaged into Milan criteria.[32] Not surprisingly, presence of tumor thrombus lowers successful downstaging to a mere 11% to 24%.[35,36]

DOWNSTAGING OUTCOMES AND FAILURE CRITERIA

There is a growing body of literature that supports the use of downstaging by demonstrating excellent outcomes among carefully selected patients under defined protocols. A systematic review evaluating outcomes of 13 downstaging studies showed a pooled post-LT HCC recurrence rate of 16%; heterogeneity in survival reporting limited pooling of data, but generally 4-year to 5-year survival was 70% to 90%.[25] A study examining national experience with downstaging demonstrated no difference in 3-year post-LT survival between UNOS-DS and within Milan criteria groups (83.2% for Milan criteria vs 79.1% for UNOS-DS; *P* = .17).[37] The lack of an absolute ceiling for downstaging in the United States is reflected in the all-comers protocol, whereby any patient with absence of vascular invasion or extrahepatic disease

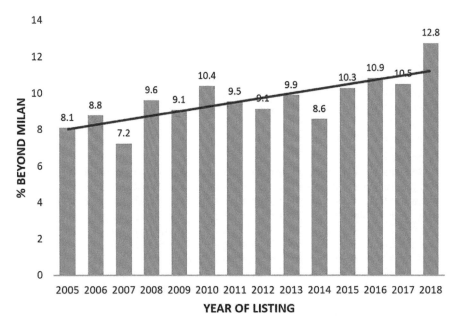

Fig. 2. Trend in listing for HCC requiring downstaging in UNOS (2005–2018). Red line represents line for trend (*P*<.001).

irrespective of tumor burden is eligible for transplantation if downstaging to within Milan criteria is achieved.[38] It is clear, however, that all-comers are unlikely to have a successful outcome with attempted downstaging, with an 80% probability of dropout in 3 years and 5-year intention to treat survival of only 21%.[38] Nationally, 3-year post-LT survival for all-comers who successfully undergo downstaging was 71%, significantly lower than the group always within Milan criteria (*P* = .04).[37] Therefore, although post-LT outcomes are encouraging among successfully downstaged patients, there likely is an upper threshold beyond which downstaging is not an ideal option and alternative treatments considered.

In addition to an upper limit, failure criteria have been proposed for those who enter the downstaging pathway to ensure standardized practice and optimize outcomes. Any patient who develops tumor burden beyond downstaging entry criteria, macrovascular invasion, or extrahepatic disease typically is excluded from LT. For those with disease progression after LRT (defined by Modified Response Evaluation Criteria in Solid Tumors (mRECIST) progression as 20% increase in diameter or development of new tumor[s]) but who remain within downstaging criteria, LT should be deferred and additional LRT applied until disease is within Milan criteria and stability is demonstrated on follow-up imaging. The same strategy applies to those who develop disease progression after successful downstaging into Milan criteria with the rationale being that tumor progression despite LRT is a clear risk factor for worse post-LT outcomes.[23,39]

FACTORS THAT INFLUENCE DOWNSTAGING OUTCOMES

Since downstaging has been established as a pathway for HCC candidates beyond Milan criterias to access LT and cure, focus has turned to fine-tuning the ability to identify those with high potential for downstaging success, low risk of dropout, and acceptable post-LT outcomes. Traditionally, tumor size and number alone have been relied on but increasing data support the incorporation of serologic and imaging biomarkers to better predict tumor biology in patients undergoing downstaging. In addition to assessing tumor-related factors, there also are several nontumor factors that could influence downstaging outcomes, including type of LRT, underlying liver disease severity, and wait time to LT.

Tumor-Related Factors

α-Fetoprotein

An established tool for HCC screening and diagnosis, AFP also correlates with pathologic grade, disease progression, and survival in patients with HCC.[22,40,41] In LT patients with HCC, higher AFP is associated with higher likelihood of dropout, more poorly differentiated tumors and microvascular invasion on explant, more post-LT recurrence and lower post-LT survival.[20,42] A very high AFP consistently has predicted poor outcomes post-LT regardless of initial tumor burden. For example, a pre-LT AFP greater than 1000 ng/mL within Milan criteria was associated a 4.5-fold increased risk of HCC recurrence and 7-fold risk of vascular invasion.[20] Lowering AFP with LRT to less than less than 500 ng/mL prior to transplantation had favorable effects on outcomes, with a 2-fold decrease in mortality and 3-fold decrease in recurrence.[43] Based on these findings, UNOS implemented as national policy in 2017 that HCC patients with an AFP greater than 1000 ng/mL are not eligible for LT until AFP is under 500 ng/mL after LRT, which also applies to downstaging candidates. To further improve precision of AFP as a selection tool, researchers have also looked at the slope of AFP prior to LT in single-center studies, with the goal of evaluating trend rather than 2 discrete time points.[44,45] In patients transplanted in a single US center, an AFP slope fitted for all AFPs (at least 3) measured prior to LT of greater than 7.5 ng/mL/mo performed better than a single AFP at LT or established AFP cutoffs for predicting HCC recurrence.[45] A majority of patients had a negative AFP slope as a result of LRT (median AFP slope was −0.15 ng/mL), which highlights that rising AFP despite LRT should serve as an indicator of poor tumor biology.

Among downstaging patients, AFP is a predictor of both waitlist dropout and post-LT outcomes. In the UNOS database, an initial AFP greater than 1000 ng/mL predicted a 5-fold risk of dropout among all-comers and 50% of all-comers with an AFP greater than 100 ng/mL at listing dropped out at 2 years.[46] AFP greater than 100 ng/mL at LT was an independent risk factor for worse post-LT survival in both UNOS-DS and all-comers groups.[37] Specifically, in patients with tumor burden beyond Milan criteria on pre-LT imaging, the 3-year post-LT survival was 59% for those with AFP greater than or equal to 100 ng/mL compared with 72% with AFP 20 ng/mL to 99 ng/mL and 81% if AFP less than 20 ng/mL. Whether more stringent AFP criteria should be applied to downstaging candidates to optimize the balance between survival benefit and post-LT outcomes, however, is not yet clear.

Other serologic tumor markers

Additional tumor markers have emerged as potential adjuncts to AFP for both diagnosis and prognosis of HCC, including -gamma-carboxyprothrombin (DCP) and Lens culinaris agglutinin–reactive fraction of AFP (AFP-L3). DCP has been utilized primarily in Asia and is thought to correlate with tumor aggressiveness. Studies have linked higher DCP to worse prognosis after both hepatectomy and radiofrequency ablation.[47,48] In a study from Japan in living donor LT (LDLT) recipients, of those with DCP greater than 7.5 ng/mL, 62% and 38% had evidence of microvascular invasion or poorly differentiated tumors on explant, respectively.[49] DCP greater than 7.5 was an independent risk factor for tumor recurrence and had superior area under the curve characteristics compared with AFP. Patients under the Kyoto expanded criteria ($\leq$10 tumors each under 5 cm and DCP <7.5 mg/mL) had equivalent outcomes compared with those within Milan criteria with very low 5-year post-LT recurrence. AFP, AFP-L3, and DCP all were retrospectively analyzed in a cohort of 127 HCC patients (32% outside Milan criteria) with available serum prior to LT, of which 41 (32%) had recurrence over 7.5 years of follow-up.[50] Using 80th percentile values as cutoffs, all biomarkers were significantly associated with HCC recurrence, although DCP greater than 7.5 mg/mL was the strongest predictor overall and AFP greater than 250 ng/mL the strongest among patients outside Milan criteria. Furthermore, a combination of DCP and AFP appeared to have an additive effect in predicting recurrence. Routine use of these additional tumor markers in clinical practice has not yet been adopted in the United States. Further studies are needed to validate their utility in DDLT as well as downstaging candidates and to establish a clear benefit beyond that of AFP alone.

Imaging and histologic biomarkers

In HCC patients outside of Milan criteria undergoing LDLT or listed in short wait time regions, FDG-PET scans and histologic grade may play a role in selection criteria, because time and response to LRT are not available surrogates for tumor biology. For example, in 123 HCC patients undergoing LDLT in Korea, a positive FDG-PET scan (signal cutoff 1.10) conferred an approximately 10-fold risk of post-LT recurrence.[51] Hong and colleagues[51] also demonstrated a striking 30-fold risk of recurrence in those with a positive FDG-PET and AFP greater than or equal to 200 ng/mL compared with the double-negative group. An LDLT study from Taiwan examining FDG-PET positivity stratified by tumor burden within and beyond UNOS-DS criteria found the lowest 5-year recurrence-free survival (30%) in those with positive PET and outside UNOS-DS and highest survival (86%) if PET-negative and within UNOS-DS.[52] The tumor-to-nontumor ratio on FDG-PET of greater than or equal to 2 also was a strong predictor of low recurrence-free survival. Prospective evaluation of the extended Toronto criteria, which excludes patients from LT on the basis of histologic grade (poorly differentiated) and/or cancer-related symptoms (weight loss, Eastern Cooperative Oncology Group performance status, and so forth) alone, reported similar 5-year post-LT survival in those beyond versus within Milan criteria, with AFP greater than 500 ng/mL a predictor of poor outcome in both groups.[14] The use of these modalities can be considered on an individualized basis in patients undergoing downstaging, particularly if the anticipated wait time to LT is short or LDLT is an option.

Non–Tumor-Related Factors

Local-regional treatment type

In terms of type of LRT, the most commonly used options for downstaging are performed transarterially, including yttrium 90 (Y-90) radioembolization, and transarterial chemoembolization (TACE). Y-90 results in profound radiation and antitumor effects but appears to cause little ischemic damage.[53,54] The PREMIERE (Prospective Randomized Study of Chemoembolization Versus Radioembolization for the Treatment of Hepatocellular Carcinoma) trial[55] was a single-center phase 2 randomized study that compared conventional TACE with Y-90. Median time to progression was significantly longer with Y-90 at greater than 26 months compared with 7 months with TACE, but there was no significant difference in radiographic response rate or median survival. Additionally, only 22% (n = 10/45) initially exceeded Milan criteria, so no comment could be made on the effectiveness of tumor downstaging with each modality. In the Multicenter Evaluation of Reduction in Tumor Size Before Liver Transplantation (MERITS-LT) prospective, nonrandomized consortium of more than 200 patients, probability of successful downstaging to within Milan criteria was approximately 90%, with TACE and Y-90 similarly efficacious in achieving tumor downstaging.[56] Therefore, the choice between Y-90 and TACE as initial LRT to achieve downstaging likely will vary by center, at least until a multicenter randomized trial comparing these 2 modalities in intermediate stage HCC is performed.

Tumor ablation (eg, radiofrequency, microwave, and andcryoablation) works well for small tumors less than 3 cm, with response rates approaching 90% but efficacy is much lower with larger lesions[57–60] and therefore, typically is not employed as initial LRT for tumor downstaging. Stereotactic body radiation therapy (SBRT) is a viable treatment option for HCC, including as a bridge to LT, especially at centers with significant experience performing SBRT.[61] In patients with intermediate-stage HCC, combination therapy (typically TACE followed by ablation) generally is safe and leads to superior outcomes compared with TACE or ablation alone.[62–64] In a retrospective analysis of 400 patients, Ren and colleagues[65] found improved progression-free survival at 5 years with TACE + ablation compared with TACE alone for patients with tumors 3.1 cm to 5 cm as well as in those with tumors greater than 5 cm.

Systemic therapy

Recent advances in systemic options for the treatment of advanced HCC have accelerated the discussion of combination LRT/systemic therapy for bridging to LT. To date, efficacy of combination LRT with conventional sorafenib has been poor, with no survival benefit in trials of adjuvant use postresection/radiofrequency ablation[66] and in combination with LRT, including TACE and Y-90,[67,68] albeit a longer time to progression was seen in the latter group. In the past few years, several promising immunotherapies and small molecule inhibitors have been approved as second-line therapy for advanced HCC (eg, nivolumab, cabozantinib, and pembrolizumab)[69,70] and now are being tested first-line and in combination with LRT in ongoing trials (eg, ClinicalTrials.gov NCT03572582). Although retrospective studies suggest pre-LT sorafenib is safe in the post-transplant setting,[71] significant safety concerns exist for immunotherapies and the risk of post-LT acute rejection and graft failure, owing to coinhibition of tumor and donor antigens, that have been reported in multiple clinical settings, including LT.[72] Successful LT without adverse outcomes, however, in patients with nivolumab exposure has been described in case reports.[73] In 9 patients who received nivolumab pre-LT at Mount Sinai Medical Center, most within 4 weeks of LT, none developed major complications, including rejection, graft failure, or death though short-term follow-up (Parissa Tabrizian, MD, unpublished data, 2020). Four of 9 patients were downstaged into Milan criteria and 8 of 9 also received LRT. Although encouraging, more data are needed to determine what role, if any, these new therapies will have among current downstaging candidates and in expanding downstaging criteria in the future. High-risk HCC patients exceeding Milan criteria should be a priority group for recruitment in prospective trials to determine whether combination LRT/systemic therapy can improve waitlist and potentially post-LT outcomes.

Liver function

In terms of severity of underlying liver disease, there are definite safety concerns related to downstaging, including hepatic decompensation after LRT. It has been proposed that only patients with adequate hepatic function (Child Pugh score A/B, bilirubin ≤3–4 mg/dL) should undergo downstaging, based on recommended guidelines for TACE.[24,74] Previous studies have identified Child Pugh score class B/C (vs A) as a significant predictor of unsuccessful downstaging.[26,32] Child Pugh class B/C patients have fewer LRT options, presumably receive less aggressive treatments given concerns of hepatic decompensation after LRT and are more likely to have liver-related death without LT regardless of whether they receive LRT. In the multicenter prospective study from UNOS Region 5, Mehta and colleagues[32] observed downstaging treatment failure in all Child B/C patients with pretreatment AFP greater than or equal to 1000 ng/mL and concluded that these patients should be excluded from attempted downstaging.

Wait time

Wait time to LT after successful downstaging also appears to influence post-LT outcome. In HCC patients not requiring tumor downstaging, a minimum observation period of up to 6 months may improve overall post-LT survival by avoiding LT in patients with aggressive tumor biology and high risk of recurrence who otherwise would have experienced waitlist dropout with longer wait time.[5,75–77] Similarly, in a recent national analysis of patients meeting UNOS-DS criteria,[37] patients from short wait and mid-wait regions (median wait times to LT of 2.6 and 6.5 months, respectively) had worse 3-year post-LT survival at less than 80% compared with patients in long wait regions (median wait time 13 months) who had a 3-year post-LT survival greater than 90%. These findings suggest an influence of longer wait time in selecting better candidates for LT after tumor downstaging. Therefore, after successful downstaging to within Milan criteria, observing disease stability for at least 3 months to 6 months before LT is recommended to minimize the risks for tumor recurrence.

PUTTING IT TOGETHER: CHOOSING THE RIGHT PATIENT

Prior to attempted downstaging, an assessment of a patient's LT candidacy should be undertaken because approximately 40% of patients with tumor burden meeting UNOS-DS criteria are not LT candidates, typically due to having medical or psychosocial contraindications to listing (**Fig. 3**).[56] Second, an assessment of liver function is needed. Patients generally should be Child-Pugh A or B with a bilirubin less than or equal to 3 mg/dL to safely undergo LRT and be effectively downstaged into Milan criteria without hepatic decompensation that would preclude further treatment. Based on very poor outcomes, patients with extrahepatic disease and/or vascular invasion should not be considered at outset at most centers, although there are emerging data suggesting reasonable outcomes with LDLT after successful downstaging in patients with tumor thrombus and favorable tumor profile.[78]

From there, the initial tumor burden and AFP are important. Although a high AFP at diagnosis (eg, >1000 ng/mL) is not a barrier to downstaging, response to LRT is of particular importance in this group. Outside of formal UNOS policy requiring an AFP less than 500 ng/mL at time of transplant for these patients, studies have demonstrated that the lower the AFP at transplant, the better the post-LT outcome, suggesting that lower AFP goals should be targeted if feasible. Additional therapy for those with rising AFP after LRT, even if under 500 ng/mL, should be considered prior to LT. Patients outside of UNOS-DS criteria and/or with high AFP should be counseled on their substantial risk of dropout. In these high-risk patients, additional testing, such as DCP or FDG-PET scan, could be considered. Ultimately, the upper threshold of tumor burden acceptable will be an individualized process for each transplant

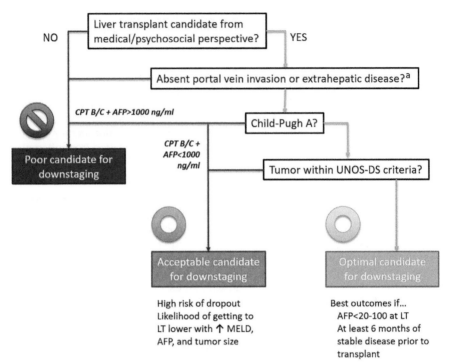

Fig. 3. Algorithm for patient selection for downstaging of HCC prior to LT. [a] LT may be considered in experienced centers after tumor/thrombus downstaging.

center, taking into account availability of LDLT, wait time, and rate of post-LT recurrence tolerated.

Last, method of downstaging, or type of LRT, based on existing data, does not appear to have an impact on likelihood of successful downstaging or post-LT outcome, but greater clarity is expected regarding this point in the future. What is vital, however, to ensuring optimal outcomes post-LT is monitoring of the trajectory of patients in the period during and after downstaging, with removal from listing if failure criteria are met. Patients with radiographic and biochemical response to LRT and stability in the 3-month to 6-month period after successful downstaging in general will have acceptable outcomes on par with HCC patients initially within Milan criteria.

HCC is a rarity as a cancer for which organ transplantation provides the best chance of cure and the rising burden of HCC dictates that HCC will remain a leading indication for LT. Pushing the boundary of the upper threshold of HCC burden has life-saving implications for the individual patient but needs to be balanced against the cost incurred by post-LT recurrence and mortality. Downstaging of carefully selected patients under established protocols, while using existing tools to select for favorable tumor biology, provides an avenue for patients with HCC initially beyond conventional LT criteria to equitably access LT. Future pathways for downstaging research include continued efforts to push limits of expanded criteria, further refinement of existing markers and development of novel markers of tumor biology, and determination of best therapeutic strategies to improve rates of downstaging success.

DISCLOSURE

N. Mehta has served on advisory boards for WAKO Diagnostics and has received institutional research funding from Wako Diagnostics, Glycotest, and Target Pharmasolutions. K. Zhou reports institutional research funding from Gilead Sciences.

REFERENCES

1. Forner A, Reig M, Bruix J. Hepatocellular carcinoma. Lancet 2018;391(10127): 1301–14.
2. White DL, Thrift AP, Kanwal F, et al. Incidence of hepatocellular carcinoma in all 50 United States, from 2000 through 2012. Gastroenterology 2017;152(4): 812–20.e5.
3. Mehta N, Dodge JL, Hirose R, et al. Increasing liver transplant waitlist dropout for hepatocellular carcinoma with widening geographical disparities: implications for organ allocation. Liver Transplantation 2018;24(10):1346–56.
4. Massie AB, Caffo B, Gentry SE, et al. MELD exceptions and rates of waiting list outcomes. Am J Transplant 2011;11(11):2362–71.
5. Halazun KJ, Patzer RE, Rana AA, et al. Standing the test of time: outcomes of a decade of prioritizing patients with hepatocellular carcinoma, results of the UNOS natural geographic experiment. Hepatology 2014;60(6):1957–62.
6. Organ procurement and transplantation Network. National Data. Liver Transplant 2017. Accessed February 15, 2020.
7. Mazzaferro V, Regalia E, Doci R, et al. Liver transplantation for the treatment of small hepatocellular carcinomas in patients with cirrhosis. N Engl J Med 1996; 334(11):693–9.
8. Mazzaferro V, Llovet JM, Miceli R, et al. Predicting survival after liver transplantation in patients with hepatocellular carcinoma beyond the Milan criteria: a retrospective, exploratory analysis. Lancet Oncol 2009;10(1):35–43.
9. Mazzaferro V, Sposito C, Zhou J, et al. Metroticket 2.0 model for analysis of competing risks of death after liver transplantation for hepatocellular carcinoma. Gastroenterology 2018;154(1):128–39.
10. Mehta N, Yao FY. Hepatocellular cancer as indication for liver transplantation: pushing beyond Milan. Curr Opin Organ Transplant 2016;21(2):91–8.
11. Yao FY, Xiao L, Bass NM, et al. Liver transplantation for hepatocellular carcinoma: validation of the UCSF-expanded criteria based on preoperative imaging. Am J Transplant 2007;7(11):2587–96.
12. Yao FY, Ferrell L, Bass NM, et al. Liver transplantation for hepatocellular carcinoma: expansion of the tumor size limits does not adversely impact survival. Hepatology 2001;33(6):1394–403.
13. Kaido T, Ogawa K, Mori A, et al. Usefulness of the Kyoto criteria as expanded selection criteria for liver transplantation for hepatocellular carcinoma. Surgery 2013;154(5):1053–60.
14. Sapisochin G, Goldaracena N, Laurence JM, et al. The extended Toronto criteria for liver transplantation in patients with hepatocellular carcinoma: a prospective validation study. Hepatology 2016;64(6):2077–88.
15. Lee SD, Lee B, Kim SH, et al. Proposal of new expanded selection criteria using total tumor size and (18)F-fluorodeoxyglucose - positron emission tomography/ computed tomography for living donor liver transplantation in patients with hepatocellular carcinoma: the National Cancer Center Korea criteria. World J Transplant 2016;6(2):411–22.

16. Toso C, Meeberg G, Hernandez-Alejandro R, et al. Total tumor volume and alpha-fetoprotein for selection of transplant candidates with hepatocellular carcinoma: a prospective validation. Hepatology 2015;62(1):158–65.

17. Clavien PA, Lesurtel M, Bossuyt PM, et al. Recommendations for liver transplantation for hepatocellular carcinoma: an international consensus conference report. Lancet Oncol 2012;13(1):e11–22.

18. Volk ML, Vijan S, Marrero JA. A novel model measuring the harm of transplanting hepatocellular carcinoma exceeding Milan criteria. Am J Transplant 2008;8(4): 839–46.

19. Lai Q, Avolio AW, Graziadei I, et al. Alpha-fetoprotein and modified response evaluation criteria in solid tumors progression after locoregional therapy as predictors of hepatocellular cancer recurrence and death after transplantation. Liver Transpl 2013;19(10):1108–18.

20. Hameed B, Mehta N, Sapisochin G, et al. Alpha-fetoprotein level > 1000 ng/mL as an exclusion criterion for liver transplantation in patients with hepatocellular carcinoma meeting the Milan criteria. Liver Transpl 2014;20(8):945–51.

21. Halazun KJ, Najjar M, Abdelmessih RM, et al. Recurrence after liver transplantation for hepatocellular carcinoma: a new MORAL to the story. Ann Surg 2017; 265(3):557–64.

22. Duvoux C, Roudot-Thoraval F, Decaens T, et al. Liver transplantation for hepatocellular carcinoma: a model including alpha-fetoprotein improves the performance of Milan criteria. Gastroenterology 2012;143(4):986–94.e3 [quiz: e14-5].

23. Otto G, Herber S, Heise M, et al. Response to transarterial chemoembolization as a biological selection criterion for liver transplantation in hepatocellular carcinoma. Liver Transpl 2006;12(8):1260–7.

24. Yao FY, Fidelman N. Reassessing the boundaries of liver transplantation for hepatocellular carcinoma: where do we stand with tumor down-staging? Hepatology 2016;63(3):1014–25.

25. Parikh ND, Waljee AK, Singal AG. Downstaging hepatocellular carcinoma: a systematic review and pooled analysis. Liver Transpl 2015;21(9):1142–52.

26. Yao FY, Mehta N, Flemming J, et al. Downstaging of hepatocellular cancer before liver transplant: long-term outcome compared to tumors within Milan criteria. Hepatology 2015;61(6):1968–77.

27. Ravaioli M, Grazi GL, Piscaglia F, et al. Liver transplantation for hepatocellular carcinoma: results of down-staging in patients initially outside the Milan selection criteria. Am J Transpl 2008;8(12):2547–57.

28. Jang JW, You CR, Kim CW, et al. Benefit of downsizing hepatocellular carcinoma in a liver transplant population. Aliment Pharmacol Ther 2010;31(3):415–23.

29. Barakat O, Wood RP, Ozaki CF, et al. Morphological features of advanced hepatocellular carcinoma as a predictor of downstaging and liver transplantation: an intention-to-treat analysis. Liver Transpl 2010;16(3):289–99.

30. Lewandowski RJ, Kulik LM, Riaz A, et al. A comparative analysis of transarterial downstaging for hepatocellular carcinoma: chemoembolization versus radioembolization. Am J Transplant 2009;9(8):1920–8.

31. De Luna W, Sze DY, Ahmed A, et al. Transarterial chemoinfusion for hepatocellular carcinoma as downstaging therapy and a bridge toward liver transplantation. Am J Transpl 2009;9(5):1158–68.

32. Mehta N, Guy J, Frenette CT, et al. Excellent outcomes of liver transplantation following down-staging of hepatocellular carcinoma to within milan criteria: a multicenter study. Clin Gastroenterol Hepatol 2018;16(6):955–64.

33. OPTN. Organ Procurement and transplantation Network (OPTN) Policies. Available at: https://optn.transplant.hrsa.gov/.

34. Bittermann T, Niu B, Hoteit MA, et al. Waitlist priority for hepatocellular carcinoma beyond milan criteria: a potentially appropriate decision without a structured approach. Am J Transplant 2014;14(1):79–87.

35. Chapman WC, Majella Doyle MB, Stuart JE, et al. Outcomes of neoadjuvant transarterial chemoembolization to downstage hepatocellular carcinoma before liver transplantation. Ann Surg 2008;248(4):617–25.

36. Pracht M, Edeline J, Lenoir L, et al. Lobar hepatocellular carcinoma with ipsilateral portal vein tumor thrombosis treated with yttrium-90 glass microsphere radioembolization: preliminary results. Int J Hepatol 2013;2013:827649.

37. Mehta N, Dodge JL, Grab JD, et al. National experience on down-staging of hepatocellular carcinoma before liver transplant: influence of tumor burden, AFP, and wait time. Hepatology 2019;71(3):943–54.

38. Sinha J, Mehta N, Dodge JL, et al. Are there upper limits in tumor burden for down-staging of HCC to liver transplant? Analysis of the all-comers protocol. Hepatology 2019;70(4):1185–96.

39. Millonig G, Graziadei IW, Freund MC, et al. Response to preoperative chemoembolization correlates with outcome after liver transplantation in patients with hepatocellular carcinoma. Liver Transpl 2007;13(2):272–9.

40. Bai DS, Zhang C, Chen P, et al. The prognostic correlation of AFP level at diagnosis with pathological grade, progression, and survival of patients with hepatocellular carcinoma. Sci Rep 2017;7(1):12870.

41. Tyson GL, Duan Z, Kramer JR, et al. Level of alpha-fetoprotein predicts mortality among patients with hepatitis C-related hepatocellular carcinoma. Clin Gastroenterol Hepatol 2011;9(11):989–94.

42. Berry K, Ioannou GN. Serum alpha-fetoprotein level independently predicts post-transplant survival in patients with hepatocellular carcinoma. Liver Transplant 2013;19(6):634–45.

43. Mehta N, Dodge JL, Roberts JP, et al. Alpha-fetoprotein decrease from > 1,000 to < 500 ng/mL in patients with hepatocellular carcinoma leads to improved post-transplant outcomes. Hepatology 2019;69(3):1193–205.

44. Lai Q, Inostroza M, Rico Juri JM, et al. Delta-slope of alpha-fetoprotein improves the ability to select liver transplant patients with hepatocellular cancer. HPB (Oxford) 2015;17(12):1085–95.

45. Giard JM, Mehta N, Dodge JL, et al. Alpha-fetoprotein slope >7.5 ng/mL per month predicts microvascular invasion and tumor recurrence after liver transplantation for hepatocellular carcinoma. Transplantation 2018;102(5):816–22.

46. Huang A, Dodge J, Yao F, et al. National experience on waitlist outcomes for down-staging of hepatocellular carcinoma to within milan criteria: high dropout rate in the "all-comers" group. Hepatology 2019;70(S1):90A.

47. Sakaguchi T, Suzuki S, Morita Y, et al. Impact of the preoperative des-gamma-carboxy prothrombin level on prognosis after hepatectomy for hepatocellular carcinoma meeting the Milan criteria. Surg Today 2010;40(7):638–45.

48. Kobayashi M, Ikeda K, Kawamura Y, et al. High serum des-gamma-carboxy prothrombin level predicts poor prognosis after radiofrequency ablation of hepatocellular carcinoma. Cancer 2009;115(3):571–80.

49. Fujiki M, Takada Y, Ogura Y, et al. Significance of des-gamma-carboxy prothrombin in selection criteria for living donor liver transplantation for hepatocellular carcinoma. Am J Transpl 2009;9(10):2362–71.

50. Chaiteerakij R, Zhang X, Addissie BD, et al. Combinations of biomarkers and Milan criteria for predicting hepatocellular carcinoma recurrence after liver transplantation. Liver Transpl 2015;21(5):599–606.

51. Hong G, Suh KS, Suh SW, et al. Preoperative alpha-fetoprotein and F-FDG PET predict tumor recurrence better than Milan criteria in living donor liver transplantation. J Hepatol 2016;64(4):852–9.

52. Hsu CC, Chen CL, Wang CC, et al. Combination of FDG-PET and UCSF criteria for predicting HCC recurrence after living donor liver transplantation. Transplantation 2016;100(9):1925–32.

53. Salem R, Mazzaferro V, Sangro B. Yttrium 90 radioembolization for the treatment of hepatocellular carcinoma: biological lessons, current challenges, and clinical perspectives. Hepatology 2013;58(6):2188–97.

54. Salem R, Lewandowski RJ, Mulcahy MF, et al. Radioembolization for hepatocellular carcinoma using Yttrium-90 microspheres: a comprehensive report of long-term outcomes. Gastroenterology 2010;138(1):52–64.

55. Salem R, Gordon AC, Mouli S, et al. Y90 radioembolization significantly prolongs time to progression compared with chemoembolization in patients with hepatocellular carcinoma. Gastroenterology 2016;151(6):1155–63.e2.

56. Mehta N, Guy J, Frenette CT, et al. Transarterial chemoembolization and radioembolization are similarly efficacious in achieving successful hepatocellular carcinoma (HCC) down-staging: results from the MERITS-LTconsortium. Abstract presented at 2020 American Transplant Congress.

57. Sala M, Llovet JM, Vilana R, et al. Initial response to percutaneous ablation predicts survival in patients with hepatocellular carcinoma. Hepatology 2004;40(6):1352–60.

58. N'Kontchou G, Mahamoudi A, Aout M, et al. Radiofrequency ablation of hepatocellular carcinoma: long-term results and prognostic factors in 235 Western patients with cirrhosis. Hepatology 2009;50(5):1475–83.

59. Lencioni R, Cioni D, Crocetti L, et al. Early-stage hepatocellular carcinoma in patients with cirrhosis: long-term results of percutaneous image-guided radiofrequency ablation. Radiology 2005;234(3):961–7.

60. Santambrogio R, Opocher E, Zuin M, et al. Surgical resection versus laparoscopic radiofrequency ablation in patients with hepatocellular carcinoma and Child-Pugh class a liver cirrhosis. Ann Surg Oncol 2009;16(12):3289–98.

61. Sapisochin G, Barry A, Doherty M, et al. Stereotactic body radiotherapy vs. TACE or RFA as a bridge to transplant in patients with hepatocellular carcinoma. An intention-to-treat analysis. J Hepatol 2017;67(1):92–9.

62. Inchingolo R, Posa A, Mariappan M, et al. Locoregional treatments for hepatocellular carcinoma: current evidence and future directions. World J Gastroenterol 2019;25(32):4614–28.

63. Yin X, Zhang L, Wang YH, et al. Transcatheter arterial chemoembolization combined with radiofrequency ablation delays tumor progression and prolongs overall survival in patients with intermediate (BCLC B) hepatocellular carcinoma. BMC Cancer 2014;14:849.

64. Chu HH, Kim JH, Yoon HK, et al. Chemoembolization combined with radiofrequency ablation for medium-Sized hepatocellular carcinoma: a Propensity-Score analysis. J Vasc Interv Radiol 2019;30(10):1533–43.

65. Ren Y, Cao Y, Ma H, et al. Improved clinical outcome using transarterial chemoembolization combined with radiofrequency ablation for patients in Barcelona clinic liver cancer stage A or B hepatocellular carcinoma regardless of tumor

size: results of a single-center retrospective case control study. BMC Cancer 2019;19(1):983.

66. Bruix J, Takayama T, Mazzaferro V, et al. Adjuvant sorafenib for hepatocellular carcinoma after resection or ablation (STORM): a phase 3, randomised, double-blind, placebo-controlled trial. Lancet Oncol 2015;16(13):1344–54.

67. Ricke J, Klumpen HJ, Amthauer H, et al. Impact of combined selective internal radiation therapy and sorafenib on survival in advanced hepatocellular carcinoma. J Hepatol 2019;71(6):1164–74.

68. Zeng J, Lv L, Mei ZC. Efficacy and safety of transarterial chemoembolization plus sorafenib for early or intermediate stage hepatocellular carcinoma: a systematic review and meta-analysis of randomized controlled trials. Clin Res Hepatol Gastroenterol 2016;40(6):688–97.

69. El-Khoueiry AB, Sangro B, Yau T, et al. Nivolumab in patients with advanced hepatocellular carcinoma (CheckMate 040): an open-label, non-comparative, phase 1/2 dose escalation and expansion trial. Lancet 2017;389(10088):2492–502.

70. Zhu AX, Finn RS, Edeline J, et al. Pembrolizumab in patients with advanced hepatocellular carcinoma previously treated with sorafenib (KEYNOTE-224): a nonrandomised, open-label phase 2 trial. Lancet Oncol 2018;19(7):940–52.

71. Frenette CT, Boktour M, Burroughs SG, et al. Pre-transplant utilization of sorafenib is not associated with increased complications after liver transplantation. Transpl Int 2013;26(7):734–9.

72. Hu B, Yang XB, Sang XT. Liver graft rejection following immune checkpoint inhibitors treatment: a review. Med Oncol 2019;36(11):94.

73. Schwacha-Eipper B, Minciuna L, Banz V, et al. Immunotherapy as a downtaging therapy for liver transplantation. Hepatology 2020. https://doi.org/10.1002/hep.31234.

74. European Association For The Study of The Liver, European Organisation For Research, Treatment of Cancer. EASL-EORTC clinical practice guidelines: management of hepatocellular carcinoma. J Hepatol 2012;56(4):908–43.

75. Samoylova ML, Dodge JL, Yao FY, et al. Time to transplantation as a predictor of hepatocellular carcinoma recurrence after liver transplantation. Liver Transpl 2014;20(8):937–44.

76. Schlansky B, Chen Y, Scott DL, et al. Waiting time predicts survival after liver transplantation for hepatocellular carcinoma: a cohort study using the United Network for Organ Sharing registry. Liver Transpl 2014;20(9):1045–56.

77. Mehta N, Heimbach J, Lee D, et al. Wait time of < 6 and > 18 Months predicts hepatocellular carcinoma recurrence after liver transplantation: Proposing a wait time "Sweet Spot. Transplantation 2017;101(9):2071–8.

78. Soin AS, Bhangui P, Kataria T, et al. Experience with LDLT in patients with hepatocellular carcinoma and portal vein tumor thrombosis postdownstaging. Transplantation 2020. https://doi.org/10.1097/TP.0000000000003162.

Locoregional Therapies for Hepatocellular Carcinoma

What Has Changed in the Past Ten Years?

Anjana A. Pillai, MD[a], Meera Ramanathan, MD[b],
Laura Kulik, MD[b],*

KEYWORDS

- HCC • Liver cancer • Locoregional therapy • Systemic therapy • TACE • TARE
- Y90

KEY POINTS

- The evolution of locoregional therapies in the last decade has allowed for broader patient selection, individualized therapy with a refined, targeted approach, and less systemic toxicity and improved patient outcomes.
- With the rapidly changing landscape of systemic therapy, the role of locoregional therapies alone or in combination for downstaging and curative intent will continue to evolve as we await this coming decade.
- The timely transition from locoregioanl therapy to systemic therapy will need to be defined.

INTRODUCTION

Hepatocellular carcinoma (HCC) is among the fastest growing cancers and is the fourth most common cause of cancer-related mortality worldwide.[1] In the last decade, treatment strategies and approaches for HCC have evolved dramatically, especially within the realm of locoregional therapies (LRT). These treatments have been shown to improve progression-free survival (PFS), disease-free survival, and overall survival (OS) in patients with HCC. LRTs can be used with curative intention, for downstaging or bridging to liver transplantation (LT) and as palliative therapy in inoperable, advanced HCCs. This review focuses on current trends in locoregional therapy as well as identifies the optimal time period to transition to systemic therapy **(Fig. 1).**[2]

[a] Department of Internal Medicine, University of Chicago Medicine, 5841 South Maryland Avenue, Chicago, IL 60687, USA; [b] Department of Internal Medicine, Northwestern Memorial Hospital, 676 North St. Clair 19th Floor, Chicago, IL 60611, USA
* Corresponding author.
E-mail address: lkulik@nm.org

Clin Liver Dis 24 (2020) 681–700
https://doi.org/10.1016/j.cld.2020.07.011
1089-3261/20/© 2020 Elsevier Inc. All rights reserved.
liver.theclinics.com

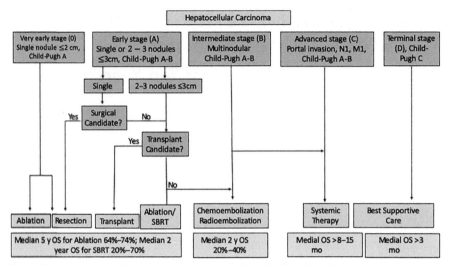

Fig. 1. Treatment algorithm and OS based on BCLC classification. (*Adapted from* Llovett J et al. Trial Design and Endpoints in HCC: AASLD consensus conference, Hepatology, 2020; with permission.)

Ablative Therapies

Image-guided tumor ablative therapies are a well-established form of local cancer treatment, with options evolving rapidly. Percutaneous ablative therapies focus on image-guided destruction of tumor tissue through direct application of either chemical- or energy-based treatment, with the benefit of offering curative intent for some patients. These treatments are typically indicated for patients with small HCCs, up to 3 lesions each ≤3 cm, Child-Pugh (CP) class A or B.[3]

Percutaneous ethanol injection

Ethanol-based ablative techniques were first described in the 1980s and previously served as the primary form of ablation. Complete tumor necrosis can be achieved in 90% of HCC nodules less than 2 cm[4]; however, for tumors greater than 2 cm, recurrence rates approached nearly 50%, likely because of incomplete necrosis achieved in larger tumors.[5] Although the technique offers low morbidity and mortality, ethanol ablation is typically no longer used as first-line treatment because of multiple randomized controlled trials (RCTs) and meta-analyses showing superiority with radiofrequency ablation (RFA) in terms of treatment response, local tumor cure rate, and OS.[3,6-12]

Radiofrequency ablation

RFA was first introduced in the treatment of HCC in the early 1990s and is the most commonly used ablative technique. This particular method uses high-frequency alternating current, converting radiofrequency energy into heat, thereby inducing damage to the tumor tissue. For early-stage HCC, RFA can be used as first-line therapy. In a recent study, RFA offered favorable long-term outcomes for patients with a single HCC lesion less than 3 cm when used as first-line therapy.[12] In this study, patients were followed for 10 years after treatment with an OS of 74.2% with prognostic factors for OS, including local tumor progression (LTP), CP class, platelet levels, intrahepatic distant recurrence, aggressive intrasegmental recurrence, and extrahepatic metastatic disease. In another study by Salmi and colleagues,[13] 5-year OS for HCC lesions less than 3.5 cm approached 64%, with a local recurrence rate of 14%. Ablative margin by RFA affects development of LTP, although data are lacking regarding the ideal size of the tumor margin. Currently, a 0.5- to 1.0-cm margin is recommended.[14]

Given the successes of RFA, head-to-head prospective RCTs have been conducted between RFA and surgical resection of localized HCC. In a study by Cucchetti and colleagues,[15] local resection of tumors was found to provide better survival outcomes in comparison to RFA for single nodules 3 to 4 cm in size; however, the treatment modalities were comparable in patients with tumors less than 2 cm and in patients with 2 to 3 small tumors ≤3 cm. Similar results were found by Fang and colleagues[16] for tumors less than 3 cm. This difference may be due to the limited ability of RFA to attain adequate tissue necrosis in larger tumors. When analyzed for cost efficacy, RFA was found to be superior for early-stage HCC and for multiple small HCCs. Given the notable survival benefit for single tumors 3 to 5 cm, surgery remained the more cost-effective option for these patients. In contrast, in a single-center RCT by Ng and colleagues[17] in 2017 comparing hepatic resection to RFA in patients with early-stage HCC, regardless of tumor size, RFA was not found to be superior to hepatectomy with regard to tumor recurrence rate and 10-year OS. RFA did allow for shorter treatment duration, less procedural blood loss, and decreased length of hospital stay. In a more recent study by Lee and colleagues,[18] local recurrence rate was higher in RFA (53% vs 26%), but OS was not significantly different between RFA and resection (86% vs 83%).

A limitation of RFA is the risk involved when lesions are too close in proximity to the liver capsule or critical structures, such as vasculature, because of what is referred to as the "heat-sink effect." Studies have shown that in these lesions, perivascular cells are not ablated effectively, increasing risk of local recurrence.[19] In addition, as previously mentioned, complete necrosis of lesions is less successful in larger lesions, increasing risk of local tumor recurrence.

In patients with very early-stage HCC, both RFA and resection are viable options. In patients who can undergo resection, this allows for pathologic examination of the tumor and subsequent risk stratification if the patient needs eventual LT.

Microwave ablation

Microwave ablation (MWA), first described in the 1970s, causes tumor destruction through hyperthermic injury via electromagnetic waves. Although prospective, randomized clinical data are limited regarding this technique, it offers certain advantages over RFA, such as shorter procedure time and less susceptibility to incomplete ablation. MWA is also less susceptible to the heat sink effect and is thus less limited by critical structures near the treatment field. Furthermore, the ability to use multiple probes during a single treatment allows for a larger treatment field, allowing for more effective treatment of larger lesions.[20] In a recent metaanalysis, similar efficacy was demonstrated by both RFA and MWA, and 1 study suggested potential superiority of MWA in larger HCCs.[21,22]

Survival probability for MWA has been shown to be greatest for lesions less than 4 cm.[23] Combination therapies for larger lesions, such as transarterial chemoembolization (TACE) followed by MWA, have shown favorable outcomes and are often used for lesions not amenable to treatment with a single modality alone.[24,25]

Cryoablation

The use of cryoablation, largely developed in the 1980s, involves the use of very low temperatures to kill tumor cells by producing intracellular and extracellular ice crystals, resulting in cell dehydration and rupture. In addition, this also induces ischemic hypoxia to the tumor owing to vascular injury. This procedure is done with intraprocedural image-based monitoring, allowing for more control over the ablation field.[3] Long-term survival analysis data are limited for cryoablation, and most ablative treatments have transitioned to the newer modalities. It is, however, still sporadically used in conjunction with other locoregional therapies. An RCT involving 360 patients comparing RFA versus cryoablation in 1 to 2 HCC lesions ≤4 cm, cryoablation resulted in lower local tumor progression, although both treatment modalities had similar 5-year survival rates and were found to be equally effective.[26]

Irreversible electroporation

Irreversible electroporation (IRE) is a newer, nonthermal technique involving delivery of short electrical pulses into a given tumor, leading to cell death owing to apoptosis by producing irreversible pores in cellular membranes.[27,28] This technique offers the benefit of preserving connective tissue, vessels, and bile ducts, making it an option for treatment of those lesions in a position that makes surgery and thermal techniques high risk, such as central liver lesions.[29] These benefits were shown in a small study by Cheng and colleagues[30] when looking at posttransplant treatment fields. Bile ducts were preserved, and treatment fields showed complete pathologic necrosis. Interestingly, however, in another study looking at ablation zones, IRE was found to have the largest transition zone between living and necrotic tissue, potentially heightening risk of local recurrence.[31] IRE does require general anesthesia, multiple electrode insertions, and muscle blocks, introducing a risk that the aforementioned treatments do not.[3] In addition, the insertion channels cannot be cauterized, potentially increasing risk of bleeding complications.[28] In a German study, a retrospective analysis showed no difference in complication grade nor rates between thermal techniques and IRE.[28] This therapy is currently recommended for very early-stage HCC, although further, large-scale studies are needed to determine its efficacy and safety in comparison to the more commonly used thermal techniques.

Stereotactic body radiotherapy

Stereotactic body radiotherapy (SBRT), also known as stereotactic ablative radiotherapy, presents an additional option for select patients with localized, unresectable HCC, used either individually or in conjunction with other treatment methods. Unlike traditional radiation therapy that involves multiple sessions of small-dose, daily radiation treatments, SBRT entails anywhere from 1 to 5 treatments at a higher biologically effective dose.[32] SBRT offers high rates of local tumor control, low toxicity, and PFS comparable to resection and RFA. In a study by Wahl and colleagues,[33] SBRT and RFA had similar success rates for tumors less than 2 cm; however, for those tumors greater than 2 cm, SBRT had improved control. Although there are no RCTs to date comparing SBRT to other accepted treatment modalities, SBRT shows promise in the management of HCC. Another arena where radiation has been examined is with the intent to bridge to transplant. The use if SBRT for bridging to transplant can be seen in centers were transarterial radioembolization (TARE) is not readily available. A single-center study from Toronto showed similar dropout rates and OS from listing/LT with external beam radiation compared with RFA or TACE,[34] suggesting that radiotherapy may offer an alternative therapy when TACE or RFA is not deemed feasible. Please refer to Chien Pong Chen's article, "Role of External Beam Radiotherapy in Hepatocellular Carcinoma," in this issue for a detailed discussion of the role for this therapy.

Catheter-Based Therapies

Both chemoembolization and radioembolization play a large role in the treatment paradigm of HCC. These 2 therapies have been refined over the last decade with broader applications and improved patient survival.

Chemoembolization

Because HCCs are uniquely supplied by the hepatic artery,[35,36] transarterial treatments have proven to be extremely effective in delivering targeted embolic therapy to the tumor while preserving and minimizing exposure to surrounding liver parenchyma, particularly when performed in a superselective manner. There are 3 types of embolization that are commonly used as intraarterial therapy for HCC: bland embolization, conventional transarterial chemoembolization (cTACE), and drug-eluting bead chemoembolization (DEB-TACE).[37]

Bland embolization or transcatheter arterial embolization (TAE) was the first generation of embolic agents used, first described in the late 1970s, and were divided into spherical and nonspherical subgroups with the goal of terminal vessel blockade.[37,38] Since its inception in the treatment of HCC, there have been conflicting data regarding its applicability compared with TACE, including results in RCTs.[39,40]

The most successful single-center data come from the Memorial Sloan Kettering group. In a retrospective analysis of 322 patients with advanced HCC treated with TAE, median OS was 21 months with a 1-year survival of 66%.[41] In patients without extrahepatic disease or vascular invasion, the OS at 1 and 3 years was 84% and 51%, respectively. A recent metaanalysis of 55 randomized controlled studies did not show any significant survival benefit with cTACE, DEB-TACE, or TARE when compared with TAE.[42]

cTACE was first performed in the 1980s as a method for targeted intraarterial delivery of chemotherapy to the tumor followed by an embolic agent.[43,44] There has been significant heterogeneity with TACE, including the chemotherapeutic agents used (cisplatin, doxorubicin, or mitomycin C either alone or in combination along with iodinated contrast and ethiodized oil),[45] as well as the embolic agent used (gelfoam, polyvinyl alcohol, or spherical embolic agents) to prevent drug washout and to increase intratumoral retention of the agents to induce cytotoxic cell death and ischemic necrosis. TACE evolved into the standard of care in patients with intermediate HCC as the result of 2 RCTs from Europe and Asia that met their primary endpoint of OS.[46,47] A systemic review of 101 studies of cTACE in 10,108 patients confirmed an objective response rate (ORR) of 52.5%, median OS of 19.4 months with 1-, 3-, and 5-year survival of 70.3%, 40.4%, and 32.4%.[48] The most common adverse event was postembolic syndrome, which was seen in almost 50% of patients, although procedure-related mortality remained low at 0.6%.

DEB-TACE or intraarterial injection of drug-eluting microspheres loaded with a chemotherapeutic agent (ie, doxorubicin) was developed in 2005.[49] DEB has allowed for predictable and sustained targeted drug delivery while minimizing plasma concentrations of chemotherapy, resulting in higher tumor retention of doxorubicin with minimal systemic absorption. In 2010, Lammer and colleagues[50] completed the first prospective, randomized controlled, multicenter study evaluating DEB-TACE versus cTACE in the treatment of advanced HCC, called the "PRECISION V study. In this study, 212 CP A/B patients were randomized to receive doxorubicin-eluting (DC) beads versus cTACE. Results were not statistically significant for primary aim of tumor response at 6 months with DC beads. Data showed complete response (CR) of 27% versus 22% and ORR of 52% versus 44% in the DC arm versus cTACE arm, respectively. However, there was a higher ORR in patients with CP B disease and bilobar/recurrent disease with DC beads. Safety profiles of both treatment arms were similar (20.4% vs 19.4%), but there was significant less serious liver toxicity in the DC arm (16%) versus cTACE (25%). These results were validated in numerous subsequent studies[51–53] and various metaanalyses with similar tumor response rates.[54–59]

Several studies have been conducted comparing cTACE or DEB-TACE with TAE. Of the 5 RCTs, three showed similar OS between modalities,[47,60,61] one showed no difference in PFS or OS between the 2 treatments arms,[62] and one showed patients receiving DEB-TACE had longer time to progression (TTP) compared with TAE.[63] Combining LRT has also been studied with variable success. In a metaanalysis of 8 RCTs of 648 patients treated with combination of TACE + RFA RFA alone, combination therapy had a significant recurrence-free survival and OS especially in patients with intermediate and large (>3 cm) HCCs[64]; there was no benefit of combination therapy in patients with small tumors. Ginsburg and colleagues[65] performed a retrospective study examining the benefit of DEB-TACE + RFA or MWA in 89 patients with small HCCs and noted a 78% initial CR, median PFS of 9 months, and median OS of 39 months. There was no significant difference between the 2 modalities in efficacy or safety; there was a 3% adverse event rate, mainly related to prolonged hospitalization. Overall, these studies suggest that there may be a role of combination therapies in select patients.

Transarterial chemoembolization + sorafenib

Since the approval of Sorafenib for unresectable HCC, there have been several phase 3 RCTs that have aimed to demonstrate an improved OS and TTP with combination of TACE/DEB with tyrosine kinase inhibitors (TKIs) by blunting of the angiogenic flare after embolization compared with TACE alone. Several of these trials were negative; however, it did demonstrate that in highly selected candidates that the median OS for TACE is approximately 26 months.[66] Trial design may in part have led to negative results, including the timing of TKI relative to TACE/DEB, dosage and duration of TKI, and early termination of trials. Of note in the SPACE trial, those randomized to DEB + Sorafenib received only 1 DEB therapy because of conservative stopping rules of which several patients had subsequent additional DEB therapy once off the trial. A more recent phase 2 trial from Japan, Transcatheter Arterial Chemoembolization Therapy in Combination With Sorafenib, reported a significantly improved PFS in those receiving TACE + Sorafenib compared with TACE alone: 25.2 versus 13.5 months, respectively (hazard ratio [HR] 0.59, 95% confidence interval [CI] 0.41–0.87; $P = .006$).[67] The approach in this trial was unique in that the presence of new intrahepatic lesions did not lead to cessation of assigned therapy, leading to longer time on Sorafenib (median 38.7 weeks) relative to prior negative phase 3 trials (median range 17.0–24.0 weeks). Results of the coprimary endpoint of OS are awaited.

Transarterial chemoembolization + radiation therapy

A metaanalysis of 25 trials from Asia showed the pooled OS was significantly higher with TACE + radiation therapy compared with TACE alone (22.7 vs TACE 13.5 months; $P<.001$); however, there were higher adverse events because of gastric/duodenal ulceration and an increase in transaminases with the combination therapy.[68]

Transarterial radioembolization

Selective internal radiation therapy or TARE is a form of brachytherapy that allows intraarterial delivery of radioactive microspheres (loaded with Yttrium 90 or Y90) to the tumor bed.[69] TARE allows for higher targeted dose of radiation therapy internally to the tumor when compared with external beam radiation and SBRT. Although TACE can cause occlusion of medium- and large-size arteries because of the size of particles used, Y90 microspheres are much smaller and target therapy within the capillary bed of the tumor delivering tumoricidal doses of radiation while sparing the surrounding liver tissue.[70] Two commercially available microspheres, glass/ceramic-based or resin-coated polystyrene, serve as delivery platforms and differ in particle size, activity, density, and composition.[71] TARE has traditionally been used in patients with intermediate or advanced disease, including those with bilobar disease or large tumors who are poor candidates for TACE, as well as those with tumors invading branch of the portal vein where TACE is contraindicated or those who progress on TACE. More recently, with a superselective approach, radiation segmentectomy has been used as potential curative therapy for smaller lesions.

Early prospective studies of TARE were mostly single-center reports (**Table 1**).[72–75] The most favorable results have been reported by the Milan group, which mostly comprised CP A patients, highlighting the competing risk of mortality related to tumor and liver failure.

Side effects include fatigue, abdominal discomfort, and nausea and vomiting. Expertise and proper angiography are imperative to avoid off-target delivery of radiation that can lead to complications.

Several studies have been performed comparing efficacy of TACE versus TARE.[76–79] In a single-center retrospective analysis of 245 patients treated with transarterial locoregional therapy (122 with TACE and 123 with TARE), TTP was significantly

Table 1
Summary of patient characteristics and outcomes with transarterial radioembolization for the treatment of hepatocellular carcinoma

	Salem et al,[72] 2010 (n = 291) Single-Center Glass	Hilgard et al,[73] 2010 (n = 108) Single-Center Glass	Sangro et al,[74] 2010 (n = 325) Multicenter Resin	Mazzaferro et al,[75] 2012 (n = 52) Single-Center Glass
Patient characteristics				
CP A/B/C (%)	45/52/3	77/22 ($\leq$7)/0	82/18/0	83/17 ($\leq$7)/0
BCLC A/B/C/D (%)	17/28/52/3	2/47/51/0	16/27/56/1	0/33/67/0
Mean tumor size (cm)	7.0	—	—	5.6
Multifocal (%)	73	—	76	69
PVT (%)	43	31	23	67
Extrahepatic mets (%)	16	30	9	—
Outcome (excluded mets)				
Overall survival (mo)	CP A: 17.2 CP B: 7.7 BCLC A: 26.9 BCLC B: 17.2 BCLC C: 7.3	CP A: 17.2 CP B: 6.0 BCLC A: — BCLC B: 16.4 BCLC C: not reached	CP A: — CP B: — BCLC A: 24.4 BCLC B: 16.9 BCLC C: 10.0	CP A: — CP B: — BCLC A: — BCLC B: 18 BCLC C: 13
TTP (mo)	7.9 CP A: 10.8 CP B: 8.4	10.0	—	11

Abbreviations: mets, metastasis.

longer with TARE than TACE (13.3 vs 8.4 months) with no difference in OS between the 2 groups.[79] Early pilot RCTs comparing TACE and TARE found no significant difference in outcomes; however, TARE was given once and TACE was performed every 6 weeks until there was CR.[80] In 2016, PREMIERE, the largest RCT to date, randomized CP A/B patients with Barcelona Clinic Liver Cancer (BCLC) A/B HCC to cTACE versus Y90 and demonstrated significant longer median TTP (>26 months) with TARE than cTACE (6.8 months). Median OS and response to therapy were similar between both groups.[81] Lewandowski and colleagues[82] retrospectively compared the efficacy of TACE versus TARE for United Network for Organ Sharing (UNOS) downstaging criteria from T3 to T2 for potential LT. In this study, 43 patients in each arm received TACE or TARE, and median tumor size was similar in both arms (5.7 cm in TACE vs 5.6 cm in TARE). Downstaging to UNOS T2 occurred in 31% of patients with TACE and 58% of patients with TARE, whereas TTP was similar between both groups. OS survival was not significant between the 2 arms, although patients in the TARE arm had greater event-free survival. In most clinical scenarios, the safety and efficacy of TACE and TARE are equivalent, and use of one in favor of the other often depends on institutional bias and availability.

Another promising outcome of radioembolization therapy is the concept of radiation lobectomy and the unintentional volumetric hypertrophy that occurs on the contralateral side of the treated tumor secondary to radiation changes. Vouche and colleagues[83] demonstrated in a group of 83 patients with right unilobar malignancies (HCC, cholangiocarcinoma, and colorectal cancer) that Y90 radiation lobectomy was safe and effective to hypertrophy future liver remnant (FLR) with volumetric changes comparable to portal vein embolization (PVE). This finding was confirmed by Garlipp and colleagues[84] in 2 centers in Germany where patients with right-sided malignancies with limited or no left-sided tumor involvement were treated by right lobar PVE (n = 141) or TARE (n = 35). The investigators concluded that radioembolization resulted in substantial contralateral hypertrophy, albeit less than PVE with therapeutic (nonlobectomy) doses. The ability to synchronously treat the tumor while allowing for hypertrophy of FLR makes TARE an effective method of treatment as a bridge to resection.

In more recent years, segmental radioembolization has also increased in popularity. Radiation segmentectomy was defined as radioembolization of 2 or fewer hepatic segments with high-dose radiation.[85] In a study of 84 patients with advanced, inoperable HCC, radiation segmentectomy proved to be safe and efficacious with a significant response in size and necrosis (in 59% and 81% of patients, respectively).[85] Mean TTP was 13.6 months, and median OS was 26.9 months.

Studies comparing segmental radioembolization versus segmental chemoembolization showed the former to be a promising method of therapy for local tumor control with no significant increase in toxicity profile.[86] Padia and colleagues,[86] in a single-center retrospective study, examined 101 patients who underwent radiation segmentectomy with 77 patients who underwent segmental DEB-TACE or cTACE. In this cohort, patients receiving chemoembolization had worse performance status and CP class, whereas those receiving radioembolization had larger, infiltrative tumors with more vascular invasion. They reported index and overall CR of 92% and 84% for Y90 versus 74% and 58% for TACE, which was statistically significant. Index tumor progression at 1 and 2 years was 8% and 15% in the Y90 arm and 30% and 42% in the TACE arm. Median PFS and OS were also statistically significant, favoring radiation segmentectomy. Biederman and colleagues[87] examined radiation segmentectomy versus TACE in a single-center retrospective study of 112 patients with unresectable, solitary HCC ≤3 cm without evidence of metastasis or vascular invasion. In this study,

55 patients underwent Y90 segmentectomy compared with 57 patients who underwent segmental TACE. Y90 segmentectomy showed superior imaging response and longer time to secondary therapy when compared with segmental TACE. In a single-center retrospective study of 70 patients with unresectable, solitary HCC ≤5 cm, not amenable to percutaneous ablation or resection, the effectiveness of radiation segmentectomy (dose of >190 Gy) was assessed for curative intent.[88] Median TTP was 2.4 years, and OS was 6.7 years. In patients with tumors ≤3 cm (n = 45), OS was significantly longer than in patients with tumors greater than 3 cm with 1-, 3- and 5-year survival of 100%, 82%, and 75%, respectively. These studies confirm that radiation segmentectomy could be a viable curative option for early-stage HCC and similar in effectiveness to percutaneous ablation or resection.

Last, TARE has been shown to be safe and effective in portal vein thrombus (PVT). It has become clear that patient selection is paramount to obtaining clinically meaningful results and to avoid hepatic decompensation. Spreafico and colleagues[89] have developed a prognostic scoring system for patients with PVT intended for therapy with TACE. This prognostic scoring system consists of 3 identified factors that were independent predictors of OS. Points are given based on these 3 factors that included the degree of PVT extension V1 to V3 (mainly PVT, V4 was excluded), bilirubin level, and tumor burden. This scoring system can be used to identify the most ideal candidates with therapy with TARE who achieved median OS 32 months and those in which TARE should not be offered because of futility. Another technical aspect regarding TARE, which impacts OS, is boosted radiation dose into the tumor. Improvement in OS and response rates, particularly in those with PVT, has been demonstrated when greater than 205 Gy is delivered to the tumor.[90,91] This personalized approach is feasible with glass microspheres. The macroaggregated albumin (MAA) before Y90 administration is used to determine the distribution of the glass microspheres and quantify delivery of radiation to the tumor that can be boosted to achieve a dose greater than 205 Gy. It is important to recognize that not all patients will be candidates for boosted radiation because of risk of toxicity; this includes cases whereby greater than 120 Gy is estimated to be delivered to nontumorous tissue or when tumor volume exceeds 70% of the total liver volume. A phase 2 RCT, conducted at 4 centers in France, showed that the use of personalized dosimetry with a target of at least 205 Gy into the tumor led to a significant increase in OS (26.7 months) compared with standard dosimetry (10.7 months).[92]

As TARE becomes more widely accepted within the treatment paradigm of HCC, studies evaluating cost and convenience are also important. Currently, TARE requires a 2-step outpatient procedure; the first procedure is a diagnostic angiogram with an MAA scan to assess degree of lung shunting and potential for off-target delivery of radiation, which may require coil embolization to prevent. The patient returns on a separate day at which time the microspheres loaded with Y90 are delivered. The feasibility of same-day Y90 was reported by a single center in 78 patients using glass microspheres (77% with HCC).[92] More recently, the same institution reported that the lung shunt in T1/T2 lesions among 448 patients (excluding patients with transjugular intrahepatic portosystemic shunt) was negligible, and therefore, the lung shunt study could be eliminated. This finding supports the notion of streamlining patients to therapy with same-day Y90 and lowering cost.[93] Another single-center study evaluated the concept of same-day mapping and treatment with Y90 in a retrospective analysis of 26 patients with either HCC or liver metastases using resin microspheres.[93] Further studies will need to be conducted to evaluate the safety, efficacy, and reproducibility of this concept.

When Do You Transition from Locoregional Therapies to Systemic Therapy?

In the advent of impressive advances in systemic therapy, specifically combination therapies, it is imperative to be mindful of when LRT should cease and systemic therapies commence. This situation is however different than foregoing LRT at the initial presentation of HCC. These 2 scenarios will be addressed separately.

The approval of Sorafenib based on the results of the SHARP study in 2007 began the era of systemic therapy in HCC. Several agents tested in first-line trials failed to show noninferiority or superiority to Sorafenib over a 10-year period. However, in the last few years there have been several agents approved in both the first and the second line as a result of positive phase 3 RCTs demonstrating improved OS. The most recent positive trial was the IMbrave150 study, which showed a significant improvement in the coprimary endpoints of OS and PFS in patients treated with atezolizumab 1200 mg intravenously plus bevacizumab 15 mg/kg compared with Sorafenib 400 mg twice a day. No new safety signals were identified with this combination compared with monotherapy with each individual agent.

Phase 3 RCTs examining the safety and efficacy of systemic agents in unresectable HCC have been conducted in a population with preserved liver function, CP A, and largely comprise patients with BCLC C disease. However, there was a subset of patients with intermediate HCC, most deemed refractory to TACE. The 16% to 21% of BCLC B patients in first-line systemic trials showed a survival benefit with these agents.

Without a potential curative therapy, the natural history of progression from intermediate to advanced disease is generally accepted to be inevitable. The increase in the availability of effective systemic options has led to a debate of the most appropriate timing to initiate in lieu of continued LRT in order to maximize exposure to and improved OS with sequential systemic therapies.[94] TACE is the most commonly used form of LRT in intermediate HCC. Overuse of TACE/Y90 can culminate in hepatic decompensation leading to a lost opportunity of meaningful benefit of tumor control with systemic agents owing to the competing risk of mortality from worsening liver disease. In addition, tumor progression with development of PVT, particularly main PVT or infiltrative tumor, can lead to rapid decline in hepatic function, making initiation of a systemic agent a safety, tolerability, and efficacy concern because of limited data in this patient population. Global Investigation of therapeutic DEcisions in hepatocellular carcinoma and Of its treatment with SorafeNib (GIDEON), a prospective observation study that collected data on the real-life experience with Sorafenib, found a significant decline in median OS per decrement in CP class (CP A: 13.6, CP B: 5.2, CP C: 2.6 months) despite no observed difference in TTP based on CP class.[95] Small studies have reported safety of Nivolumab in CP B with a median OS of 5.9 and 7.6 months in 2 separate cohorts.[96,97]

Although TACE is the recommended therapy for BCLC B patients, this group constitutes one that is quite heterogeneous, and not all in aggregate are suitable for TACE. Systemic therapy should ideally be started at time of TACE refractoriness or in BCLC B patients in whom TACE is unlikely to benefit, while liver function remains preserved. The Japan Society of Hepatology has defined TACE refractoriness as the inability to control a treated lesion or lesions (>50% viable lesion) and/or development of new tumors after ≥2 consecutive sessions of chemoembolization, continuous elevation in tumor markers, or appearance of extrahepatic spread or vascular invasion.[98] OPTIMIS was a global observational prospective trial that aimed to characterize TACE utilization and outcomes in a real-world setting of patients with BCLC stage B HCC or higher.[99] A total of 1650 patients were treated with TACE of whom 32% were BCLC C, 7% had extrahepatic spread, and 7% had portal vein invasion. Response rates declined with each subsequent TACE, whereas progressive disease increased. At inclusion, 39% met TACE ineligibility criteria, and during the course of the study, 31% became TACE ineligible with less than 10% receiving Sorafenib at that time. Improved OS has been demonstrated in patients who were started on Sorafenib at the time of TACE refractoriness compared with those who continued to receive TACE.[100,101] This real-world study highlights the crucial need for defining consensus on when LRT no longer provides benefit and allows a timely transition to systemic therapy.

However, despite an accepted consensus on transitioning to systemic therapy once TACE refractoriness develops, approximately one-quarter of patients have already declined to CP B/C, thereby jeopardizing initiation and potential benefit of systemic agents.[99,101,102] The GIDEON trial found that the proportion of patients who were CP B at the time of starting Sorafenib was higher in those who received ≥6 TACE sessions.[103]

A nationwide database in Japan used α-fetoprotein (AFP), AFP-L3, and Desgamma-carboxy prothrombin (DCP) levels before TACE in 1306 treatment-naïve patients with intermediate-stage HCC and preserved liver function.[104] A point was given for each marker if ≥100 ng/mL (AFP), greater than 10% (AFP-L3), and greater than 100 mAU/mL (DCP) to determine a tumor marker score. As the score increased, median OS diminished: 0, 1, ≥2 = 4.8, 3.8, 3.2 years, respectively; $P<.01$. A score ≥2 was an independent predictor of mortality; as such, the investigators concluded the tumor marker score could be used to prognosticate which patients with intermediate HCC will have a suboptimal response to TACE and predict TACE refractoriness.

A newer proposed term, TACE unsuitability, encompasses circumstances that predispose to one of the 3 scenarios associated with TACE: becoming TACE refractory, decline to CP B, or unlikely chance of tumor response.[105] Tumor burden beyond up-to-7 criteria is a predictor of TACE refractoriness as well as TACE leading to decline in liver function.[100] Initiation of TACE in those with albumin-bilirubin grade 2 is another group at high risk for reduction in hepatic reserve after TACE.[106] There are several identified situations that predict to TACE resistance, such as massive tumors, poorly differentiated HCC, multifocal intrahepatic metastasis, and sarcomatous changes induced by TACE. Such morphologic changes in HCC can occur when residual viable tumor is influenced by the hypoxia-induced angiogenic surge associated with TACE.[107]

A study of CP A patients beyond up-to-7 criteria reported improved OS in a propensity-matched TACE-naïve cohort treated with Lenvatinib (LEN) followed by on demand selective TACE (70%) compared with patients who received TACE (37.9 vs 21 months, respectively; HR 0.48; 95% CI 0.16–0.79).[105] The improved OS in the LEN-TACE group was ascribed to preservation of liver function allowing a longer treatment period with full-dose LEN and high tumor response rates associated with LEN. LEN has been reported to demonstrate high response rates in poorly differentiated HCC, a subgroup that historically had the worse prognosis. LEN-TACE sequential therapy in patients with TACE unsuitability is a shift in the paradigm of HCC therapy, and although reports of its efficacy are promising, additional studies are required to validate this approach as a standard of care. Another study from Japan reported real-life experience with LEN.[108] A total of 116 patients with BCLC B tumor, the vast majority CP A, were treated with systemic therapy as first-line therapy with 61% treated with LEN as initial therapy and the remainder treated with LEN as second- or third-line systemic therapy. Median OS was not reached, whereas median PFS was 14 months.

Earlier use of systemic therapy in patients with intermediate HCC guided by prognostic models with data supporting improved OS may lead to a paradigm shift in treatment in a subset of the BCLC B group. Consideration for an earlier initiation of systemic therapy needs to be balanced against the use of LRT for the intended purpose of downstaging to Milan criteria (MC). Some patients may not meet acceptable criteria for LRT because of the presence of ascites, performance status, or CP B; however, successful downstaging could allow access to transplantation, which offers the best chance for long-term OS in HCC. In addition, the ceiling of tumor burden for the accepted downstaging protocol adopted by UNOS includes tumor burden (1 lesion >5 cm and ≤8 cm, 2 or 3 lesions each less than 5 cm and total diameter of all lesions ≤8 cm, or 4 or 5 lesions each less than 3 cm and total diameter of all lesions ≤8 cm) that exceeds the up-to-7 criteria. Although guidelines have advocated for restriction in eligibility criteria for candidates for downstaging based on initial tumor burden in order to optimize chance of successful downstaging to MC, other single-center studies reported a 30% success rate in downstaging to the MC followed by LT with no limit on initial tumor size and number, including the presence of non–main PVT.[109] OS and recurrence rates were similar to those downstaged and those who met MC. The investigators concluded that patients exceeding the MC who are otherwise candidates for LT should undergo aggressive attempts at downstaging without an a priori exclusion. During the time period that this study was conducted, Sorafenib was the only systemic therapy approved for advanced HCC.

Combination therapy with TACE + radiation therapy has been compared with Sorafenib in an RCT in patients with CP A HCC with PVT (58.9% had unilateral disease) without metastatic disease.[110] TACE occurred every 6 weeks, and radiotherapy (RT; planned total dose of 45 Gy) was started after the first TACE. The combination group demonstrated a significantly longer 12-week PFS compared with Sorafenib 86.7% versus 34.3% retrospectively (P<.001). Independent of macroscopic vascular invasion extent, 24-week PFS remained significantly higher in the TACE-RT group. In addition, median TTP and OS were superior in the combination group (TTP: 31.0 vs 11.7 weeks; OS: 55 vs 43 weeks, respectively). Crossover owing to tumor progression was higher at 24 weeks in the Sorafenib group, 90.7%, compared with 23% in TACE/RT group. Of note, this study was conducted in a primarily hepatitis B virus population and therefore its applicability to other populations is not known.

With a decrease in priority for LT in HCC, it is expected that the use of living donor liver transplantation (LDLT) will continue to expand in HCC. A multicenter trial of LDLT in HCC exceeding the MC reported that the only independent predictor of OS was meeting the MC at time of LT.[111] The response to LRT to downstage both tumor burden and AFP levels has been shown to portend favorable long-term results and highlights that LRT can be used to gain insight into the biological aggressiveness of a tumor and serve as an important selection tool. Therefore, desertion of LRT in an otherwise appropriate LT candidate other than tumor burden and AFP could result in a potential lost chance for LT. Additional research is required to know if use of systemic therapy, specifically LEN with higher response rates, can lead to successful downstaging alone or in combination with LRT resulting in LT. Of note, an RCT of TACE + Sorafenib versus TACE in patients awaiting LT reported no significant difference in the primary endpoint of TTP; however, all patients within this trial met MC.[112]

Locoregional therapies + immune oncology
Immunotherapy is being studied in combination with LRT. The hope is to augment the immune response by causing release of neoantigens induced by LRT-associated

tumor necrosis and hence improve OS. The first proof-of-concept study used TACE or RFA in 32 patients (BCLC B/C with progressive disease at enrollment, 75% Sorafenib experienced) followed by tremelimumab, an anti-CLLA-4 antibody, resulting in a partial response in 26%, TTP of 7.4 months, and OS of 12.3 months.[113]

SUMMARY

The evolution of LRT in the last decade has allowed for broader patient selection, individualized therapy with a refined, targeted approach and less systemic toxicity, and improved patient outcomes. With the rapidly changing landscape of systemic therapy, the role of LRT alone or in combination for downstaging and curative intent will continue to evolve as we await this coming decade.

DISCLOSURE

Guarantor of the article: L. Kulik. Specific author contributions: A.A. Pillai, M. Ramanathan, and L. Kulik drafted and revised and approved the article. Financial support: None. Potential competing interests: None. A.A. Pillai is on the speakers bureau for Simply Speaking Hepatitis and Eisai Inc, and on the Medical Advisory Board for Exelixis, Eisai and Genentech. M. Ramanathan has nothing to declare. L. Kulik is on the Speaker's Bureau for Eisai Inc and serves as a consultant for Merck on the medical advisory board for BMS, Eisai Bayer, and research support is for Target HCC.

REFERENCES

1. Kanwal F, Singal AG. Surveillance for hepatocellular carcinoma: current best practice and future direction. Gastroenterology 2019;157(1):54–64.
2. Llovet JM, Villanueva A, Marrero JA, et al. Trial design and endpoints in hepatocellular carcinoma: AASLD consensus conference. Hepatology 2020. [Epub ahead of print].
3. Shiina S, Sato K, Tateishi R, et al. Percutaneous ablation for hepatocellular carcinoma: comparison of various ablation techniques and surgery. Can J Gastroenterol Hepatol 2018;2018:4756147.
4. Sala M, Llovet JM, Vilana R, et al. Initial response to percutaneous ablation predicts survival in patients with hepatocellular carcinoma. Hepatology 2004;40(6): 1352–60.
5. Pompili M, De Matthaeis N, Saviano A, et al. Single hepatocellular carcinoma smaller than 2 cm: are ethanol injection and radiofrequency ablation equally effective? Anticancer Res 2015;35(1):325–32.
6. Giorgio A, Di Sarno A, De Stefano G, et al. Percutaneous radiofrequency ablation of hepatocellular carcinoma compared to percutaneous ethanol injection in treatment of cirrhotic patients: an Italian randomized controlled trial. Anticancer Res 2011;31(6):2291–5.
7. Bouza C, López-Cuadrado T, Alcázar R, et al. Meta-analysis of percutaneous radiofrequency ablation versus ethanol injection in hepatocellular carcinoma. BMC Gastroenterol 2009;9:31.
8. Germani G, Pleguezuelo M, Gurusamy K, et al. Clinical outcomes of radiofrequency ablation, percutaneous alcohol and acetic acid injection for hepatocellular carcinoma: a meta-analysis. J Hepatol 2010;52(3):380–8.
9. Lin SM, Lin CJ, Lin CC, et al. Randomised controlled trial comparing percutaneous radiofrequency thermal ablation, percutaneous ethanol injection, and

percutaneous acetic acid injection to treat hepatocellular carcinoma of 3 cm or less. Gut 2005;54(8):1151–6.

10. Shiina S, Teratani T, Obi S, et al. A randomized controlled trial of radiofrequency ablation with ethanol injection for small hepatocellular carcinoma. Gastroenterology 2005;129(1):122–30.

11. Brunello F, Veltri A, Carucci P, et al. Radiofrequency ablation versus ethanol injection for early hepatocellular carcinoma: a randomized controlled trial. Scand J Gastroenterol 2008;43(6):727–35.

12. Cho YK, Kim JK, Kim MY, et al. Systematic review of randomized trials for hepatocellular carcinoma treated with percutaneous ablation therapies. Hepatology 2009;49(2):453–9.

13. Salmi A, Turrini R, Lanzani G, et al. Efficacy of radiofrequency ablation of hepatocellular carcinoma associated with chronic liver disease without cirrhosis. Int J Med Sci 2008;5(6):327–32.

14. Ahmed M, Solbiati L, Brace CL, et al. Image-guided tumor ablation: standardization of terminology and reporting criteria–a 10-year update. Radiology 2014; 273(1):241–60.

15. Cucchetti A, Piscaglia F, Cescon M, et al. Cost-effectiveness of hepatic resection versus percutaneous radiofrequency ablation for early hepatocellular carcinoma. J Hepatol 2013;59(2):300–7.

16. Fang Y, Chen W, Liang X, et al. Comparison of long-term effectiveness and complications of radiofrequency ablation with hepatectomy for small hepatocellular carcinoma. J Gastroenterol Hepatol 2014;29(1):193–200.

17. Ng KKC, Chok KSH, Chan ACY, et al. Randomized clinical trial of hepatic resection versus radiofrequency ablation for early-stage hepatocellular carcinoma. Br J Surg 2017;104(13):1775–84.

18. Lee HW, Lee JM, Yoon JH, et al. A prospective randomized study comparing radiofrequency ablation and hepatic resection for hepatocellular carcinoma. Ann Surg Treat Res 2018;94(2):74–82.

19. Bhardwaj N, Strickland AD, Ahmad F, et al. A comparative histological evaluation of the ablations produced by microwave, cryotherapy and radiofrequency in the liver. Pathology 2009;41(2):168–72.

20. Wright AS, Lee FT Jr, Mahvi DM. Hepatic microwave ablation with multiple antennae results in synergistically larger zones of coagulation necrosis. Ann Surg Oncol 2003;10(3):275–83.

21. Facciorusso A, Di Maso M, Muscatiello N. Microwave ablation versus radiofrequency ablation for the treatment of hepatocellular carcinoma: a systematic review and meta-analysis. Int J Hyperthermia 2016;32(3):339–44.

22. Poulou LS, Botsa E, Thanou I, et al. Percutaneous microwave ablation vs radiofrequency ablation in the treatment of hepatocellular carcinoma. World J Hepatol 2015;7(8):1054–63.

23. Liang P, Dong B, Yu X, et al. Prognostic factors for survival in patients with hepatocellular carcinoma after percutaneous microwave ablation. Radiology 2005; 235(1):299–307.

24. Xu LF, Sun HL, Chen YT, et al. Large primary hepatocellular carcinoma: transarterial chemoembolization monotherapy versus combined transarterial chemoembolization-percutaneous microwave coagulation therapy. J Gastroenterol Hepatol 2013;28(3):456–63.

25. Zhang R, Shen L, Zhao L, et al. Combined transarterial chemoembolization and microwave ablation versus transarterial chemoembolization in BCLC stage B hepatocellular carcinoma. Diagn Interv Radiol 2018;24(4):219–24.

26. Wang C, Wang H, Yang W, et al. Multicenter randomized controlled trial of percutaneous cryoablation versus radiofrequency ablation in hepatocellular carcinoma. Hepatology 2015;61(5):1579–90.
27. Tameez Ud Din A, Tameez-Ud-Din A, Chaudhary FMD, et al. Irreversible electroporation for liver tumors: a review of literature. Cureus 2019;11(6):e4994.
28. Verloh N, Jensch I, Lürken L, et al. Similar complication rates for irreversible electroporation and thermal ablation in patients with hepatocellular tumors. Radiol Oncol 2019;53(1):116–22.
29. Sutter O, Calvo J, N'Kontchou G, et al. Safety and efficacy of irreversible electroporation for the treatment of hepatocellular carcinoma not amenable to thermal ablation techniques: a retrospective single-center case series. Radiology 2017;284(3):877–86.
30. Cheng RG, Bhattacharya R, Yeh MM, et al. Irreversible electroporation can effectively ablate hepatocellular carcinoma to complete pathologic necrosis. J Vasc Interv Radiol 2015;26(8):1184–8.
31. Cornelis FH, Durack JC, Kimm SY, et al. A comparative study of ablation boundary sharpness after percutaneous radiofrequency, cryo-, microwave, and irreversible electroporation ablation in normal swine liver and kidneys. Cardiovasc Intervent Radiol 2017;40(10):1600–8.
32. Lin TA, Lin JS, Wagner T, et al. Stereotactic body radiation therapy in primary hepatocellular carcinoma: current status and future directions. J Gastrointest Oncol 2018;9(5):858–70.
33. Wahl DR, Stenmark MH, Tao Y, et al. Outcomes after stereotactic body radiotherapy or radiofrequency ablation for hepatocellular carcinoma. J Clin Oncol 2016;34(5):452–9.
34. Sapisochin G, Barry A, Doherty M, et al. Stereotactic body radiotherapy vs. TACE or RFA as a bridge to transplant in patients with hepatocellular carcinoma. An intention-to-treat analysis. J Hepatol 2017;67(1):92–9.
35. Kerbel RS. Tumor angiogenesis. N Engl J Med 2008;358(19):2039–49.
36. Breedis C, Young G. The blood supply of neoplasms in the liver. Am J Pathol 1954;30(5):969–77.
37. Kritzinger J, Klass D, Ho S, et al. Hepatic embolotherapy in interventional oncology: technology, techniques, and applications. Clin Radiol 2013;68(1):1–15.
38. Tadavarthy SM, Knight L, Ovitt TW, et al. Therapeutic transcatheter arterial embolization. Radiology 1974;112(1):13–6.
39. Bruix J, Castells A, Montanyà X, et al. Phase II study of transarterial embolization in European patients with hepatocellular carcinoma: need for controlled trials. Hepatology 1994;20(3):643–50.
40. Bruix J, Llovet JM, Castells A, et al. Transarterial embolization versus symptomatic treatment in patients with advanced hepatocellular carcinoma: results of a randomized, controlled trial in a single institution. Hepatology 1998;27(6):1578–83.
41. Maluccio MA, Covey AM, Porat LB, et al. Transcatheter arterial embolization with only particles for the treatment of unresectable hepatocellular carcinoma. J Vasc Interv Radiol 2008;19(6):862–9.
42. Katsanos K, Kitrou P, Spiliopoulos S, et al. Comparative effectiveness of different transarterial embolization therapies alone or in combination with local ablative or adjuvant systemic treatments for unresectable hepatocellular carcinoma: a network meta-analysis of randomized controlled trials. PLoS One 2017;12(9):e0184597.

43. Kajanti M, Rissanen P, Virkkunen P, et al. Regional intra-arterial infusion of cisplatin in primary hepatocellular carcinoma. A phase II study. Cancer 1986; 58(11):2386–8.

44. Sasaki Y, Imaoka S, Kasugai H, et al. A new approach to chemoembolization therapy for hepatoma using ethiodized oil, cisplatin, and gelatin sponge. Cancer 1987;60(6):1194–203.

45. Bruix J, Sala M, Llovet JM. Chemoembolization for hepatocellular carcinoma. Gastroenterology 2004;127(5 Suppl 1):S179–88.

46. Lo CM, Ngan H, Tso WK, et al. Randomized controlled trial of transarterial lipiodol chemoembolization for unresectable hepatocellular carcinoma. Hepatology 2002;35(5):1164–71.

47. Llovet JM, Real MI, Montaña X, et al. Arterial embolisation or chemoembolisation versus symptomatic treatment in patients with unresectable hepatocellular carcinoma: a randomised controlled trial. Lancet 2002;359(9319):1734–9.

48. Lencioni R, de Baere T, Soulen MC, et al. Lipiodol transarterial chemoembolization for hepatocellular carcinoma: a systematic review of efficacy and safety data. Hepatology 2016;64(1):106–16.

49. Hong K, Khwaja A, Liapi E, et al. New intra-arterial drug delivery system for the treatment of liver cancer: preclinical assessment in a rabbit model of liver cancer. Clin Cancer Res 2006;12(8):2563–7.

50. Lammer J, Malagari K, Vogl T, et al. Prospective randomized study of doxorubicin-eluting-bead embolization in the treatment of hepatocellular carcinoma: results of the PRECISION V study. Cardiovasc Intervent Radiol 2010; 33(1):41–52.

51. van Malenstein H, Maleux G, Vandecaveye V, et al. A randomized phase II study of drug-eluting beads versus transarterial chemoembolization for unresectable hepatocellular carcinoma. Onkologie 2011;34(7):368–76.

52. Sacco R, Bargellini I, Bertini M, et al. Conventional versus doxorubicin-eluting bead transarterial chemoembolization for hepatocellular carcinoma. J Vasc Interv Radiol 2011;22(11):1545–52.

53. Golfieri R, Giampalma E, Renzulli M, et al. Randomised controlled trial of doxorubicin-eluting beads vs conventional chemoembolisation for hepatocellular carcinoma. Br J Cancer 2014;111(2):255–64.

54. Gao S, Yang Z, Zheng Z, et al. Doxorubicin-eluting bead versus conventional TACE for unresectable hepatocellular carcinoma: a meta-analysis. Hepatogastroenterology 2013;60(124):813–20.

55. Facciorusso A, Di Maso M, Muscatiello N. Drug-eluting beads versus conventional chemoembolization for the treatment of unresectable hepatocellular carcinoma: a meta-analysis. Dig Liver Dis 2016;48(6):571–7.

56. Zou JH, Zhang L, Ren ZG, et al. Efficacy and safety of cTACE versus DEB-TACE in patients with hepatocellular carcinoma: a meta-analysis. J Dig Dis 2016;17(8): 510–7.

57. Chen P, Yuan P, Chen B, et al. Evaluation of drug-eluting beads versus conventional transcatheter arterial chemoembolization in patients with unresectable hepatocellular carcinoma: a systematic review and meta-analysis. Clin Res Hepatol Gastroenterol 2017;41(1):75–85.

58. Xie ZB, Wang XB, Peng YC, et al. Systematic review comparing the safety and efficacy of conventional and drug-eluting bead transarterial chemoembolization for inoperable hepatocellular carcinoma. Hepatol Res 2015;45(2):190–200.

59. Huang K, Zhou Q, Wang R, et al. Doxorubicin-eluting beads versus conventional transarterial chemoembolization for the treatment of hepatocellular carcinoma. J Gastroenterol Hepatol 2014;29(5):920–5.

60. Kawai S, Okamura J, Ogawa M, et al. Prospective and randomized clinical trial for the treatment of hepatocellular carcinoma–a comparison of lipiodol-transcatheter arterial embolization with and without adriamycin (first cooperative study). The Cooperative Study Group for Liver Cancer Treatment of Japan. Cancer Chemother Pharmacol 1992;31(Suppl):S1–6.

61. Chang JM, Tzeng WS, Pan HB, et al. Transcatheter arterial embolization with or without cisplatin treatment of hepatocellular carcinoma. A randomized controlled study. Cancer 1994;74(9):2449–53.

62. Brown KT, Do RK, Gonen M, et al. Randomized trial of hepatic artery embolization for hepatocellular carcinoma using doxorubicin-eluting microspheres compared with embolization with microspheres alone. J Clin Oncol 2016; 34(17):2046–53.

63. Malagari K, Pomoni M, Kelekis A, et al. Prospective randomized comparison of chemoembolization with doxorubicin-eluting beads and bland embolization with BeadBlock for hepatocellular carcinoma. Cardiovasc Intervent Radiol 2010; 33(3):541–51.

64. Chen QW, Ying HF, Gao S, et al. Radiofrequency ablation plus chemoembolization versus radiofrequency ablation alone for hepatocellular carcinoma: a systematic review and meta-analysis. Clin Res Hepatol Gastroenterol 2016;40(3): 309–14.

65. Ginsburg M, Zivin SP, Wroblewski K, et al. Comparison of combination therapies in the management of hepatocellular carcinoma: transarterial chemoembolization with radiofrequency ablation versus microwave ablation. J Vasc Interv Radiol 2015;26(3):330–41.

66. Kudo M, Arizumi T. Transarterial chemoembolization in combination with a molecular targeted agent: lessons learned from negative trials (post-TACE, BRISK-TA, SPACE, ORIENTAL, and TACE-2). Oncology 2017;93(Suppl 1): 127–34.

67. Kudo M, Ueshima K, Ikeda M, et al. Randomized, open label, multicenter, phase II trial comparing transarterial chemoembolization (TACE) plus sorafenib with TACE alone in patients with hepatocellular carcinoma (HCC): TACTICS trial. J Clin Oncol 2018;36(4_suppl):206.

68. Huo YR, Eslick GD. Transcatheter arterial chemoembolization plus radiotherapy compared with chemoembolization alone for hepatocellular carcinoma: a systematic review and meta-analysis. JAMA Oncol 2015;1(6):756–65.

69. Brown DB, Gould JE, Gervais DA, et al. Transcatheter therapy for hepatic malignancy: standardization of terminology and reporting criteria. J Vasc Interv Radiol 2009;20(7 Suppl):S425–34.

70. Sangro B, Bilbao JI, Boan J, et al. Radioembolization using 90Y-resin microspheres for patients with advanced hepatocellular carcinoma. Int J Radiat Oncol Biol Phys 2012;66(3):792–800.

71. Murthy R, Nunez R, Szklaruk J, et al. Yttrium-90 microsphere therapy for hepatic malignancy: devices, indications, technical considerations, and potential complications. Radiographics 2005;25(Suppl 1):S41–55.

72. Salem R, Lewandowski RJ, Mulcahy MF, et al. Radioembolization for hepatocellular carcinoma using yttrium-90 microspheres: a comprehensive report of long-term outcomes. Gastroenterology 2010;138(1):52–64.

73. Hilgard P, Hamami M, Fouly AE, et al. Radioembolization with yttrium-90 glass microspheres in hepatocellular carcinoma: European experience on safety and long-term survival. Hepatology 2010;52(5):1741–9.

74. Sangro B, Carpanese L, Cianni R, et al. Survival after yttrium-90 resin microsphere radioembolization of hepatocellular carcinoma across Barcelona clinic liver cancer stages: a European evaluation. Hepatology 2011;54(3):868–78.

75. Mazzaferro V, Sposito C, Bhoori S, et al. Yttrium-90 radioembolization for intermediate-advanced hepatocellular carcinoma: a phase 2 study. Hepatology 2013;57(5):1826–37.

76. Lance C, McLennan G, Obuchowski N, et al. Comparative analysis of the safety and efficacy of transcatheter arterial chemoembolization and yttrium-90 radioembolization in patients with unresectable hepatocellular carcinoma. J Vasc Interv Radiol 2011;22(12):1697–705.

77. Kooby DA, Egnatashvili V, Srinivasan S, et al. Comparison of yttrium-90 radioembolization and transcatheter arterial chemoembolization for the treatment of unresectable hepatocellular carcinoma. J Vasc Interv Radiol 2010;21(2):224–30.

78. Carr BI, Kondragunta V, Buch SC, et al. Therapeutic equivalence in survival for hepatic arterial chemoembolization and yttrium 90 microsphere treatments in unresectable hepatocellular carcinoma: a two-cohort study. Cancer 2010; 116(5):1305–14.

79. Salem R, Lewandowski RJ, Kulik L, et al. Radioembolization results in longer time-to-progression and reduced toxicity compared with chemoembolization in patients with hepatocellular carcinoma. Gastroenterology 2011;140(2): 497–507.e2.

80. Kolligs FT, Bilbao JI, Jakobs T, et al. Pilot randomized trial of selective internal radiation therapy vs. chemoembolization in unresectable hepatocellular carcinoma. Liver Int 2015;35(6):1715–21.

81. Salem R, Gordon AC, Mouli S, et al. Y90 radioembolization significantly prolongs time to progression compared with chemoembolization in patients with hepatocellular carcinoma. Gastroenterology 2016;151(6):1155–63.e2.

82. Lewandowski RJ, Kulik LM, Riaz A, et al. A comparative analysis of transarterial downstaging for hepatocellular carcinoma: chemoembolization versus radioembolization. Am J Transplant 2009;9(8):1920–8.

83. Vouche M, Lewandowski RJ, Atassi R, et al. Radiation lobectomy: time-dependent analysis of future liver remnant volume in unresectable liver cancer as a bridge to resection. J Hepatol 2013;59(5):1029–36.

84. Garlipp B, de Baere T, Damm R, et al. Left-liver hypertrophy after therapeutic right-liver radioembolization is substantial but less than after portal vein embolization. Hepatology 2014;59(5):1864–73.

85. Riaz A, Gates VL, Atassi B, et al. Radiation segmentectomy: a novel approach to increase safety and efficacy of radioembolization. Int J Radiat Oncol Biol Phys 2011;79(1):163–71.

86. Padia SA, Johnson GE, Horton KJ, et al. Segmental yttrium-90 radioembolization versus segmental chemoembolization for localized hepatocellular carcinoma: results of a single-center, retrospective, propensity score-matched study. J Vasc Interv Radiol 2017;28(6):777–85.e1.

87. Biederman DM, Titano JJ, Korff RA, et al. Radiation segmentectomy versus selective chemoembolization in the treatment of early-stage hepatocellular carcinoma. J Vasc Interv Radiol 2018;29(1):30–7.e2.

88. Lewandowski RJ, Gabr A, Abouchaleh N, et al. Radiation segmentectomy: potential curative therapy for early hepatocellular carcinoma. Radiology 2018; 287(3):1050–8.

89. Spreafico C, Sposito C, Vaiani M, et al. Development of a prognostic score to predict response to Yttrium-90 radioembolization for hepatocellular carcinoma with portal vein invasion. J Hepatol 2018;68(4):724–32.

90. Garin E, Lenoir L, Edeline J, et al. Boosted selective internal radiation therapy with 90Y-loaded glass microspheres (B-SIRT) for hepatocellular carcinoma patients: a new personalized promising concept. Eur J Nucl Med Mol Imaging 2013;40(7):1057–68.

91. Garin E, Rolland Y, Pracht M, et al. High impact of macroaggregated albumin-based tumour dose on response and overall survival in hepatocellular carcinoma patients treated with (90) Y-loaded glass microsphere radioembolization. Liver Int 2017;37(1):101–10.

92. Gari E. Major impact of personalized dosimetry using 90Y loaded glass microspheres SIRT in HCC: Final overall survival analysis of a multicenter randomized phase II study (DOSISPHERE-01). Journal of Clinical Oncology 38(4_suppl):516.

93. Li MD, Chu KF, DePietro A, et al. Same-day yttrium-90 radioembolization: feasibility with resin microspheres. J Vasc Interv Radiol 2019;30(3):314–9.

94. Finn RS, Merle P, Granito A, et al. Outcomes with sorafenib (SOR) followed by regorafenib (REG) or placebo (PBO) for hepatocellular carcinoma (HCC): results of the international, randomized phase 3 RESORCE trial. J Clin Oncol 2017;35(4_suppl):344.

95. Marrero JA, Kudo M, Venook AP, et al. Observational registry of sorafenib use in clinical practice across Child-Pugh subgroups: the GIDEON study. J Hepatol 2016;65(6):1140–7.

96. Kambhampati S, Bauer KE, Bracci PM, et al. Nivolumab in patients with advanced hepatocellular carcinoma and Child-Pugh class B cirrhosis: safety and clinical outcomes in a retrospective case series. Cancer 2019;125(18): 3234–41.

97. Kudo M, Matilla A, Santoro A, et al. Checkmate-040: nivolumab (NIVO) in patients (pts) with advanced hepatocellular carcinoma (aHCC) and Child-Pugh B (CPB) status. J Clin Oncol 2019;37(4_suppl):327.

98. Kudo M, Matsui O, Izumi N, et al. JSH consensus-based clinical practice guidelines for the management of hepatocellular carcinoma: 2014 update by the Liver Cancer Study Group of Japan. Liver Cancer 2014;3(3–4):458–68.

99. Peck-Radosavljevic M, Kudo M, Raoul J-L, et al. Outcomes of patients (pts) with hepatocellular carcinoma (HCC) treated with transarterial chemoembolization (TACE): global OPTIMIS final analysis. J Clin Oncol 2018;36(15_suppl):4018.

100. Arizumi T, Minami T, Chishina H, et al. Time to transcatheter arterial chemoembolization refractoriness in patients with hepatocellular carcinoma in Kinki criteria stages B1 and B2. Dig Dis 2017;35(6):589–97.

101. Ogasawara S, Chiba T, Ooka Y, et al. Efficacy of sorafenib in intermediate-stage hepatocellular carcinoma patients refractory to transarterial chemoembolization. Oncology 2014;87(6):330–41.

102. Arizumi T, Ueshima K, Minami T, et al. Effectiveness of sorafenib in patients with transcatheter arterial chemoembolization (TACE) refractory and intermediate-stage hepatocellular carcinoma. Liver Cancer 2015;4(4):253–62.

103. Kudo M, Ikeda M, Takayama T, et al. Safety and efficacy of sorafenib in Japanese patients with hepatocellular carcinoma in clinical practice: a subgroup analysis of GIDEON. J Gastroenterol 2016;51(12):1150–60.

104. Hiraoka A, Michitaka K, Kumada T, et al. Prediction of prognosis of intermediate-stage HCC patients: validation of the tumor marker score in a nationwide database in Japan. Liver Cancer 2019;8(5):403–11.

105. Kudo M. A new treatment option for intermediate-stage hepatocellular carcinoma with high tumor burden: initial lenvatinib therapy with subsequent selective TACE. Liver Cancer 2019;8(5):299–311.

106. Hiraoka A, Kumada T, Michitaka K, et al. Newly proposed ALBI grade and ALBI-T score as tools for assessment of hepatic function and prognosis in hepatocellular carcinoma patients. Liver Cancer 2019;8(5):312–25.

107. Kojiro M, Sugihara S, Kakizoe S, et al. Hepatocellular carcinoma with sarcomatous change: a special reference to the relationship with anticancer therapy. Cancer Chemother Pharmacol 1989;23(Suppl):S4–8.

108. Tsuchiya K, Kurosaki M, Kaneko S, et al. A nationwide multicenter study in patients with unresectable hepatocellular carcinoma treated with lenvatinib in real world practice in Japan. J Clin Oncol 2019;37(4_suppl):364.

109. Chapman WC, Garcia-Aroz S, Vachharajani N, et al. Liver transplantation for advanced hepatocellular carcinoma after downstaging without up-front stage restrictions. J Am Coll Surg 2017;224(4):610–21.

110. Yoon SM, Ryoo BY, Lee SJ, et al. Efficacy and safety of transarterial chemoembolization plus external beam radiotherapy vs sorafenib in hepatocellular carcinoma with macroscopic vascular invasion: a randomized clinical trial. JAMA Oncol 2018;4(5):661–9.

111. Llovet JM, Pavel M, Rimola J, et al. Pilot study of living donor liver transplantation for patients with hepatocellular carcinoma exceeding Milan Criteria (Barcelona Clinic Liver Cancer extended criteria). Liver Transpl 2018;24(3):369–79.

112. Hoffmann K, Ganten T, Gotthardtp D, et al. Impact of neo-adjuvant Sorafenib treatment on liver transplantation in HCC patients - a prospective, randomized, double-blind, phase III trial. BMC Cancer 2015;15:392.

113. Kudo M. Immuno-oncology in hepatocellular carcinoma: 2017 update. Oncology 2017;93(Suppl 1):147–59.

Role of External Beam Radiotherapy in Hepatocellular Carcinoma

Chien Peter Chen, MD, PhD

KEYWORDS

- Hepatocellular carcinoma • Radiotherapy • Radiation
- Stereotactic body radiotherapy • External beam radiotherapy
- Particle beam radiotherapy

KEY POINTS

- EBRT can provide comparable outcomes with similar safety profile as other loco-regional treatments for both resectable and unresectable HCC.
- For resectable HCC cases, EBRT can bridge patients to transplantation.
- In unresectable HCC patients, EBRT can provide high local control rates.
- EBRT can offer effective palliation in the metastatic HCC setting.
- Consideration of EBRT in the management of HCC should occur with a multidisciplinary treatment team.

INTRODUCTION

Liver cancer is the second leading cause of cancer death in men and sixth leading cause of cancer death in women.[1] The most common type of primary liver cancer globally is hepatocellular carcinoma (HCC) and causes include viral and nonviral etiologies, such as nonalcoholic fatty liver disease/nonalcoholic steatohepatitis and alcohol use.[2,3] Cases of HCC are expected to increase and effective treatments are imperative.

Patients with limited disease are eligible for liver transplantation. Due to limited availability of donor organs and strict criteria of liver transplantation, however, a significant proportion of HCC patients is not eligible for upfront curative treatments. Locoregional modalities with or without systemic therapies can help bridge patients to transplant. As for locally advanced and metastatic cases, radiotherapy and systemic therapies have improved and can offer effective palliation.[4] Systemic therapy options include molecular targeted agents.[5–11] Additionally, immune checkpoint modulators may have a role in HCC.[12–14]

Department of Radiation Oncology, Scripps Radiation Therapy Center, 10670 John Jay Hopkins Drive, San Diego, CA 92121, USA
E-mail address: chen.chienpong@scrippshealth.org

Clin Liver Dis 24 (2020) 701–717
https://doi.org/10.1016/j.cld.2020.07.006
1089-3261/20/© 2020 Elsevier Inc. All rights reserved.

liver.theclinics.com

As systemic therapies improve, local therapies have become more relevant. Local therapies for HCC include minimally invasive procedures, such as transarterial chemoembolization (TACE), radiofrequency ablation (RFA), microwave ablation, highly focused ultrasound, and irreversible electroporation.[15–17] For locally advanced cases, however, minimally invasive procedures can be limited by impaired portal-vein blood flow due to portal-vein thrombus, untreatable arteriovenous fistula, impaired renal function, bleeding diathesis, and tumor location (ie, protruding from the liver surface).[18–23]

Another local therapy, either alone or in combination with other locoregional and systemic therapies, is external beam radiotherapy (EBRT). Historically, EBRT had a limited role in treating the liver due to risk of radiation-induced liver disease (RILD). Classic RILD, which occurs within 4 months following radiotherapy, can present with fatigue, anicteric ascites, and hepatomegaly, with relatively normal liver function tests and normal bilirubin. Nonclassic RILD, which can occur within 3 months following radiotherapy, can present with jaundice and/or significant elevation of serum transaminases. Patients with underlying liver disease are at higher risk for nonclassic RILD.[24] Various technological advances have allowed for more precise and dose-escalated treatment regimens using radiotherapy. Given these developments, treatment guidelines for HCC have been updated. This review discusses the role of EBRT for HCC.

EXTERNAL BEAM RADIOTHERAPY TECHNIQUES

EBRT modalities include photon and particle beam radiation (**Table 1**). Photon-based EBRT involve x-rays whereas particle-based EBRT uses subatomic particles, such as protons, or heavier charged particles, such as carbon ions. Photon-based EBRT techniques include 2-dimensional radiotherapy (2DRT), 3-dimensional conformal radiotherapy (3DCRT), intensity-modulated radiotherapy (IMRT), and stereotactic body radiotherapy (SBRT). Particle-based EBRT techniques include 3DCRT and intensity-modulated proton therapy.

2DRT uses x-ray films to determine the appropriate positioning of radiation treatment fields via bony landmarks. Because no CT simulation is done, neither target volume nor critical organs at risk (OARs) are explicitly delineated. 2DRT allows for rapid treatment planning and treatment initiation. 2DRT is ideal for palliative situations.

Fig. 1 demonstrates the difference in dose distribution for the various EBRT techniques.

Although 2DRT planning does not employ CT-based planning, to better illustrate the dosimetric differences among the various EBRT approaches, a 2DRT plan is superimposed on a planning CT scan of an example HCC patient. The dose distribution of a 2DRT plan involves higher relative dose (yellow) deposition not only in the target lesion but also in a significant proportion of the liver.

In 3DCRT, the tumor target and critical OARs are delineated on a planning CT. Multiple x-ray treatment fields are used and arranged around the target to optimize coverage of the target while minimizing dose to critical OARs, such as the liver, kidneys, and spinal cord. Each of the x-ray treatment fields can be shaped by collimators to block out critical OARs. Each treatment field has uniform radiation intensity. The shape and radiation dose rate of each x-ray field typically are fixed. **Fig. 1** illustrates a more conformal dose distribution in the 3DCRT plan compared with the 2DRT plan. Additionally, less of the critical OARs receives high dose, which can reduce toxicity.

IMRT represents a more advanced form of 3DCRT. IMRT plans involve delineation of a target and critical OARs. Multiple x-ray fields are used and collimators are utilized

Table 1
Comparison of external beam radiotherapy techniques

Technique	Pros	Cons
2DRT	Ease of planning Least expensive	Difficult to spare liver and other nearby critical organs Palliative in intent
3DCRT	Conformal dose distribution Some critical organ sparing Inexpensive	Longer treatment regimen (multiple weeks of treatment)
IMRT	More conformal dose distribution than 2DRT/3DCRT Higher LC than 2DCRT/3DCRT Potentially more sparing of critical structures than 3DCRT	Complicated planning Can involve patient immobilization, tumor tracking, image guidance Longer treatment regimen (multiple weeks of treatment) More expensive technique than 2DRT/3DCRT
SBRT	High fractional dose that can lead to LC than 2DRT/3DCRT/IMRT Superior dose distribution and thus potential decreased liver toxicity Short treatment regimen (2–5 fractions)	Complicated planning Requires patient immobilization, tumor tracking, image guidance More expensive technique than 2DRT/3DCRT
Proton/heavy ion (particle)	High LC Decreased integral dose that may lead to decreased liver toxicity	More susceptible to tissue heterogeneity and range uncertainty Significant financial and spatial investment required for particle therapy program High cost for particle therapy treatment package (most expensive of all EBRT options) Longer treatment regimen (multiple weeks of treatment)

to shape each treatment field. IMRT, however, uses nonuniform radiation intensity by modulating the shape of the treatment fields and utilizes inverse planning.[25] IMRT thus can achieve even more conformal dosimetric plans, which translates into less volume of critical OARs receiving high dose than with 3DCRT plans, as shown in **Fig. 1**. Due to the complexity of generating IMRT plans, IMRT does require more time for treatment planning and quality assurance.

SBRT is characterized by careful delineation of target and critical OARs, tight target margins, and strict dose constraints for OARs. SBRT uses potentially ablative doses in short treatment regimens. SBRT plans deliver high fractional doses, such as 500 cGy to 1000 cGy, often over 2 to 5 fractions. In contrast, fractionated EBRT treatment modalities, including 2DRT, 3DCRT, and IMRT, deliver lower doses per daily fraction, where typical daily doses are in the 180-cGy to 300-cGy range, over 2 weeks to 6 weeks. **Fig. 1** shows the superior dose distribution of SBRT over other photon-based modalities. Additionally, given the high fractional dose, SBRT can offer ablative potential and thus offer high local tumor control.[26] Due to the tight target margins, however, careful patient immobilization, advanced tumor tracking, image guidance, and respiratory management are critical for accurate delivery of SBRT plans.[27–29]

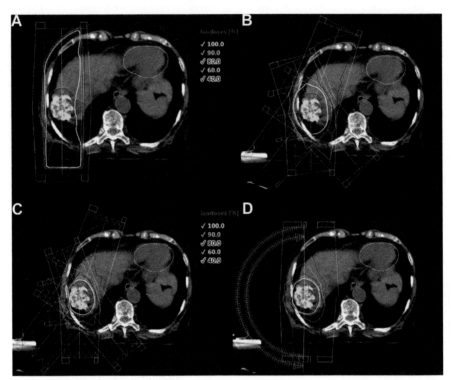

Fig. 1. Comparison of dose distribution for various EBRT techniques. Target is designated in red translucent color. Isodose lines represented by percent of total dose. (*A*). 2DRT (*B*). 3DCRT. (*C*) IMRT. (*D*) SBRT.

Similar to photon-based EBRT, charged particle therapy, such as proton beam therapy (PBT), can utilize 3-dimensional conformal and intensity-modulated approaches. Particle beam therapy, however, offers potential dosimetric advantages over some photon-based EBRT techniques. Charged particles have a finite range dependent on the initial charged particle energy. Particle EBRT uses simpler beam arrangements than photon EBRT. Particle EBRT thus can achieve decreased integral dose compared with photon EBRT. The effect of tissue heterogeneity and of range uncertainty, however, can negate or at least minimize the clinical advantages of particle-based radiotherapy. Additionally, particle EBRT requires significant financial and spatial investment, which have led to its limited availability and high cost.[30]

DOSE CONSTRAINTS

Regardless of the type of EBRT, whether photon based or particle based, dose constraints for the liver and nearby OARs must be respected. Early work on whole-liver radiation tolerance in patients treated for liver metastases was performed in the Radiation Therapy Oncology Group (RTOG) 76-09 and RTOG 84-05 trials. The whole liver could be treated safely to 2100 cGy in 7 daily fractions or 3000 cGy in 20 fractions delivered twice daily.[31,32] Partial-liver treatment, however, allowed for radiation dose escalation.[33] In 1991, Emami and coworkers[34] suggested baseline partial-liver tolerances. The whole-liver radiation dose associated with a 5% risk of RILD is 3000 cGy whereas a dose of 5000 cGy to one-third of the liver is associated with the same 5% risk.[34] Models for RILD were developed and demonstrated that doses as high as 7260 cGy were safe if delivered to less than a third of the liver. normal tissue complication probability modeling showed that a mean dose of 5660 cGy was associated with a complication rate of approximately 5%. Additionally, the liver radiation tolerance was lower with patients with HCC versus those with liver metastases.[35–38] These studies suggested that focal radiation techniques could offer local disease control with relatively low risk for RILD.

Current dose constraints limit liver mean dose to less than 2800 cGy to achieve less than 5% risk of RILD for fractionated EBRT regimens. For SBRT, the quantitative analysis of normal tissue effects in the clinic constraints suggest keeping at least 700 cm^3 of liver receiving less than 1500 cGy for a 3-fraction SBRT regimen to achieve less than 5% risk of RILD. The American Association of Physicists in Medicine (AAPM) Task Group 101 constraints indicate at least 700 cm^3 of liver should receive less than 2100 cGy for 5-fraction SBRT regimens and less than 1920 cGy for a 3-fraction SBRT regimens.[39,40]

Evaluation for RILD includes Child-Pugh score (increase by 2 or more) and appropriate laboratory markers assessment, such as elevation of alkaline phosphatase (more than twice the upper limit of normal), of transaminases (greater than 5 times the upper limit of normal), and of total bilirubin as well as decrease in albumin and prothrombin time. Patients who may be inappropriate for radiation treatment include patients with liver reserve less than 700 cm^3, with active RILD, or with active connective tissue disorders, such as inflammatory bowel disease.

CURRENT GUIDELINES ON ROLE OF EXTERNAL BEAM RADIOTHERAPY FOR HEPATOCELLULAR CARCINOMA

Despite improved understanding and reduction of RILD risk with EBRT, many current guidelines suggest a limited role for radiation. The European Association for the Study of the Liver, American Association for the Study of Liver Diseases, and Japan Society of Hepatology guidelines do not include EBRT as a routine treatment of HCC.[41–43] In contrast, the Asian Pacific Association for the Study of the Liver guidelines indicates SBRT and charged particle therapy as reasonable options for patients who have failed other local therapies and could be considered for symptomatic bony metastases.[44] The Korean Liver Cancer Association guidelines indicates EBRT as an option in multiple settings, including HCC patients with portal vein tumor thrombus (PVTT), HCC patients with incomplete response to TACE, and HCC patients with symptomatic metastases.[45] The most liberal indications of radiotherapy occur in the Chinese guidelines, which suggests EBRT in multiple settings including adjuvant therapy for select patients with close margins.[46]

The discrepancy of recommendations for the role of EBRT is due partly to the lack of inclusion of radiation oncologists in the committees that develop treatment guidelines. With more recent evidence highlighting the efficacy of radiotherapy in HCC, the updated National Comprehensive Cancer Network guidelines includes radiotherapy as a treatment modality for HCC patients as follows[47]:

- Potentially resectable/transplantable patients with Child-Pugh class A or class B without portal hypertension but with adequate liver reserve
- Tumors 2 cm to 5 cm in diameter or 2 to 3 tumors less than or equal to 3 cm each without macrovascular invasion and no extrahepatic disease that are ineligible for transplant
- Unresectable HCC patients who are ineligible for transplant

- Inoperable patients, due to performance status or comorbidity, having local disease only or local disease with minimal extrahepatic disease
- Symptom control in the metastatic setting

COMPARATIVE OUTCOMES AMONG EXTERNAL BEAM RADIOTHERAPY MODALITIES
Three-Dimensional Conformal Radiotherapy and Intensity-Modulated Radiotherapy

3DCRT and IMRT are the main modalities used for fractionated EBRT regimens to treat HCC.

In the unresectable setting, including cases of PVTT, 3DCRT or IMRT provides good local control (LC) either alone or in combination with TACE or concurrent systemic therapy. The objective relative response (RR) ranged from 43% to 74% and the overall survival (OS) rate at 2 years ranged from 23% to 69%. Grade 3 hepatotoxicity was observed in 0% to 13%. Combined treatments tended to increase severe toxicity.[48–56] **Fig. 2** presents an unresectable, locally advanced HCC case treated with a combination of IMRT and sorafenib. Additionally, EBRT can be effective for inferior vena cava invasion.[57] In the resectable setting, adjuvant radiation has been considered in resectable or transplantable cases due to recurrence rates as high as 30%.[58–61] Microvascular invasion reduces disease-free and OS.[62] Postoperative radiotherapy has shown benefit in select scenarios. In posthepatectomy patients with tumors close to major vessels and close margins (<1 cm), adjuvant radiation significantly improved 3-year OS compared with patients who had close margin but did not receive radiation (OS, 64% vs 52%, respectively). The results of the adjuvant radiation group were comparable to results in patients who received wide margins (>1 cm).[63] Similarly, HCC patients with microvascular invasion receiving adjuvant radiation had improved relapse-free survival (RFS) and OS compared with TACE or conservative

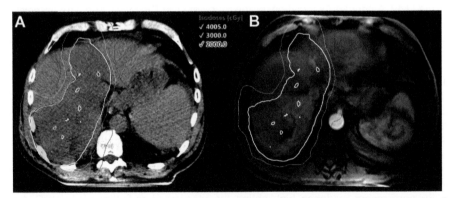

Fig. 2. IMRT for unresectable HCC. A 64-year-old man with a history of hepatis C–related cirrhosis developed an HCC with portal vein involvement and an AFP of 19,497 ng/mL. He was Child-Pugh A and was treated with IMRT (4005 cGy in 15 fractions) and sorafenib in 2014. (A) IMRT plan on planning CT. Isodose lines represented in absolute dose (cGy). (B) IMRT plan projected on pretreatment MRI abdomen. His AFP nadired to 6 and remained low with no recurrent disease until about 2 years post-treatment. His AFP increased to 19 and he underwent another course of IMRT in late 2016. He had control for another few years but ultimately progressed and went on nivolumab. He completed a third course of EBRT in 2019. Although, his HCC has since progressed locally, he remains alive as of August 2020.

management. The 3-year RFS rates for the adjuvant radiation, adjuvant TACE, and conservative management groups were 45%, 27%, and 11%, respectively. The 3-year OS rates for the adjuvant radiation, adjuvant TACE, and conservative management groups were 73%, 44%, and 28%, respectively.[64] Lastly, radiation can palliate symptoms from bone metastases and even lymph node metastases with response rates above 73%.[65–68]

Due to more conformal dose distribution and potential for dose escalation, IMRT can offer higher LC and OS rates than 3DCRT. LC rates (3-year 47% vs 28%, respectively) and OS rates (3-year 33% vs 14%, respectively) were in favor of IMRT. Toxicity rates were similar between 3DCRT and IMRT with RILD rates in 5% or less.[69,70] As for dose escalation, an IMRT simultaneous integrated boost approach achieved better objective RR (100% vs 62%, respectively; $P = .039$), LC at 2 years (86% vs 59%, respectively; $P = .119$), and OS at 2 years (83% vs 44%, respectively; $P = .037$) in the higher-dose group.[71] In cases of large liver tumors greater than 6 cm to 8 cm, however, IMRT can have higher integral dose whereby more volume of normal liver receives a low dose.[72,73] Depending on the size and location of the HCC target, careful selection of the appropriate EBRT modality is necessary.

Overall, fractionated 3DCRT or IMRT, either alone or when combined with other treatments, can offer good LC in unresectable HCC, including those with major vascular involvement, and can improve LC in select postoperative scenarios with microvascular invasion or close margins. In metastatic cases, EBRT can offer good palliation.

Stereotactic Body Radiotherapy

Recent studies have demonstrated the efficacy of SBRT in both resectable HCC and unresectable HCC.

Chen[4] recently presented a review of select SBRT studies and showed that SBRT offered 3 year LC as high as 90% and 3 year OS as high as 70%. SBRT also can serve as a bridge to transplantation in early-stage inoperable HCC, with doses ranging from 3000 cGy to 5400 cGy using a median fractional dose of 600 cGy. Post-SBRT liver explant revealed 27% complete response and 54% partial response.[74] **Fig. 3** presents a patient with cT1N0M0 HCC whereby SBRT served as a bridge to liver transplantation.

For HCC not eligible for transplant, SBRT provides high LC.[75,76] For small HCCs ineligible for resection or ablation, SBRT alone achieved a 2-year OS and PFS of 79% and 49%, respectively, compared with 80% and 43%, respective, with SBRT plus TACE.[77] **Fig. 4** presents a case of a patient ineligible for transplantation but had a small HCC who underwent definitive SBRT. Overall, SBRT alone or in combination with other treatments can offer high control rates for both resectable and unresectable HCC cases.

Particle External Beam Radiotherapy

Most particle-based EBRT experience for HCC has been with PBT. A large retrospective series of HCCs treated with hypofractionated regimens demonstrated 5-year LC of 87% with 5-year OS of 23%.[78] Other recent studies, including a recent review of PBT for HCC, reported 3-year LC 70% to 88% and a 3-year OS ranging from 45% to 65%.[79–81] As for heavy charged particles, such as carbon ions, they can offer higher radiobiological effectiveness and linear energy transfer than conventional x-rays and even protons. Carbon ion therapy for HCC can provide 5-year LC rates of 81% to 96%, with late grade 3 toxicity in 3% to 4% range.[82,83] A recent review of charged particle therapy reported actuarial LC rages ranging from 71% to 95% at 3 years and OS

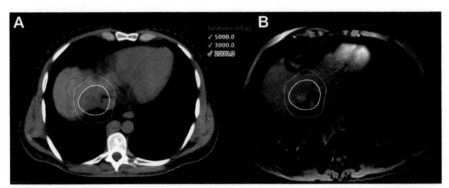

Fig. 3. SBRT as bridge to transplantation. A35-year-old man with a history of Budd-Chiari–related cirrhosis who developed a cT1N0M0 HCC next to the right liver dome. AFP was 1872. He underwent TACE in 7/2018 but subsequent imaging and post-TACE AFP of 1613 indicated residual disease. He completed a course of SBRT involving 5000 cGy in 5 fractions. (A) SBRT plan on planning CT. Isodose lines represented in absolute dose (cGy). (B) SBRT plan projected on pretreatment MRI abdomen. The patient's AFP nadired to 2.8 in June, 2019, and he underwent transplant on June 26, 2019. Post-transplant pathology showed 100% necrosis with complete response.

at 5 years ranging from 25% to 42%. Late grade 3 or higher adverse events occurred in only 2% of patients.[84] A meta-analysis comparing charged particles and SBRT, however, showed that comparable outcomes with no advantage in survival or LC with particle therapy.[85] Despite the similar outcomes, given the significant cost associated with construction and operations of particle beam facilities, particle EBRT for HCC may be appropriate in select cases, such as previously irradiated patients.

COMPARATIVE OUTCOMES OF EXTERNAL BEAM RADIOTHERAPY AND OTHER LOCOREGIONAL TREATMENTS

EBRT provides at least equivalent outcomes and safety profiles as other locoregional treatments for HCC (**Table 2**).[4] As a bridging modality to transplantation, SBRT, TACE,

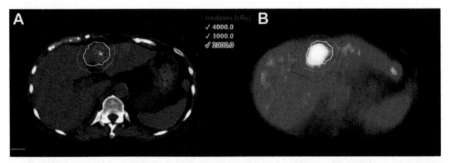

Fig. 4. SBRT for HCC ineligible for transplantation. A 74-year-old woman with NASH cirrhosis developed a left liver lobe HCC with AFP of 736. She completed TACE followed by SBRT (4000 cGy in 5 fractions) in March, 2016. (A) SBRT plan on planning CT. Isodose lines represented in absolute dose (cGy). (B) SBRT plan projected on pretreatment PET, which demonstrated an FDG (Fluorodeoxyglucose [^{18}F]) avid HCC. The patient's AFP normalized by 6 months post-treatment and has remained in the normal range.

Table 2
Select studies comparing stereotactic body radiotherapy to other locoregional treatments for hepatocellular carcinoma

Study	n	Stage	Modalities Compared	Stereotactic Body Radiotherapy Details	Outcomes	Toxicities (Grade 3 +)
Sapir et al,[105] 2018	209	NR	SBRT vs TACE	Median BED, 100 Gy	SBRT: 2-y LC, 91%; 2-y OS, 55% TACE: 2-y LC, 23%; 2-y OS, 35%	SBRT, 8%, vs TACE, 13% ($P = .05$)
Su et al,[90] 2017	117	BCLC A, 93% BCLC B, 7%	SBRT vs resection	42–48 Gy in 3–5 fractions	SBRT: 5-y OS, 70%; 5-y PFS, 41% Resection: 5-y OS, 64%; 5-y PFS, 40%	SBRT, 3% (nausea, weight loss); resection, 25% (hepatic pain, hepatic hemorrhage, weight loss)
Wahl et al,[87] 2016	224	Mostly TNM stage I/II	SBRT vs RFA	Median BED, 100 Gy	SBRT: 2-y FFLP, 84%; 2-y OS, 46% RFA: 2-y FFLP, 80%; 2-y OS, 53%	SBRT, 5% RFA, 11%
Mohamed et al,[106] 2016	60	IM, 78% OM, 22%	SBRT vs TACE vs RFA vs Y90 as bridge to transplant	Median, 50 Gy (range 45–60 Gy); Y90, average dose, 109 Gy	SBRT: PD, 4%; NN, 14% TACE: PD, 5.5%; NN, 4% RFA: PD, 0%; NN, 20% Y90: PD, 11%; NN, 0%	SBRT, 0% TACE, 11% RFA, 22% Y90, 0%

Abbreviations: BED, biological equivalent dose; BCLC, Barcelona clinic liver cancer; CP, Child-Pugh; CR, complete response; IM, inside Milan; NN, no necrosis on pathologic response; NR, not reported; OM, outside Milan; PD, progressive disease; PFS, progression-free survival; PR, partial response; SD, stable disease; Y90, radioembolization.

and RFA had comparable outcomes for 5-year actuarial survival.[86] For inoperable HCC cases treated with either SBRT to RFA, SBRT provided higher 2-year freedom from local progression (FFLP) (97% vs 84%, respectively) despite the SBRT group having more patients with unfavorable factors, such as lower pretreatment Child-Pugh scores, higher pretreatment α-fetoprotein (AFP) levels, and greater number of prior liver-directed treatments. Larger tumor size was a predictor for FFLP for RFA but not with SBRT. Acute grade 3 or higher complication rate was lower for SBRT (5% vs 11%, respectively). Two-year OS was comparable (46% vs 53%, respectively).[87] Similarly, the LC rate in HCC patients receiving TACE versus SBRT was comparable for LC, OS, and 1-year mortality.[88] When EBRT is combined with other locoregional treatments, higher OS can be achieved. A meta-analysis of 25 trials demonstrated that TACE plus EBRT had a 5-year survival OR of 3.98 compared with TACE alone. There was increased risk for gastroduodenal ulcers, however, in the combined modality, with an OR of 12.8.[89] Even in resectable cases, EBRT can offer favorable outcomes as resection. Su and colleagues[90] compared SBRT versus resection, and 5-year OS and PFS were virtually identical.

Selective internal radiation therapy (SIRT) has been useful in treating large lesions and tumors with vascular invasion.[91] Adverse events, however, including radiation pneumonitis, pulmonary fibrosis due to hepatopulmonary shunts, postradioembolization syndrome, and radioembolization-induced liver disease, have been observed.[92,93] In patients with PVTT, the pooled response rates for SIRT were 33% versus 51% for 3DCRT and 71% for SBRT. The pooled 1-year OS rates also was higher for EBRT modalities.[94] In another recent study comparing SIRT to EBRT involving unresectable HCC, there was no difference in OS or disease-specific survival.[95] Hence, proper patient selection is paramount for SIRT compared with EBRT approaches.

SUMMARY

With advancements in technology, including improved image guidance and dose escalation with partial-liver treatments, high LC rates with relatively low toxicity have been achieved with various EBRT modalities. As systemic therapies improve, locoregional therapies, such as EBRT, will become more relevant. Multiple clinical trials utilizing EBRT alone or in combination with other treatment modalities, which include systemic or local therapies, are under way.[96]

In regard to the future role of EBRT in HCC management, accurate tumor localization and visualization techniques may allow for further dose escalation and better outcomes. Magnetic resonance (MR)-based strategies, such as gadolinium ethoxybenzyl diethylenetriaminepentaacetic acid (Gd-EOB-DTPA)-enhanced MRIs, can offer more precise EBRT targeting and assessment of treatment accuracy.[97] MR linear accelerators (MR-linacs), which couple an magnetic resonance imaging (MRI) scanner and linear accelerator, can track and visualize tumors in real time. Because MRIs can better delineate HCCs compared with planning CT-based images, MR-linacs, with real-time tracking, can allow for tighter tumor margins, lower OAR doses, and dose escalation. In a recent multi-institutional study, MR-guided liver SBRT was performed using a median delivered dose of 5000 cGy in 5 fractions. With a median follow-up of 21.2 months, the freedom from local progression was 100% for HCC. No grade 4 or greater gastrointestinal toxicities were observed.[98–100] SBRT, especially MR-based SBRT, may help expand the role of radiotherapy in HCC treatment.

Neoadjuvant therapy has been used to downstage disease and to evaluate treatment response prior to resection for other solid malignancies. For HCC, transarterial radioembolization, and TACE, systemic therapy have been suggested as possible neoadjuvant approaches.[101] In a recent randomized, multicenter study involving patients with resectable HCC and PVTT, neoadjuvant radiotherapy involving 3DCRT of 1800 cGy in 6 fractions resulted in a significantly improved 2-year OS of 27% versus 9% in hepatectomy alone.[102] As for the safety of preoperative EBRT, Hasan and colleagues[103] showed that preoperative EBRT (median of 4000 cGy in 5 fractions) resulted in 39% complete response with no increase in postoperative mortality or length of stay after transplant. Neoadjuvant EBRT presents another potential indication for EBRT in the management of HCC.

Due to the increased evidence of efficacy and safety of EBRT for HCC, treatment algorithms have started to incorporate EBRT.[47,104–106] There remain many guidelines that continue to ignore EBRT as a treatment modality of HCC. Given the variability of recommendations from different guidelines, a multidisciplinary team involving hepatology, surgical oncology, medical oncology, and radiation oncology ideally should convene to make the appropriate treatment recommendations for each HCC patient.

ACKNOWLEDGMENTS

The author would like to thank colleagues, Dr Catherine Frenette and Richard Seier.

DISCLOSURE

The authors have nothing to disclose.

REFERENCES

1. Bray F, Ferlay J, Soerjomataram I, et al. Global cancer statistics 2018: GLOBOCAN estimates of incidence and mortality worldwide for 36 cancers in 185 countries. CA Cancer J Clin 2018;68(6):394–424.

2. Ghouri YA, Mian I, Rowe JH. Review of hepatocellular carcinoma: epidemiology, etiology, and carcinogenesis. J Carcinog 2017;16:1.

3. Akinyemiju T, Abera S, Ahmed M, et al. The burden of primary liver cancer and underlying etiologies from 1990 to 2015 at the global, regional, and National level: results from the global burden of disease study 2015. JAMA Oncol 2017;3(12):1683–91.

4. Chen CP. Role of radiotherapy in the treatment of hepatocellular carcinoma. J Clin Transl Hepatol 2019;7(2):183–90.

5. Cheng AL, Kang YK, Chen Z, et al. Efficacy and safety of sorafenib in patients in the Asia-Pacific region with advanced hepatocellular carcinoma: a phase III randomised, double-blind, placebo-controlled trial. Lancet Oncol 2009;10(1): 25–34.

6. Llovet JM, Ricci S, Mazzaferro V, et al. Sorafenib in advanced hepatocellular carcinoma. N Engl J Med 2008;359(4):378–90.

7. Kudo M. Systemic therapy for hepatocellular carcinoma: latest advances. Cancers (Basel) 2018;10(11):412.

8. Kudo M, Finn RS, Qin S, et al. Lenvatinib versus sorafenib in first-line treatment of patients with unresectable hepatocellular carcinoma: a randomised phase 3 noninferiority trial. Lancet 2018;391(10126):1163–73.

9. Abou-Alfa GK, Meyer T, Cheng AL, et al. Cabozantinib in patients with advanced and progressing hepatocellular carcinoma. N Engl J Med 2018; 379(1):54–63.

10. Bruix J, Qin S, Merle P, et al. Regorafenib for patients with hepatocellular carcinoma who progressed on sorafenib treatment (RESORCE): a randomised, double-blind, placebo-controlled, phase 3 trial. Lancet 2017;389(10064):56–66.

11. Zhu AX, Kang YK, Yen CJ, et al. REACH-2: a randomized, double-blind, placebocontrolled phase 3 study of ramucirumab versus placebo as second-line treatment in patients with advanced hepatocellular carcinoma (HCC) and elevated baseline alphafetoprotein (AFP) following first-line sorafenib. J Clin Oncol 2018;36:4003.

12. Zhu AX, Finn RS, Edeline J, et al. Pembrolizumab in patients with advanced hepatocellular carcinoma previously treated with sorafenib (KEYNOTE-224): a nonrandomised, open-label phase 2 trial. Lancet Oncol 2018;19(7):940–52.

13. El-Khoueiry AB, Sangro B, Yau T, et al. Nivolumab in patients with advanced hepatocellular carcinoma (CheckMate 040): an open-label, non-comparative, phase ½ dose escalation and expansion trial. Lancet 2017;389(10088): 2492–502.

14. Cheng AL, Qin S, Ikeda M, et al. LBA3 – Imbrave150: efficacy and safety results from a ph III study evaluating atezolizumab (atezo) + bevacizumab (bev) vs sorafenib (Sor) as first treatment (tx) for patients (pts) with unresectable hepatocellular carcinoma (HCC). Ann Oncol 2019;30(Supplement 9):ix186–7.

15. Daher S, Massarwa M, Benson AA, et al. Current and future treatment of hepatocellular carcinoma: an updated comprehensive review. J Clin Transl Hepatol 2018;6(1):69–78.

16. Maluccio MA, Covey AM, Porat LB, et al. Transcatheter arterial embolization with only particles for the treatment of unresectable hepatocellular carcinoma. J Vasc Interv Radiol 2008;19(6):862–9.

17. Kudo M, Ueshima K, Torimura T, et al. Randomized, open label, multicenter, phase II trial of transcatheter arterial chemoembolization (TACE) in combination with sorafenib as compared with TACE alone in patients with hepatocellular carcinoma: TACTICS trial. J Clin Oncol 2018;36:206.

18. Raoul JL, Sangro B, Forner A, et al. Evolving strategies for the management of intermediate-stage hepatocellular carcinoma: available evidence and expert opinion on the use of transarterial chemoembolization. Cancer Treat Rev 2011;37(3):212–20.

19. Forner A, Gilabert M, Bruix J, et al. Treatment of intermediate-stage hepatocellular carcinoma. Nat Rev Clin Oncol 2014;11(9):525–35.

20. Benoist S, Nordlinger B. Radiofrequency ablation in liver tumours. Ann Oncol 2004;15(Suppl 4):iv313–7.

21. de Baere T, Bessoud B, Dromain C, et al. Percutaneous radiofrequency ablation of hepatic tumors during temporary venous occlusion. AJR Am J Roentgenol 2002;178(1):53–9.

22. Lau WY, Leung TW, Yu SC, et al. Percutaneous local ablative therapy for hepatocellular carcinoma: a review and look into the future. Ann Surg 2003;237(2): 171–9.

23. Liang P, Yu J, Lu MD, et al. Practice guidelines for ultrasound-guided percutaneous microwave ablation for hepatic malignancy. World J Gastroenterol 2013; 19(33):5430–8.

24. Guha C, Kavanagh BD. Hepatic radiation toxicity: avoidance and amelioration. Semin Radiat Oncol 2011;21(4):256–63.

25. Intensity Modulated Radiation Therapy Collaborative Working Group. Intensity-modulated radiotherapy: current status and issues of interest. Int J Radiat Oncol Biol Phys 2001;51(4):880–914.

26. Fuss M, Thomas CR Jr. Stereotactic body radiation therapy: an ablative treatment option for primary and secondary liver tumors. Ann Surg Oncol 2004; 11(2):130–8.

27. Guckenberger M, Sweeney RA, Wilbert J, et al. Image-guided radiotherapy for liver cancer using respiratory-correlated computed tomography and cone-beam computed tomography. Int J Radiat Oncol Biol Phys 2008;71(1):297–304.

28. Kubo HD, Hill BC. Respiration gated radiotherapy treatment: a technical study. Phys Med Biol 1996;41(1):83–91.

29. Shimohigashi Y, Toya R, Saito T, et al. Tumor motion changes in stereotactic body radiotherapy for liver tumors: an evaluation based on four-dimensional cone-beam computed tomography and fiducial markers. Radiat Oncol 2017; 12(1):61.

30. Mitin T, Zeitman AL. Promises and pitfalls of heavy-particle therapy. J Clin Oncol 2014;32(26):2855–63.

31. Russell AH, Clyde C, Wasserman TH, et al. Accelerated hyperfractionated hepatic irradiation in the management of patients with liver metastases: results of the RTOG dose escalating protocol. Int J Radiat Oncol Biol Phys 1993; 27(1):117–23.

32. Borgelt BB, Gelber R, Brady LW, et al. The palliation of hepatic metastases: results of the Radiation Therapy Oncology Group pilot study. Int J Radiat Oncol Biol Phys 1981;7(5):587–91.

33. Austin-Seymour MM, Chen GT, Castro JR, et al. Dose volume histogram analysis of liver radiation tolerance. Int J Radiat Oncol Biol Phys 1986;12(1):31–5.

34. Emami B, Lyman J, Brown A, et al. Tolerance of normal tissue to therapeutic irradiation. Int J Radiat Oncol Biol Phys 1991;21(1):109–22.

35. Dawson LA, Ten Haken RK. Partial volume tolerance of the liver to radiation. Semin Radiat Oncol 2005;15(4):279–83.

36. Dawson LA, Normolle D, Balter JM, et al. Analysis of radiation-induced liver disease using the Lyman NTCP model. Int J Radiat Oncol Biol Phys 2002;53(4): 810–21.

37. Robertson JM, Lawrence TS, Walker S, et al. The treatment of colorectal liver metastases with conformal radiation therapy and regional chemotherapy. Int J Radiat Oncol Biol Phys 1995;32(2):445–50.

38. McGinn CJ, Ten Haken RK, Ensminger WD, et al. Treatment of intrahepatic cancers with radiation doses based on a normal tissue complication probability model. J Clin Oncol 1998;16(6):2246–52.

39. Pan CC, Kavanagh BD, Dawson LA, et al. Radiation associated liver injury. Int J Radiat Oncol Biol Phys 2010;76(3):S94–100.

40. Benedict SH, Yenice KM, Followill D, et al. Stereotactic body radiation therapy: the report of AAPM Task Group 101. Med Phys 2010;37(8):4078–101.

41. EASL Clinical Practice Guidelines: Management of hepatocellular carcinoma. J Hepatol 2018;69:182–236.

42. Heimbach JK, Kulik LM, Finn RS, et al. AASLD guidelines for the treatment of hepatocellular carcinoma. Hepatology 2018;67(1):358–80.

43. Kudo M, Matsui O, Izumi N, et al. JSH Consensus-based clinical practice guidelines for the management of hepatocellular carcinoma: 2014 update by the liver cancer study group of Japan. Liver Cancer 2014;3(3–4):458–68.

44. Omata M, Cheng AL, Kokudo N, et al. Asia-Pacific clinical practice guidelines on the management of hepatocellular carcinoma: a 2017 update. Hepatol Int 2017;11(4):317–70.

45. Korean Liver Cancer Study Group (KLCSG);National Cancer Center Korea (NCC). 2014 Korean liver cancer study group-National cancer Center Korea practice guideline for the management of hepatocellular carcinoma. Korean J Radiol 2015;16(3):465–522.

46. Zhou J, Sun HC, Wang Z, et al. Guidelines for Diagnosis and treatment of primary liver cancer in China (2017 edition). Liver Cancer 2018;7(3):235–60.

47. National Comprehensive Cancer Network. Hepatobiliary cancers (Version 4.2019). Available at: https://www.nccn.org/professionals/physician_gls/pdf/hepatobiliary.pdf. Accessed February 11,2020.

48. Kang MK, Kim MS, Kim SK, et al. High-dose radiotherapy with intensity-modulatedradiation therapy for advanced hepatocellular carcinoma. Tumori 2011;97(6):724–31.

49. Zhang T, Zhao YT, Wang Z, et al. Efficacy and safety of intensity-modulated radiotherapy following transarterial chemoembolization in patients with unresectable hepatocellular carcinoma. Medicine (Baltimore) 2016;95(21):e3789.

50. McIntosh A, Hagspiel KD, Al-Osaimi AM, et al. Accelerated treatment using intensity-modulated radiation therapy plus concurrent capecitabine for unresectable hepatocellular carcinoma. Cancer 2009;115(21):5117–25.

51. Chi KH, Liao CS, Chang CC, et al. Angiogenic blockade and radiotherapy in hepatocellular carcinoma. Int J Radiat Oncol Biol Phys 2010;78(1):188–93.

52. Kong M, Hong SE, Choi WS, et al. Treatment outcomes of helical intensity modulated radiotherapy for unresectable hepatocellular carcinoma. Gut Liver 2013; 7(3):343–51.

53. Kim JY, Yoo EJ, Jang JW, et al. Hypofractionated radiotheapy using helical tomotherapy for advanced hepatocellular carcinoma with portal vein tumor thrombosis. Radiat Oncol 2013;8:15.

54. Huang CM, Huang MY, Tang JY, et al. Feasibility and efficacy of helical tomotherapy in cirrhotic patients with unresectable hepatocellular carcinoma. World J Surg Oncol 2016;13:201.

55. Wang PM, Hsu WC, Chung NN, et al. Radiotherapy with volumetric modulated arc therapy for hepatocellular carcinoma patients ineligible for surgery or ablative treatments. Strahlenther Onkol 2013;189(4):301–7.

56. Chen SW, Lin LC, Kuo YC, et al. Phase 2 study of combined sorafenib and radiation therapy in patients with advanced hepatocellular carcinoma. Int J Radiat Oncol Biol Phys 2014;88(5):1041–7.

57. Rim CH, Kim CY, Yang DS, et al. External beam radiation therapy to hepatocellular carcinoma involving inferior vena cava and/or right atrium: a metaanalysis and systemic review. Radiother Oncol 2018;129(1):123–9.

58. Lai EC, Fan ST, Lo CM, et al. Hepatic resection for hepatocellular carcinoma. An audit of 343 patients. Ann Surg 1995;221(3):291–8.

59. Schwarz RE, Smith DD. Trends in local therapy for hepatocellular carcinoma and survival outcomes in the US population. Am J Surg 2008;195(6):829–36.

60. Liang W, Wu L, Ling X, et al. Living donor liver transplantation versus deceased donor liver transplantation for hepatocellular carcinoma: a meta-analysis. Liver Transpl 2012;18(10):1226–36.

61. Grant RC, Sandhu L, Dixon PR, et al. Living vs. deceased donor liver transplantation for hepatocellular carcinoma: a systematic review and meta-analysis. Clin Transpl 2013;27(1):140–7.

62. Rodriguez-Peralvarez M, Luong TV, Andreana L, et al. A systematic review of microvascular invasion in hepatocellular carcinoma: diagnostic and prognostic variability. Ann Surg Oncol 2013;20(1):325–39.

63. Wang WH, Wang Z, Wu JX, et al. Survival benefit with IMRT following narrow margin hepatectomy in patients with hepatocellular carcinoma close to major vessels. Liver Int 2015;35(12):2603–10.

64. Wang L, Wang W, Yao X, et al. Postoperative adjuvant radiotherapy is associated with improved survival in hepatocellular carcinoma with microvascular invasion. Oncotarget 2017;8(45):79971–81.

65. He J, Zeng ZC, Tang ZY, et al. Clinical features and prognostic factors in patients with bone metastases from hepatocellular carcinoma receiving external beam radiotherapy. Cancer 2009;115(12):2710–20.

66. Hayashi S, Tanaka H, Hoshi H. Palliative external-beam radiotherapy for bone metastases from hepatocellular carcinoma. World J Hepatol 2014;6(12):923–9.

67. Bhatia R, Ravulapati S, Befeler A, et al. Hepatocellular carcinoma with bone metastases: incidence, prognostic significance, and management-Single-Center experience. J Gastrointest Cancer 2017;48(4):321–5.

68. Rim CH, Kim CY, Yang DS, et al. The role of external beam radiotherapy for hepatocellular carcinoma patients with lymph node metastasis: a meta-analysis of observational studies. Cancer Manag Res 2018;10:3305–15.

69. Hou JZ, Zeng ZC, Wang BL, et al. High dose radiotherapy with image-guided hypo-IMRT for hepatocellular carcinoma with portal vein and/or inferior vena cava tumor thrombi is more feasible and efficacious than conventional 3D-CRT. Jpn J Clin Oncol 2016;46(4):357–62.

70. Yoon HI, Lee IJ, Han KH, et al. Improved oncologic outcomes with image guided intensity-modulated radiation therapy using helical tomotherapy in locally advanced hepatocellular carcinoma. J Cancer Res Clin Oncol 2014;140(9):1595–605.

71. Kim TH, Park JW, Kim YJ, et al. Simultaneous integrated boost-intensity modulated radiation therapy for inoperable hepatocellular carcinoma. Strahlenther Onkol 2014;190(10):882–90.

72. Bae SH, Jang WI, Park HC. Intensity-modulated radiotherapy for hepatocellular carcinoma: dosimetric and clinical results. Oncotarget 2017;8(35):59965–76.

73. Chen D, Wang R, Meng X, et al. A comparison of liver protection among 3-D conformal radiotherapy, intensity-modulated radiotherapy and RapidArc for hepatocellular carcinoma. Radiat Oncol 2014;9:48.

74. Moore A, Cohen-Naftaly M, Tobar A, et al. Stereotactic body radiation therapy (SBRT) for definitive treatment and as a bridge to liver transplantation in early stage inoperable Hepatocellular carcinoma. Radiat Oncol 2017;12(1):163.

75. Qiu H, Moravan MJ, Milano MT, et al. SBRT for hepatocellular carcinoma: 8-year experience from a regional transplant Center. J Gastrointest Cancer 2018;49(4):463–9.

76. Gerum S, Heinz C, Belka C, et al. Stereotactic body radiation therapy (SBRT) in patients with hepatocellular carcinoma and oligometastatic liver disease. Radiat Oncol 2018;13(1):100.

77. Kimura T, Aikata H, Doi Y, et al. Comparison of stereotactic body radiation therapy combined with or without transcatheter arterial chemoembolization for patients with small hepatocellular carcinoma ineligible for resection or ablation therapies. Technol Cancer Res Treat 2018;17. 1533033818783450.

78. Chiba T, Tokuuye K, Matsuzaki Y, et al. Proton beam therapy for hepatocellular carcinoma: a retrospective review of 162 patients. Clin Cancer Res 2005;11(10):3799–805.

79. Sugahara S, Nakayama H, Fukuda K, et al. Proton-beam therapy for hepatocellular carcinoma associated with portal vein tumor thrombosis. Strahlenther Onkol 2009;185(12):782–8.
80. Kawashima M, Furuse J, Nishio T, et al. Phase II study of radiotherapy employing proton beam for hepatocellular carcinoma. J Clin Oncol 2005;23(9): 1839–46.
81. Yoo GS, Yu JI, Park HC. Proton therapy for hepatocellular carcinoma: current knowledges and future perspectives. World J Gastroenterol 2018;24(28): 3090–100.
82. Kato H, Tsujii H, Miyamoto T, et al. Results of the first prospective study of carbon ion radiotherapy for hepatocellular carcinoma with liver cirrhosis. Int J Radiat Oncol Biol Phys 2004;59(5):1468–76.
83. Komatsu S, Fukumoto T, Demizu Y, et al. Clinical results and risk factors of proton and carbon ion therapy for hepatocellular carcinoma. Cancer 2011;117(21): 4890–904.
84. Igaki H, Mizumoto M, Okumura T, et al. A systematic review of publications on charged particle therapy for hepatocellular carcinoma. Int J Clin Oncol 2018; 23(3):423–33.
85. Qi WX, Fu S, Zhang Q, et al. Charged particle therapy versus photon therapy for patients with hepatocellular carcinoma: a systematic review and meta-analysis. Radiother Oncol 2015;114(3):289–95.
86. Sapisochin G, Barry A, Doherty M, et al. Stereotactic body radiotherapy vs. TACE or RFA as a bridge to transplant in patients with hepatocellular carcinoma. An intention-to treat analysis. J Hepatol 2017;67(1):92–9.
87. Wahl DR, Stenmark MH, Tao Y, et al. Outcomes after stereotactic body radiotherapy or radiofrequency ablation for hepatocellular carcinoma. J Clin Oncol 2016;34(5):452–9.
88. Bettinger D, Gkika E, Schultheiss M, et al. Comparison of local tumor control in patients with HCC treated with SBRT or TACE: a propensity score analysis. BMC Cancer 2018;18(1):807.
89. Huo YR, Eslick GD. Transcatheter arterial chemoembolization plus radiotherapy compared with chemoembolization alone for hepatocellular carcinoma: a systematic review and meta-analysis. JAMA Oncol 2016;1(6):756–65.
90. Su TS, Liang P, Liang J, et al. Long-term survival analysis of stereotactic ablative radiotherapy versus liver resection for small hepatocellular carcinoma. Int J Radiat Oncol Biol Phys 2017;98:639–46.
91. Wang EA, Broadwell SR, Bellavia RJ, et al. Selective internal radiation therapy with SIR-Spheres in hepatocellular carcinoma and cholangiocarcinoma. J Gastrointest Oncol 2017;8(2):266–78.
92. Riaz A, Lewandowski RJ, Kulik LM, et al. Complications following radioembolization with yttrium-90 microspheres: a comprehensive literature review. J Vasc Interv Radiol 2009;20(9):1121–30 [quiz: 1131].
93. Wright CL, Werner JD, Tran JM, et al. Radiation pneumonitis following yttrium-90 radioembolization: case report and literature review. J Vasc Interv Radiol 2012; 23(5):669–74.
94. Rim CH, Kim CY, Yang DS, et al. Comparison of radiation therapy modalities for hepatocellular carcinoma with portal vein thrombosis: a meta-analysis and systematic review. Radiother Oncol 2018;129(1):112–22.
95. Oladeru OT, Miccio JA, Yang J, et al. Conformal external beam radiation or selective internal radiation therapy-a comparison of treatment outcomes for hepatocellular carcinoma. J Gastrointest Oncol 2016;7(3):433–40.

96. Rim CH, Yoon WS. Leaflet manual of external beam radiation therapy for hepatocellular carcinoma: a review of the indications, evidences, and clinical trials. Onco Targets Ther 2018;11:2865–74.

97. Jung J, Kim H, Yoon SM, et al. Targeting accuracy of image-guided stereotactic body radiation therapy for hepatocellular carcinoma in real-life clinical practice: in vivo assessment using hepatic Parenchymal changes on Gd-EOB-DTPA-Enhanced magnetic resonance images. Int J Radiat Oncol Biol Phys 2018; 102(4):867–74.

98. Rosenberg SA, Henke LE, Shaverdian N, et al. A multi-institutional experience of MR-Guided liver stereotactic body radiation therapy. Adv Radiat Oncol 2018; 4(1):142–9.

99. Al-Ward S, Wronski M, Ahmad SB, et al. The radiobiological impact of motion tracking of liver, pancreas and kidney SBRT tumors in a MR-linac. Phys Med Biol 2018;63(21):215022.

100. Fast M, van de Schoot A, van de Lindt T, et al. Tumor trailing for liver SBRT on the MR-Linac. Int J Radiat Oncol Biol Phys 2019;103(2):468–78.

101. Akateh C, Black SM, Conteh L, et al. Neoadjuvant and adjuvant treatment strategies for hepatocellular carcinoma. World J Gastroenterol 2019;25(28): 3704–21.

102. Wei X, Jiang Y, Zhang X, et al. Neoadjuvant three-dimensional conformal radiotherapy for resectable hepatocellular carcinoma with portal vein tumor thrombus: a randomized, open-label, multicenter controlled study. J Clin Oncol 2019;37(24):2141–51.

103. Hasan S, Abel S, Uemura T, et al. Liver transplant mortality and morbidity following preoperative radiotherapy for hepatocellular carcinoma. HPB (Oxford) 2020;22(5):770–8.

104. Sayan M, Yegya-Raman N, Greco SH, et al. Rethinking the role of radiation therapy in the treatment of unresectable hepatocellular carcinoma: a Data Driven treatment algorithm for optimizing outcomes. Front Oncol 2019;9:345.

105. Sapir E, Tao Y, Schipper MJ, et al. Stereotactic body radiation therapy as an alternative to transarterial chemoembolization for hepatocellular carcinoma. Int J Radiat Oncol Biol Phys 2018;100(1):122–30.

106. Mohamed M, Katz AW, Mohamedtaki AJ, et al. Comparison of outcomes between SBRT, yttrium-90 radioembolization, transarterial chemoembolization, and radiofrequency ablation as bridge to transplant for hepatocellular carcinoma. Adv Radiat Oncol 2016;1(1):35–42.

Tyrosine Kinase Inhibitors and Hepatocellular Carcinoma

Leonardo G. da Fonseca, MD[a], Maria Reig, MD, PhD[b,c],
Jordi Bruix, MD, PhD[b,c],*

KEYWORDS

- Hepatocellular carcinoma • Tyrosine kinase • Systemic treatment • Sorafenib
- Lenvatinib • Cabozantinib • Regorafenib

KEY POINTS

- Tyrosine kinase inhibitors (TKIs) opened the era of systemic treatment of hepatocellular carcinoma (HCC). Currently, TKIs represent one of the cornerstones of HCC management.
- Novel TKIs beyond sorafenib are currently available. TKIs sequences reached unprecedented outcomes for patients with HCC.
- Combination of TKIs with immune-oncology agents are under active research with encouraging results.
- There is a need to establish criteria on how to best assess response, as well as biomarkers to predict response.

INTRODUCTION
The Role of Kinases in Cancer Treatment

Kinases are a group of enzymes that transfer a phosphate group from adenosine triphosphate (ATP) to threonine, serine, or tyrosine domains of specific proteins in response to an extracellular stimulus. Broadly, this process regulates diverse cellular regulatory functions. Tyrosine kinases have a crucial role in regulating growth factors signaling and can be divided into receptor and nonreceptor tyrosine kinases.[1]

The tyrosine kinase receptors are membrane surface proteins with an extracellular N-terminal region that binds to a ligand (usually a growth factor) and a C-terminal region that presents a binding domain for tyrosine proteins. The binding of a ligand to the extracellular portion results in autophosphorylation of the cytoplasmic domains to

a Clinical Oncology, Instituto do Cancer do Estado de São Paulo, University of São Paulo, Av. Dr. Arnaldo, 251-Cerqueira Cesar, São Paulo, São Paulo CEP 01246-000, Brazil; b Barcelona Clinic Liver Cancer (BCLC) Group, Liver Unit, Hospital Clinic Barcelona, IDIBAPS, Villarroel 170, Barcelona 08036, Spain; c University of Barcelona, Centro de Investigación Biomédica en Red de Enfermedades Hepáticas y Digestivas (CIBERehd), Barcelona, Spain
* Corresponding author. Barcelona Clinic Liver Cancer (BCLC) Group, Liver Unit, Hospital Clinic Barcelona, IDIBAPS, Villarroel 170, Barcelona 08036, Spain.
E-mail address: jbruix@clinic.cat

Clin Liver Dis 24 (2020) 719–737
https://doi.org/10.1016/j.cld.2020.07.012
1089-3261/20/© 2020 Elsevier Inc. All rights reserved.

liver.theclinics.com

activate kinase activity and, consequently, intracellular signaling pathways are triggered. The nonreceptor tyrosine kinases relay intracellular signals from membrane receptor to the nucleus, promoting cell proliferation and survival.[2] The abnormal overexpression or activation of kinases are intimately linked to oncogenesis and tumoral progression.[3]

Hereof, the set of protein kinases (named kinome) has become a central issue in drug development. Kinase inhibitors are recognized as effective tools against cancer cells and have motivated intensive research in Oncology. The inhibition of distinct kinase signaling pathways can be less cytotoxic to nontumoral cells, priming the selective killing of tumor cells with lower toxic manifestations to normal tissues.[4] This concept changed the paradigm of anticancer treatment in the early 2000s, opening the possibility to offer a selective therapy with a lower risk of producing treatment-related adverse events.

Specific oncogenic kinase targets include BRAF, epidermal growth factor receptor (EGFR), vascular endothelial growth factor receptor (VEGFR), human epidermal growth factor receptor 2 (HER2), Kit, platelet-derived growth factor receptor (PDGFR), mammalian target of rapamycin (mTOR), hepatocyte growth factor (HGF)/c-mesenchymal epithelial transition factor (c-Met), fibroblast growth factor receptor (FGFR), and others.[4] These proteins are associated with hallmarks of carcinogenesis, such as sustaining proliferative signaling, inducing angiogenesis, antiapoptotic mechanisms, activating invasion and metastasis.[5]

The idea of kinase inhibition in Oncology arose in the 1970s, when the oncogene SRC was found to be a protein kinase.[6] In the following years, the first protein kinase inhibitors, the naphthalene sulfonamides, were synthetized and gave support for developing further molecules.[7] However, the major breakthrough occurred in 2001, when imatinib was approved for the treatment of chronic myeloid leukemia.[8] Posteriorly, single and multikinase inhibitors showed clinical benefit in patients with renal cell carcinoma, gastro-intestinal stromal tumor, subtypes of non-small cell lung cancer, and hepatocellular carcinoma (HCC).[9–11]

Targeting Hepatocarcinogenesis with Kinases Inhibition

Hepatocarcinogenesis is driven by abnormal activation of different intracellular pathways, which involves the role of receptors and nonreceptors of tyrosine kinase proteins. Some notable observations encouraged the study of tyrosine kinase inhibitors (TKIs) in HCC:

- Intracellular pathways are found to be deregulated in HCC, including those related to EGFR, PDGFR, VEGFR, HGF/c-Met, and FGFR. The activation of these receptors triggers further cascades of intracellular RAS/RAF/MEK/ERK protein kinase signalling.[12] Turning these mediators on has the ability to induce liver tumors in experimental models.[13]
- Knockdown experiments showed that inactivating these kinases may have antitumoral effects, as a proof of principle that pathway blockade is a potential goal to achieve control of HCC.[14]
- Overexpression of VEGF/VEGFR and high vascularization are found in HCC.[15]
- VEGF levels correlate with angiogenic activity, microvessel density, and poorer prognosis.[15]
- Activation of the MAPK kinase pathway enhances HCC cell growth and prevents apoptosis.[16]

Together with a deeper knowledge of molecular hallmarks that drive cancer progression, the use of TKIs opened the era of systemic treatment of HCC in the

2000s. At that time, no other class (such as cytotoxic chemotherapy or antihormones) had been shown to impact positively in this malignancy. Currently, a handful of TKIs for HCC are incorporated and this class of drugs currently represents one of the cornerstones of systemic treatment (**Fig. 1, Table 1**).

THE STARTING POINT
Sorafenib: A Proof of Concept that Succeeded to Clinical Benefit

Sorafenib, an oral multi-TKI, disrupts Raf/MEK/ERK signaling at the level of Raf kinase and exerts an antiangiogenic effect by targeting VEGFR-2, -3, and PDGFR. In a phase 1 trial, including a limited number of patients with HCC, a signal of activity was observed in this subgroup.[17] This prompted a phase 2 study to evaluate efficacy, toxicity, and pharmacokinetics of sorafenib in advanced HCC. Of 137 patients treated, 72% were classified as Child-Pugh A, and 28% were classified as Child-Pugh B. Three (2.2%) patients achieved partial response and 46 (33.6%) had stable disease lasting at least 16 weeks. Median time-to-progression (TTP) was 4.2 months, median overall survival (OS) was 9.2 months, and the toxicity profile was considered manageable.[18] Although radiologic response rate was low, the results of OS and TTP warranted the design of phase 3 placebo-controlled trials in the first-line setting. The SHARP trial

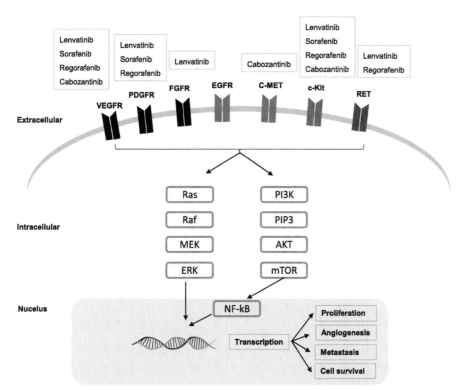

Fig. 1. Tyrosine kinases receptors and key signaling pathways in the pathogenesis of hepatocellular carcinoma. The binding of growth factors to the receptors leads to activation of the signal transduction cascades, such as the PI3K/PIP3/Akt/mTOR and Ras/Raf/MEK/ERK(-MAPK) pathways. The kinase inhibitors used for treating hepatocellular carcinoma are disposed in the figure according to the spectrum of targets.

Table 1
Tyrosine kinase inhibitors approved for hepatocellular carcinoma: molecular structure, posology, and mechanism of action

Drug	Sorafenib	Lenvatinib	Cabozantinib	Regorafenib
Molecular structure				
Posology	400 mg po bid	12 mg po qd if ≥60 kg or 8 mg po qd if <60 kg	60 mg po qd	160 mg po qd (21 d on/7 d off)
Targets	c-Raf, b-Raf, V600E b-Raf, KIT, Flt3, VEGFR2-3, and PDGFRβ	VEGFR, FGFR, PDGFRα, KIT, and RET	VEGFR1-3, MET, and AXL	VEGFR1-3, TIE2, KIT, RET, RAF-1, BRAF, BRAFV600E, PDGFR, and FGFR

Abbreviations: bid, twice a day; FGFR, fibroblast growth factor receptor; PDGFR, platelet-derived growth factor receptor; po, orally; qd, daily; VEGFR, vascular endothelial growth factor receptor.

demonstrated an OS benefit of sorafenib (10.7 versus 7.9 months; hazard ratio [HR] = 0.69; 95% CI, 0.55–0.87; P<.001) and an increment in median time to radiologic progression (2.8–5.5 months; P<.001).[10] Similar benefit was reported in a trial conducted in the Asia-Pacific region (6.5 versus 4.2 months; HR = 0.68; 95% CI, 0.50–0.93; P = .014).[19] Subgroup analyses have shown that sorafenib had consistent positive effects irrespective of background features, such as etiology, tumor burden, performance status, and tumor stage.[20,21] Based on these results, sorafenib became the first systemic agent approved for advanced HCC and remained the sole systemic treatment of this malignancy for almost a decade.

In clinical practice, the efficacy of sorafenib across HCC subgroups varies. Reduction in tumor burden is reported in only 2% to 10% of the cases.[10,22] In this sense, efforts were carried out to establish prognostic markers that would support decision making:

- A worldwide in-field observational study showed that performance status, Child-Pugh class, and Barcelona Clinic Liver Cancer (BCLC) stage were related to worse prognosis in patients under sorafenib treatment.[23]
- A pooled exploratory analysis found that macrovascular invasion, high alpha-fetoprotein (AFP), and high neutrophil-to-lymphocyte ratio were associated with poorer OS.[20]
- Greater OS sorafenib benefit over placebo was observed in patients without extrahepatic spread, with hepatitis C virus, and high neutrophil-to-lymphocyte ratio.[20]
- Angiogenesis markers, such as angiopoietin 2 and VEGF, predict prognosis, although none of them are predictors of treatment response to sorafenib.[21]
- A decline of greater than 20% from the baseline AFP level within 4 weeks of treatment is suggested to be associated with longer OS.[24]
- Imaging techniques, such as computed tomography perfusion and contrast-enhanced ultrasonography seems to be useful for identifying early responders to sorafenib.[25]

Sorafenib-related adverse events include fatigue, arterial hypertension, diarrhea, and dermatologic reactions, such as rash and hand–foot skin reaction. Early dermatologic reactions occurring within 60 days of sorafenib initiation were shown to correlate with longer TTP and OS.[26,27] Also, patients who present complete radiologic response to sorafenib are more likely to present early dermatologic events.[28] The mechanism behind the occurrence of dermatologic events is unknown, but it is hypothesized to be associated with antiangiogenic effects on the skin or to an immune modulation induced by sorafenib.

Besides the cytotoxic and angiogenic effects due to inhibition of kinases, additional immunomodulation by sorafenib has been described.[29] Macrophages are key for antitumor effects in HCC. When exposed to sorafenib, macrophages are shown to induce pyroptosis, and promote activation of natural killer (NK) cell function.[30] Both NK cells and macrophages are components of the innate immune system, which seems to be correlated with survival in patients with HCC. In addition, sorafenib was found to downregulate major histocompatibility complex class I in tumor cells, which may impair immune checkpoint inhibitor activity and favor the innate immune system.[29,30]

This wide spectrum of mechanisms targeted by sorafenib indicates that the apparent ceiling in efficacy was not reached. With the recent incorporation of immune-oncology agents and combination strategies, the role of sorafenib as the sole first-line therapy will be replaced by a continuum of care involving timing and sequencing of different strategies with different mechanisms and balancing risks and benefits of more intensive treatments. This issue is discussed in "Where Will Tyrosine Kinase Inhibitors Be Placed in the Current Landscape of Hepatocellular Carcinoma?" section.

Negative Trials After Sorafenib

Despite the advances in HCC treatment using inhibiting mechanisms mediated by kinases, other TKIs with similar mechanisms of action did not enable superior results. Even with promising results in early-phase trials, a list of TKIs failed to show superiority over sorafenib or to prolong survival after sorafenib discontinuation. The reasons for these failures may include:

- Toxicity concerns: some TKIs may be related to a critical profile of adverse events resulting in early discontinuation or clinical deterioration.
- Absence of patient selection based on molecular markers, because no predictive factor is known to determine the benefit of any specific drug in HCC.
- Trial design: stratification by relevant prognostic factors, such as tumor burden and pattern of progression, may facilitate capture of drug activity.
- Inclusion criteria: selection based on the registration of the last tumor progression can avoid biological heterogeneity in the population included.
- Molecular heterogeneity: an analysis with whole-exome sequencing from 158 resected HCCs reported that no single protein kinase has more than a 5% frequency within a tumor and some TKIs are predominantly selective in their molecular targets, which impairs the activity against heterogeneous disease.[31]
- Lower efficacy: some TKIs may simply be less effective and not reach superiority in comparative trials.

Sunitinib, a multitargeted TKI against VEGFR, PDGFR, c-KIT, and FLT-3, was tested in a phase 3 trial designed to prove both superiority and noninferiority versus sorafenib. The phase 2 trial had already anticipated that the survival with sunitinib was not superior to historical control. The study enrolled 1073 patients with advanced-stage HCC primarily from Asia. The median OS was 8 months for the sunitinib arm versus 10 months for sorafenib (HR = 1.31; 95% CI, 1.13–1.52; P = .0019). The trial was stopped early by an independent data monitoring committee because of futility and safety concerns.[32]

Brivanib, a VEGF and FGF inhibitor, was evaluated in a phase 2 trial that enrolled 55 patients, with a median OS of 10 months and a rate of progression-free survival (PFS) after 6 months of 18.2%. Two separate phase 3 studies with brivanib in first- and second-line therapy were carried out. In the first-line, 1155 patients were randomized and brivanib did not meet noninferiority to sorafenib (median OS = 9.9 versus 9.5 months, HR = 1.06; 95% CI, 0.92–1.22; P = .3730).[33] In the second-line setting, brivanib was investigated after progression or intolerance to sorafenib. The background justification is that the phenotypic resistance to VEGFR inhibition could activate alternative angiogenic pathways by way of the FGF family. In a phase 2 study with 46 patients, the median OS in patients who had failed previous therapy was 9.8 months. The phase 3 study compared brivanib to placebo in 395 patients. Again, the study did not meet its primary endpoint of OS (9.4 versus 8.2 months, P = .3307).[34]

Linifanib, a PDGF and VEGF inhibitor, provided median OS of 9.7 months in a prospective phase 2 with 44 patients. However, a phase 3 trial with more than 1000 patients failed to show survival improvement with linifanib over sorafenib (9.1 months for linifanib versus 9.8 months for sorafenib). Also, adverse events leading to treatment discontinuation and interruptions were more frequent with linifanib.[35]

An attempt to use a biomarker-driven strategy was addressed with tivantinib, a selective MET inhibitor, in a phase 3 METIV trial. This trial included patients with high

MET expression who were previously treated with sorafenib. MET, which is the receptor for HGF, activates the MAPK and phosphatidylinositol 3-kinase-AKT pathways. MET expression was an adverse prognostic factor and it is more frequently overexpressed in tumor tissue after sorafenib exposure. A phase 2 trial showed that tivantinib improved survival in patients with MET-high. Despite this background, the METIV trial was negative.[36] The possible causes for these results include differences between the phase 2 and III designs: sample size, tivantinib formulation, different laboratories evaluating MET expression, number of biopsies obtained before and after sorafenib, number of patients with MET-high tumors, and the protocol-specified requirement for biopsy results to be available before enrollment in the phase 3. As a collateral result, the METIV trial proved that tumor biopsy before trial entry is feasible and with marginal risk.

NEW PLAYERS: COMBINATIONS AND NOVEL TYROSINE KINASE INHIBITORS
Combination Strategies

The negative list of TKIs with preclinical activity that failed in phase 3 trials grounded the use of combination therapies that targeted molecular pathways at different sites and targets.

- TACE plus sorafenib: in patients with intermediate-stage disease (BCLC B), the recommended treatment is transarterial chemoembolization (TACE). The local hypoxia caused by the TACE procedure induces expression of hypoxia-inducible factors and increase levels of VEGF.[37] Thus, a strategy combining TACE and a TKIs can improve outcomes in intermediate stage. However, none of the trials that addressed TACE plus TKIs succeeded in demonstrating convincing impact.[38,39] The TACTICs trial, that randomized patients to sorafenib plus TACE versus TACE, suggested that sorafenib significantly prolonged PFS (25.2 versus 13.6 months, HR = 0.59; 95% CI, 0.41–0.67; P = .006), but survival data were not mature as only 73.6% of the OS events had been reached.[40] It has to be noted that TACTICS used a different set of definitions for progression registration and treatment interruption. Hence, the PFS are to be seen as vulnerable until establishing the refined PFS as proposed years ago by the BCLC as a proper surrogate for OS.[41] In the STAH trial, 339 patients with advanced HCC were randomized to TACE plus sorafenib versus sorafenib. The median OS for the combination was 12.8 versus 10.8 months (HR = 0.91; 95% CI, 0.69–1.21; P = .290), with no survival improvement by adding TACE in advanced stage disease.[42]
- SIRT plus sorafenib: the SORAMIC trial included 424 patients with unresectable HCC not considered for TACE to receive sorafenib versus sorafenib plus selective internal radiotherapy (SIRT). The median OS was 12.1 months in the SIRT plus sorafenib arm and 11.5 months in the sorafenib arm (HR = 1.01; 95% CI, 0.82–1.25; P = .93). A post-hoc subgroup analysis of the per-protocol population in this study suggested a survival benefit of SIRT plus sorafenib for patients ≤65 years, nonalcoholic etiology of cirrhosis, and not cirrhotic, but this requires prospective validation. Adverse events grade 3 or higher were reported in 72.3% patients in the SIRT plus sorafenib arm and in 68.5% patients in the sorafenib arm.[43] Despite the subgroup analysis, there is no clear place for SIRT in advanced HCC, but further studies may identify patients with potential benefit.
- Sorafenib plus cytotoxic chemotherapy: this is based on a theoretic adaptation of tumor cells to minimize its dependency on antiangiogenic stimulus. Doxorubicin combined with sorafenib is hypothesized to dismantle the Ask1-RAF dimer,

which releases ASK1 back to the cytoplasm, thus helping the apoptotic effect of doxorubicin. A phase 2 trial in patients with advanced HCC showed that the combination of doxorubicin plus sorafenib improved median OS (13.7 versus 6.5 months; $P = .006$).[44] However, the phase 3 trial CALGB 80802 did not confirm the superiority of doxorubicin plus sorafenib. This multigroup study randomized 356 patients to doxorubicin plus sorafenib versus sorafenib alone, with a median OS of 9.3 months in the combination arm versus 9.4 months in the sorafenib arm (HR = 1.05; 95% CI, 0.83–1.31). It was noteworthy that grade 3 and 4 neutropenia was observed in 37% of the patients who received the combination therapy.[45] Thus, in addition to the absence of survival benefit, the combination also impaired safety.

- Combining TKIs: this strategy may have synergistic or additive effects, as demonstrated in preclinical models.[43] Nevertheless, the EGFR inhibitor erlotinib did not improve survival when added to sorafenib compared with sorafenib alone in treatment-naïve patients with advanced HCC.[46] Erlotinib in combination with bevacizumab, an anti-VEGF antibody, yielded encouraging PFS, OS, and response rate in phase 2 data,[47] but another comparative phase 2 study showed that it reached similar survival outcomes to sorafenib alone.[48] The modest results with a combination of targeted therapies may be justified by a higher rate of significant adverse events leading to early discontinuation, or even by the lack of synergist effect of different targets in vivo.

- TKIs plus immunotherapy: the focus is currently being placed in combinations of TKI with immune-oncology agents, especially immune checkpoint inhibitors directed to PD1/PDL-1 blockage. VEGF may boost the activity of regulatory T cells and myeloid-derived suppressor cells. Cytokines released by these cells inhibit NK cells and CD8+ T cytotoxic cells.[49] In murine models, TKIs have decreased the population of immunosuppressive tumor-associated macrophages and increased interferon-producing CD8+ T cells.[50] Ongoing clinical trials are currently evaluating cabozantinib plus atezolizumab (NCT03755791), regorafenib plus nivolumab (NCT04170556), and lenvatinib plus pembrolizumab (NCT03713593). The latter regimen has received breakthrough therapy designation by the Food and Drug Administration after phase 1b results, with an objective response rate of 44.8% and a median duration of response of 18.7 months.[49] Of note, such response was reported using modified response evaluation criteria in solid tumors (mRECIST), running a risk of overestimation in reported response rate due to the antiangiogenic effect of lenvatinib.[51,52]

Sequencing Tyrosine Kinase Inhibitors

After almost a decade of disappointing results with TKIs, another targeted therapy has been established in the first-line setting for patients with advanced HCC. Lenvatinib is an oral TKI directed to kinase receptors involved in angiogenesis and proliferation, such as VEGFR-1, -2, and -3, FGFR1, -2, -3, and -4, PDGFR, KIT, and RET. A single-arm phase 2 study in patients with HCC treated with lenvatinib reported a median TTP of 7.4 months and a median OS of 18.7 months,[49] which prompted a phase 3 study. The REFLECT trial was a noninferiority study that randomized 954 systemic treatment-naive patients to sorafenib or lenvatinib until disease progression or limiting toxicity. The study did not include patients with greater than 50% of liver invasion, biliary tract invasion, and main portal vein invasion. The noninferiority margin was set at 1.08 and the trial succeeded in demonstrating that lenvatinib is a noninferior option with an HR of 0.92 (95% CI, 0.79–1.06), and with a median OS of 13.6 months for lenvatinib and 12.3 months for sorafenib. The secondary endpoints of PFS, TTP, and response rate favored the lenvatinib arm. However, lenvatinib was associated with a higher rate of grade 3 to 4 treatment-related adverse events, particularly arterial hypertension.[22]

A subanalysis of the REFLECT trial showed that 25.3% of the patients allocated to receive lenvatinib were treated with sorafenib after progression, and 11.8% received sorafenib beyond progression in the sorafenib arm. Around 33.6% of the patients received conventional chemotherapy (known to lack efficacy and likely bear associated toxicity) after progression in the sorafenib arm compared with 18.4% in lenvatinib arm. Sequencing therapies revealed favorable survival outcomes: the median OS for patients who received poststudy medication was 20.9 and 17.0 months in the lenvatinib and sorafenib arms, respectively,[53] there being a need to retain the impact of postprogression agents with favorable or detrimental impact.

Between 2016 and 2019, there were data published on 3 agents that prolonged survival in patients with HCC after sorafenib progression. Two of them belong to the TKI class (regorafenib and cabozantinib) and the other is the monoclonal antibody ramucirumab.

- Regorafenib: in preclinical data, regorafenib was shown to be a potent inhibitor of Raf-1 and of several receptor tyrosine kinases involved in neovascularization and tumor progression, including VEGFR-2 and -3, PDGFR, Flt-3, and c-KIT. In xenograft models, this drug enabled inhibition of tumor growth inhibition of extracellular signal-regulated kinase phosphorylation, which could be proven by an expressive reduction in microvessel density within the tumor area.[54] Besides a distinct molecular profile, regorafenib had more potent pharmacologic activity than sorafenib.[55] A phase 2 study with 36 patients with HCC showed an acceptable tolerability and evidence of antitumor activity, with a median TTP of 4.3 months and a median OS of 13.8 months.[55] These findings led the design of the RESORCE trial, which was a phase 3 placebo-controlled study including patients who progressed on sorafenib, but had tolerated ≥400 mg/d for ≥20 of the last 28 days of treatment. The investigators set that the last dose of sorafenib must have been received within the last 10 weeks before randomization, and a 2-week washout from the last dose of sorafenib was required before regorafenib initiation. This timeframe was critical to homogenize the sample in terms of biological behavior, avoiding the inclusion of indolent and rapidly progressive disease. For the first time, a systemic agent provided better OS in the second-line setting, with a median OS of 10.6 versus 7.8 months for placebo (HR = 0.63; 95% CI, 0.50–0.79; $P<.0001$). Grades 3 and 4 adverse events were reported: hypertension, hand–foot skin reaction, fatigue, and diarrhea were the most common.[56] An exploratory analysis of the RESORCE trial reported that patients who received the sequence sorafenib–regorafenib reached an unprecedented outcome, with a median OS of 26 months. Moreover, this analysis demonstrated that regorafenib conferred a clinical benefit regardless of the last dose of sorafenib or TTP on sorafenib. No biomarker associated to improved outcome was identified, and again there was an association between dermatologic adverse events and enhanced survival.[57]
- Cabozantinib: this agent inhibits VEGFR1-3, MET, and AXL, which are closely linked to tumor hypoxia, as previously explored in preclinical models.[58] Sorafenib-exposed HCC cell lines showed induction of HGF, which activates c-MET kinase, suggesting a compensatory upregulation of MET in sorafenib resistance.[59]

The CELESTIAL trial was a phase 3 placebo-controlled study that randomized patients who had been previously exposed to sorafenib to receive placebo or cabozantib. Most of the patients had been exposed to only 1 line of systemic treatment, but 28.1% had received ≥2 lines before cabozantinib. Unlike the RESORCE trial, it included patients who had progression or intolerance to sorafenib. The cabozantinib arm showed a significantly longer median OS of 10.2 versus 8.0 months (HR = 0.76; 95% CI, 0.63–0.92; P = .005). PFS and response rate also favored cabozantinib. The most common grade 3 to 4 adverse events with cabozantinib were hand–foot skin reaction, hypertension, fatigue, and increased transaminases.

- Ramucirumab: this monoclonal antibody exerts its antiangiogenic property by binding exclusively the extracellular domain of VEGFR-2, whereas TKIs are small molecules that bind intracellular kinase domains of this and other receptors.[60] Ramucirumab as second-line therapy in HCC was investigated in the REACH trial, a placebo-controlled phase 3 study in sorafenib-treated patients. Although the primary endpoint of OS was not met in the intention-to-treat population, a prespecified analysis with patients with AFP ≥400 ng/ml has shown a significant improvement in OS.[61] This hypothesis-generating finding led to a REACH-2 trial, which randomized 292 sorafenib-experienced patients with AFP ≥400 ng/mL to receive placebo or ramucirumab. Median OS was significantly improved for ramucirumab (8.5 versus 7.3 months, HR = 0.71; 95% CI, 0.53–0.95; P = .0199), with an acceptable safety profile.[62] A preplanned pooled analysis with patients showing AFP ≥400 ng/mL from REACH confirmed the survival benefit of ramucirumab in the second-line.[63] Despite being a prognostic marker, high AFP as a biomarker-driven approach raises the question of why ramucirumab benefits only this specific subgroup. AFP levels are a continuum, so that a distinction of outcomes based on a fixed threshold is biologically cumbersome to translate into practice. AFP is suggested to correlate with a distinct phenotype marked by VEGFR overexpression and increased angiogenesis, which might provide a background for the REACH-2 trial in future research.

The above-mentioned results initiated the idea of sequencing therapies as a strategy to increase survival in HCC (**Fig. 2**). Obviously, this was a great advance for the

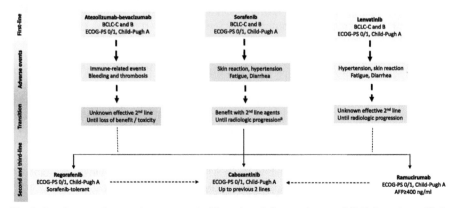

Fig. 2. Landscape of systemic treatment of hepatocellular carcinoma. BCLC, Barcelona Clinic Liver Cancer; ECOG PS, Eastern Cooperative Oncology Group performance status. [a] Pivotal trials allowed treatment until radiologic and/or clinical progression.

field. On the other hand, new challenges were posed. The selection of an agent when more than one option is available can be supported by:

- Matching individual and trial population baseline features: included population varies between trials in the same setting (**Table 2**). For instance, the REFLECT trial[22] excluded patients using more than 1 antihypertensive drug, which prevents any conclusion of the safety and efficacy of lenvatinib in this population. Similarly, there are no safety data on regorafenib in patients who did not tolerate sorafenib because this subgroup was not included in the RESORCE trial.[56]
- Toxicity profile: although sorafenib and regorafenib may be associated to dermatologic events, lenvatinib and cabozantinib were more associated with arterial hypertension. Comorbidities and each patients' lifestyle should be taken into account when selecting an agent (**Table 3**).
- Local issues and context: increasing cost and availability are important limitations because HCC has a high incidence in low- and middle-income countries. The care provider should evaluate this context when choosing the most suitable strategy.
- Prediction on treatment course based on key events: signals of liver decompensation or rapidly progressive disease (with a dismal patterns of progression[52]) may indicate treatment failure and a need to switch to a subsequent line. On the other hand, growth of preexisting lesions in the absence of significant changes in other baseline features suggests that treatment beyond progression is a reasonable alternative.

Furthermore, another question is how and when to switch to a subsequent agent. The concepts of drug resistance, treatment failure or intolerance are not uniform between trials and might hamper a direct applicability in real-life practice. The final

Table 2
Main results of efficacy from phase 1, 2, and 3 data of tyrosine kinase inhibitors approved for hepatocellular carcinoma

	Phase 1		Phase 2			Phase 3		
	Target Population		Target Population			Target Population		
	MTD	DCR	ORR	mTTP	mOS	ORR	mTTP	mOS
Sorafenib	Advanced refractory solid tumors (n = 69)		Advanced HCC, CP A-B, 1st line (n = 137)			Advanced HCC, CP A, 1st line (n = 602)		
	400 mg bid	57.8%	2.2%	4.2 mo	9.2 mo	2%	5.5 mo	10.7 mo
Lenvatinib	Advanced HCC, CP A (n = 20)		Advanced HCC, CP A (n = 46)			Advanced HCC, CP A, 1st line (n = 954)		
	12 mg qd	85%	37%	7.4 mo	18.7 mo	18.8%	7.3 mo	13.6 mo
Regorafenib	Advanced refractory solid tumors (n = 53)		Advanced HCC, CP A (n = 36)			Advanced HCC, CP A, 2nd line, sorafenib-tolerant (n = 843)		
	160 mg 21/28 d	66%	2.8%	4.3 mo	13.8 mo	11%	3.2 mo	10.6 mo
Cabozantinib	Advanced solid tumors (n = 85)		Advanced HCC, CP A, 1st and 2nd line (n = 41)			Advanced HCC, CP A, 2nd and 3rd line, after sorafenib (n = 707)		
	175 mg qd	94%	5%	NR	11.5 mo	4%	NR	10.2 mo

Abbreviations: CP, Child-Pugh; DCR, disease control rate; HCC, hepatocellular carcinoma; mo, months; mOS, median overall survival; MTD, maximum tolerated dose; mTTP, median time-to-progression; NR, nonreported; ORR, objective response rate.

Table 3
Incidence of grade 3–4 adverse events reported in phase 3 trials with tyrosine kinase inhibitors in hepatocellular carcinoma

Adverse Event	Sorafenib (%)	Lenvatinib (%)	Regorafenib (%)	Cabozantinib (%)
Any grade 3–4 adverse event	49	57	67	68
Diarrhea	4	4	3	11
Hand-foot skin reaction	11	3	13	17
Fatigue	4	4	9	10
Nausea	1	1	1	2
Hypertension	14	23	16	17
Rash	<1	0	NA	1
Vomiting	1	1	1	1
Decreased appetite	1	5	3	6
Weight loss	3	8	2	1

Descriptive data/direct comparison between trials are not appropriate.
Abbreviation: NA, nonavailable.

sections of this text are aimed at a more critical view on issues that ground decision making in advanced HCC.

Tyrosine Kinase Inhibitors Resistance

In both clinical trials and clinical practice, most patients receiving systemic treatment of advanced stage HCC will die because of tumor progression or tumor-related complications. Therefore, mechanisms of resistance in the tumor microenvironment are eventually expected at some point during the course of treatment. These mechanisms ultimately translate into macroscopic spread, organ dysfunction, clinical deterioration, and death. Resistance to targeted therapies can be innate or acquired. Some of these mechanisms have been already explored in preclinical studies, but none has a direct applicability[64]:

- Altered signaling pathways and crosstalk (eg, mTOR);
- Gene driver mutations (eg, CTNNB1, VEGFA, and KRAS);
- Epithelial–mesenchymal transition (eg, activation of MET);
- Cancer stem cells;
- Disabling of proapoptotic signals.

In the METIV trial, MET expression in tumor tissues was assessed by immunohistochemistry, and some patients provided both pre-sorafenib and post-sorafenib treatment samples. In this subgroup, 61% who were MET-low before sorafenib converted to MET-high.[36] This suggests dynamic changes in oncogenic pathways during sorafenib therapy, although the treatment with the MET inhibitor tivantinib has not shown to positively impact on OS in this study.

In vitro treatment with sorafenib is suggested to induce epithelial–mesenchymal transition via activation of the phosphatidylinositol 3-kinase-AKT-snail pathway and activation of c-MET.[59,65] Similarly, experimental models suggested that tumors resistant to sorafenib are enriched in FGF, insulin-like growth factor signaling,[65] and higher expression of p-STAT3 and Janus kinases 1 and 2.[66]

It is likely that TKIs influence clonal redistribution of tumor cells and emergence of resistance. In this sense, the search for strategies aimed to overcome resistance is warranted. The successful incorporation of second-line targeted therapies up to now, such as regorafenib and cabozantinib, are more likely to impact on a broad spectrum of molecular targets instead of blocking a specific mechanism of acquired resistance.

Challenges in Assessing Response to Tyrosine Kinase Inhibitors in Hepatocellular Carcinoma

Early identification of patients who will or will not obtain clinical benefit from treatment has key advantages: patients could be saved from toxicities, physicians have justification to maintaining or switching treatment, and there are potential cost savings. Assessing tumor burden by imaging techniques is a commonly used surrogate to discriminate between treatment benefit or failure.

However, assessment of radiologic response to TKIs remains a challenge. It is well established that response according to conventional response evaluation criteria in solid tumors (RECIST) are far lower than the proportion of patients who derive real benefit from these therapies.[67] Substantial tumor necrosis may occur as a consequence of the antiangiogenic effect of TKIs, resulting in a change in tumor cell burden but little overall size change. This feature is not taken into account by RECIST, and alternative concepts to assess TKI activity are still needed.

In HCC, an attempt to refine the assessment of response came with mRECIST, which combined the RECIST definitions for progression with the evaluation of necrosis or viable enhancing tumor.[68] Although mRECIST and EASL criteria[69] seem adequate for locoregional modalities such as intra-arterial chemotherapy or ablation, they may not be a precise method for HCC under TKI therapy.

TKIs are antiangiogenics and may induce vasoconstriction that reduces mesenteric inflow, hepatic artery supply, and ultimately arterial contrast uptake by the tumor.[70] This may lead to an overestimation of response by wrongly reading that the reduced contrast uptake represents necrosis.

A weak correlation between response and survival is evident when analyzing the pivotal trials of sorafenib in HCC, in which a survival benefit was reached despite a low response rate of less than 5%.[71] On the other hand, the rate of overall tumor control was noteworthy, which highlights that absence of progression is potentially a more accurate predictor of effectiveness of TKIs in HCC.

Another challenge is that progression on TKIs according to conventional criteria was shown to be associated with different outcomes. The pattern of progression with the onset of new extrahepatic lesions carries a worse prognosis compared with other patterns, such as growth of preexisting lesions or new intrahepatic nodules.[41] This suggests that TKIs exert their benefit in HCC by delaying dismal patterns of progressions, rather than reducing tumor burden.

Where Will Tyrosine Kinase Inhibitors Be Placed in the Current Landscape of Hepatocellular Carcinoma?

The landscape of HCC treatment changed substantially in the past few years. New agents, including immunotherapy and novel TKIs, have extended survival far beyond what was reported previously. Moreover, the concept of treatment stage migration highlights that the use of systemic agents may benefit patients even in earlier stages.

Since the successful incorporation of regorafenib in second-line treatment, the idea of sequencing therapies was established as the standard approach. In the future, combinations, including different classes of drugs will be part of the armamentarium. For example, the combination of atezolizumab and bevacizumab was reported to be superior to sorafenib in terms of OS and will probably become the upfront standard of care[72] for patients fitting the clinical profile as per selection criteria for entry into the trial.

However, combinations of agents naturally increase toxicities over monotherapy. This is particularly important in patients with HCC because limiting toxicities may accompany progressive liver dysfunction and clinical deterioration.

This increasing landscape and extended survival will probably replace the idea of successive lines of single therapies to an idea of continuum of care, which means an individualized planning tailored to every specific clinical situation. Potential roles of TKIs that should be explored in future trials include (**Fig. 3**):

- Patients who have increased risk of specific toxicities and immune-related events, eg, risk of major bleeding with bevacizumab, autoimmune disorders, transplanted patients.
- After achieving a major response with a combination regimen, some patients could be considered for a maintenance monotherapy with TKIs. These patients could be further rechallenged with the initial combination in the case of disease progression.
- Upfront TKIs with intermittent addition of immunotherapy according to longitudinal biomarker measurements. This hypothetical situation requires the identification of dynamic biomarkers that would drive an "on–off" approach.

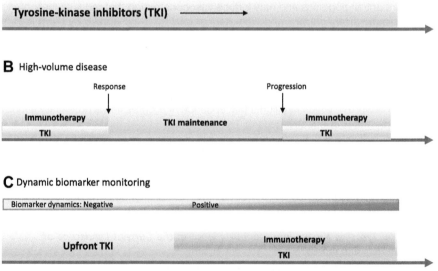

Fig. 3. Potential roles of TKIs to be explored in future trials: (*A*) subgroups with increased risk of specific toxicities and immune-related events, for example, risk of major bleeding with bevacizumab, autoimmune disorders, transplanted patients. (*B*) Add-on strategy: after achieving a major response with a combination regimen, patients could switch to TKI as a maintenance and be further rechallenged with the initial combination in case of disease progression. (*C*) Upfront TKIs with addition of immunotherapy according to potential longitudinal biomarker measurements.

FINAL CONSIDERATIONS

The use of TKIs opened up the concept that systemic treatment could benefit patients with HCC in the advanced stage. The accumulated knowledge on how to manage this class of drugs and the incorporation of novel therapies extended survival to the point that advanced HCC is no longer an acutely fatal disease in a substantial proportion of patients. Maximizing drug activity must be balanced with minimizing toxicity. This requires the development of strategies that join novel therapies with the currently used drugs, such as TKIs, to keep moving ahead with providing better outcomes to patients with HCC.

DISCLOSURE

L.G. da Fonseca—lecture fees from Bayer and Roche. M. Reig—Consultancy: Bayer-Shering Pharma, BMS, Roche, Ipsen, AstraZeneca, Lilly, BTG/Paid conferences: Bayer-Shering Pharma, BMS, Gilead, Lilly/Research Grants: Bayer-Shering Pharma, Ipsen. J. Bruix—Consultancy: AbbVie, ArQule, Astra, Basilea, Bayer, BMS, Daiichi Sankyo, GlaxoSmithKline, Gilead, Kowa, Lilly, Medimune, Novartis, Onxeo, Polaris, Quirem, Roche, Sanofi-Aventis, Sirtex, Terumo/Grants: Bayer and Ipsen.

REFERENCES

1. Arora A, Scholar EM. Role of tyrosine kinase inhibitors in cancer therapy. J Pharmacol Exp Ther 2005;315(3):971–9.
2. Coussens L, Parker PJ, Rhee L, et al. Multiple, distinct forms of bovine and human protein kinase C suggest diversity in cellular signaling pathways. Science 1986;233(4766):859–66.
3. Maurer G, Tarkowski B, Baccarini M. Raf kinases in cancer-roles and therapeutic opportunities. Oncogene 2011;30(32):3477–88.
4. Kittler H, Tschandl P. Driver mutations in the mitogen-activated protein kinase pathway: the seeds of good and evil. Br J Dermatol 2018;178(1):26–7.
5. Hanahan D, Weinberg A. Hallmarks of cancer: the next generation. Cell 2011; 144(5):646–74.
6. Collett MS, Erikson RL. Protein kinase activity associated with the avian sarcoma virus src gene product. Proc Natl Acad Sci U S A 1978;75(4):2021–4.
7. Hidaka H, Inagaki M, Kawamoto S, et al. Isoquinolinesulfonamides, novel and potent inhibitors of cyclic nucleotide dependent protein kinase and protein kinase C. Biochemistry 1984;23(21):5036–41.
8. Hopkin MD, Baxendale IR, Ley SV. A flow-based synthesis of Imatinib: the API of Gleevec. Chem Commun 2010;46(14):2450–2.
9. Motzer RJ, Hoosen S, Bello CL, et al. Sunitinib malate for the treatment of solid tumours: a review of current clinical data. Expert Opin Investig Drugs 2006; 15(5):553–61.
10. Llovet JM, Ricci S, Mazzaferro V, et al. Sorafenib in advanced hepatocellular carcinoma. N Engl J Med 2008;359(4):378–90.
11. Medical Advisory Secretariat. Epidermal growth factor receptor mutation (EGFR) testing for prediction of response to EGFR-targeting tyrosine kinase inhibitor (TKI) drugs in patients with advanced non-small-cell lung cancer: an evidence-based analysis. Ont Health Technol Assess Ser 2010;10(24):1–48.
12. Villanueva A. Hepatocellular carcinoma. N Engl J Med 2019;380(15):1450–62.
13. Paschalis G, Dimitrios G. Experimental models of hepatocellular carcinoma in mice. Surg Chronicles 2013;18(3):134–8.

14. Villanueva A, Chiang DY, Newell P, et al. Pivotal role of mTOR signaling in hepatocellular carcinoma. Gastroenterology 2008;135(6). https://doi.org/10.1053/j.gastro.2008.08.008.

15. Chao Y, Li CP, Chau GY, et al. Prognostic significance of vascular endothelial growth factor, basic fibroblast growth factor, and angiogenin in patients with resectable hepatocellular carcinoma after surgery. Ann Surg Oncol 2003;10(4): 355–62.

16. Huynh H, Thanh T, Nguyen T, et al. Kinase (MEK)-MAPK in hepatocellular carcinoma: its role in tumor progression and apoptosis. BMC Gastroenterol 2003; 19(3):1–21.

17. Strumberg D, Richly H, Hilger RA, et al. Phase I clinical and pharmacokinetic study of the novel raf kinase and vascular endothelial growth factor receptor inhibitor BAY 43-9006 in patients with advanced refractory solid tumors. J Clin Oncol 2005;23(5):965–72.

18. Abou-Alfa GK, Schwartz L, Ricci S, et al. Phase II study of sorafenib in patients with advanced hepatocellular carcinoma. J Clin Oncol 2006;24(26):4293–300.

19. Cheng A-L, Kang Y-K, Chen Z, et al. Efficacy and safety of sorafenib in patients in the Asia-Pacific region with advanced hepatocellular carcinoma: a phase III randomised, double-blind, placebo-controlled trial. Lancet Oncol 2009;10(1):25–34.

20. Bruix J, Cheng AL, Meinhardt G, et al. Prognostic factors and predictors of sorafenib benefit in patients with hepatocellular carcinoma: analysis of two phase III studies. J Hepatol 2017;67(5):999–1008.

21. Llovet JM, Pena CEA, Lathia CD, et al. Plasma biomarkers as predictors of outcome in patients with advanced hepatocellular carcinoma. Clin Cancer Res 2012;18(8):2290–300.

22. Kudo M, Finn RS, Qin S, et al. Lenvatinib versus sorafenib in first-line treatment of patients with unresectable hepatocellular carcinoma: a randomised phase 3 noninferiority trial. Lancet 2018;391(10126):1163–73.

23. Marrero JA, Kudo M, Venook AP, et al. Observational registry of sorafenib use in clinical practice across Child-Pugh subgroups: the GIDEON study. J Hepatol 2016;65(6):1140–7.

24. Shao YY, Lin ZZ, Hsu C, et al. Early alpha-fetoprotein response predicts treatment efficacy of antiangiogenic systemic therapy in patients with advanced hepatocellular carcinoma. Cancer 2010;116(19):4590–6.

25. Zocco MA, Garcovich M, Lupascu A, et al. Early prediction of response to sorafenib in patients with advanced hepatocellular carcinoma: the role of dynamic contrast enhanced ultrasound. J Hepatol 2013;59(5):1014–21.

26. Reig M, Torres F, Rodriguez-Lope C, et al. Early dermatologic adverse events predict better outcome in HCC patients treated with sorafenib. J Hepatol 2014; 61(2). https://doi.org/10.1016/j.jhep.2014.03.030.

27. Díaz-González Á, Sanduzzi-Zamparelli M, Sapena V, et al. Systematic review with meta-analysis: the critical role of dermatological events in patients with hepatocellular carcinoma treated with sorafenib. Aliment Pharmacol Ther 2019;49(5): 482–91.

28. Rimola J, Díaz-González Á, Darnell A, et al. Complete response under sorafenib in patients with hepatocellular carcinoma: relationship with dermatologic adverse events. Hepatology 2018;67(2):612–22.

29. Zhao X, Cao M, Lu Z, et al. Small-molecule inhibitor sorafenib regulates immunoreactions by inducing survival and differentiation of bone marrow cells. Innate Immun 2016;22(7):493–502.

30. Hage C, Hoves S, Strauss L, et al. Sorafenib induces pyroptosis in macrophages and triggers natural killer cell-mediated cytotoxicity against hepatocellular carcinoma. Hepatology 2019;70(4):1280–97.
31. Guichard C, Amaddeo G, Imbeaud S, et al. Integrated analysis of somatic mutations and focal copy-number changes identifies key genes and pathways in hepatocellular carcinoma. Nat Genet 2012;44(6):694–8.
32. Cheng A-L, Kang Y-K, Lin D-Y, et al. Sunitinib versus sorafenib in advanced hepatocellular cancer: results of a randomized phase III trial. J Clin Oncol 2013; 31(32):4067–75.
33. Johnson PJ, Qin S, Park JW, et al. Brivanib versus sorafenib as first-line therapy in patients with unresectable, advanced hepatocellular carcinoma: results from the randomized phase III BRISK-FL study. J Clin Oncol 2013;31(28):3517–24.
34. Llovet JM, Decaens T, Raoul JL, et al. Brivanib in patients with advanced hepatocellular carcinoma who were intolerant to sorafenib or for whom sorafenib failed: results from the randomized phase III BRISK-PS study. J Clin Oncol 2013;31(28):3509–16.
35. Cainap C, Qin S, Huang W-T, et al. Linifanib versus sorafenib in patients with advanced hepatocellular carcinoma: results of a randomized phase III trial. J Clin Oncol 2015;33(2):172–9.
36. Rimassa L, Assenat E, Peck-Radosavljevic M, et al. Tivantinib for second-line treatment of MET-high, advanced hepatocellular carcinoma (METIV-HCC): a final analysis of a phase 3, randomised, placebo-controlled study. Lancet Oncol 2018; 19(5):682–93.
37. Wang B, Xu H, Gao ZQ, et al. Increased expression of vascular endothelial growth factor in hepatocellular carcinoma after transcatheter arterial chemoembolization. Acta Radiol 2008;49(5):523–9.
38. Lencioni R, Llovet JM, Han G, et al. Sorafenib or placebo plus TACE with doxorubicin-eluting beads for intermediate stage HCC: the SPACE trial. J Hepatol 2016;64(5):1090–8.
39. Kudo M, Han G, Finn RS, et al. Brivanib as adjuvant therapy to transarterial chemoembolization in patients with hepatocellular carcinoma: a randomized phase III trial. Hepatology 2014;60(5):1697–707.
40. Kudo M, Ueshima K, Ikeda M, et al. Randomised, multicentre prospective trial of transarterial chemoembolisation (TACE) plus sorafenib as compared with TACE alone in patients with hepatocellular carcinoma: TACTICS trial. Gut 2019. https://doi.org/10.1136/gutjnl-2019-318934.
41. Reig M, Rimola J, Torres F, et al. Postprogression survival of patients with advanced hepatocellular carcinoma: rationale for second-line trial design. Hepatology 2013;58(6):2023–31.
42. Park JW, Kim YJ, Kim DY, et al. Sorafenib with or without concurrent transarterial chemoembolization in patients with advanced hepatocellular carcinoma: the phase III STAH trial. J Hepatol 2019;70(4):684–91.
43. Ricke J, Sangro B, Amthauer H, et al. The impact of combining Selective Internal Radiation Therapy (SIRT) with Sorafenib on overall survival in patients with advanced hepatocellular carcinoma: the Soramic trial palliative cohort. J Hepatol 2018;68:S102.
44. Abou-Alfa GK, Johnson P, Knox JJ, et al. Doxorubicin plus sorafenib vs doxorubicin alone in patients with advanced hepatocellular carcinoma. JAMA 2010; 304(19):2154.
45. Abou-Alfa GK, Shi Q, Knox JJ, et al. Assessment of treatment with sorafenib plus doxorubicin vs sorafenib alone in patients with advanced hepatocellular

carcinoma: phase 3 CALGB 80802 randomized clinical trial. JAMA Oncol 2019; 5(11):1582–8.

46. Zhu AX, Rosmorduc O, Evans TRJ, et al. SEARCH: a phase III, randomized, double-blind, placebo-controlled trial of sorafenib plus erlotinib in patients with advanced hepatocellular carcinoma. J Clin Oncol 2015;33(6):559–66.

47. Kaseb AO, Garrett-Mayer E, Morris JS, et al. Efficacy of bevacizumab plus erlotinib for advanced hepatocellular carcinoma and predictors of outcome: final results of a phase II trial. Oncology 2012;82(2):67–74.

48. Thomas MB, Garrett-Mayer E, Anis M, et al. A randomized phase II open label multi-institution study of the combination of bevacizumab (B) and erlotinib (E) compared to sorafenib (S) in the first-line treatment of patients (pts) with advanced hepatocellular carcinoma (HCC). J Clin Oncol 2015;33(3_suppl):337.

49. Voron T, Marcheteau E, Pernot S, et al. Control of the immune response by pro-angiogenic factors. Front Oncol 2014. https://doi.org/10.3389/fonc.2014.00070.

50. Kato Y, Tabata K, Kimura T, et al. Lenvatinib plus anti-PD-1 antibody combination treatment activates CD8+ T cells through reduction of tumor-associated macrophage and activation of the interferon pathway. PLoS One 2019;14(2):e0212513.

51. Bruix J, Reig M, Sangro B. Assessment of treatment efficacy in hepatocellular carcinoma: response rate, delay in progression or none of them. J Hepatol 2017;66(6):1114–7.

52. Bruix J, da Fonseca LG, Reig M. Insights into the success and failure of systemic therapy for hepatocellular carcinoma. Nat Rev Gastroenterol Hepatol 2019; 16(10):617–30.

53. Ikeda K, Kudo M, Kawazoe S, et al. Phase 2 study of lenvatinib in patients with advanced hepatocellular carcinoma. J Gastroenterol 2017;52(4):512–9.

54. Wilhelm SM, Carter C, Tang LY, et al. BAY 43-9006 exhibits broad spectrum oral antitumor activity and targets the RAF/MEK/ERK pathway and receptor tyrosine kinases involved in tumor progression and angiogenesis. Cancer Res 2004; 64(19):7099–109.

55. Wilhelm SM, Dumas J, Adnane L, et al. Regorafenib (BAY 73-4506): a new oral multikinase inhibitor of angiogenic, stromal and oncogenic receptor tyrosine kinases with potent preclinical antitumor activity. Int J Cancer 2011;129(1):245–55.

56. Bruix J, Qin S, Merle P, et al. Regorafenib for patients with hepatocellular carcinoma who progressed on sorafenib treatment (RESORCE): a randomised, double-blind, placebo-controlled, phase 3 trial. Lancet 2017;389(10064):56–66.

57. Bruix J, Merle P, Granito A, et al. Hand-foot skin reaction (HFSR) and overall survival (OS) in the phase 3 RESORCE trial of regorafenib for treatment of hepatocellular carcinoma (HCC) progressing on sorafenib. J Clin Oncol 2018; 36(4_suppl):412.

58. Rankin EB, Giaccia AJ. The receptor tyrosine kinase AXL in cancer progression. Cancers (Basel) 2016;8(11). https://doi.org/10.3390/cancers8110103.

59. Firtina Karagonlar Z, Koc D, Iscan E, et al. Elevated hepatocyte growth factor expression as an autocrine c-Met activation mechanism in acquired resistance to sorafenib in hepatocellular carcinoma cells. Cancer Sci 2016;107(4):407–16.

60. Vennepureddy A, Singh P, Rastogi R, et al. Evolution of ramucirumab in the treatment of cancer—a review of literature. J Oncol Pharm Pract 2017;23(7):525–39.

61. Zhu AX, Park JO, Ryoo BY, et al. Ramucirumab versus placebo as second-line treatment in patients with advanced hepatocellular carcinoma following first-line therapy with sorafenib (REACH): a randomised, double-blind, multicentre, phase 3 trial. Lancet Oncol 2015;16(7):859–70.

62. Zhu AX, Kang Y-K, Yen C-J, et al. Ramucirumab after sorafenib in patients with advanced hepatocellular carcinoma and increased α-fetoprotein concentrations (REACH-2): a randomised, double-blind, placebo-controlled, phase 3 trial. Lancet Oncol 2019;20(2):282–96.

63. Llovet JM, Yen C-J, Finn RS, et al. Ramucirumab (RAM) for sorafenib intolerant patients with hepatocellular carcinoma (HCC) and elevated baseline alpha fetoprotein (AFP): outcomes from two randomized phase 3 studies (REACH, REACH2). J Clin Oncol 2019;37(15_suppl):4073.

64. Chen S, Cao Q, Wen W, et al. Targeted therapy for hepatocellular carcinoma: challenges and opportunities. Cancer Lett 2019;460:1–9.

65. Hu G, Zhang Y, Ouyang K, et al. In vivo acquired sorafenib-resistant patient-derived tumor model displays alternative angiogenic pathways, multi-drug resistance and chromosome instability. Oncol Lett 2018;16(3):3439–46.

66. Tai W-T, Cheng A-L, Shiau C-W, et al. Dovitinib induces apoptosis and overcomes sorafenib resistance in hepatocellular carcinoma through SHP-1-mediated inhibition of STAT3. Mol Cancer Ther 2012;11(2):452–63.

67. Morgan RL, Camidge DR. Reviewing RECIST in the era of prolonged and targeted therapy. J Thorac Oncol 2018;13(2):154–64.

68. Lencioni R, Llovet J. Modified RECIST (mRECIST) assessment for hepatocellular carcinoma. Semin Liver Dis 2010;30(01):052–60.

69. Galle PR, Forner A, Llovet JM, et al. EASL clinical practice guidelines: management of hepatocellular carcinoma. J Hepatol 2018;69(1):182–236.

70. Bosch J, Abraldes JG, Fernández M, et al. Hepatic endothelial dysfunction and abnormal angiogenesis: new targets in the treatment of portal hypertension. J Hepatol 2010;53(3):558–67.

71. Huang L, De Sanctis Y, Shan M, et al. Weak correlation of overall survival and time to progression in advanced hepatocellular carcinoma. J Clin Oncol 2017;35(4_suppl). abstract 233.

72. Finn RS, Qin S, Ikeda M, et al. Atezolizumab plus Bevacizumab in Unresectable Hepatocellular Carcinoma. N Engl J Med 2020;382(20):1894–905.

Immuno-oncology for Hepatocellular Carcinoma

The Present and the Future

Samantha A. Armstrong, MD, Aiwu Ruth He, MD, PhD*

KEYWORDS

- Hepatocellular carcinoma • Immunotherapy • Checkpoint inhibitor

KEY POINTS

- Systemic immunotherapy is expanding and changing the landscape of treatment for advanced-stage hepatocellular carcinoma.
- Frontline combination immunotherapy using synergistic mechanisms is proving to extend patient lives by bringing about increased and prolonged antitumor response.
- The role of immunotherapy in the setting of liver transplant remains uncertain; resolution of the potential lack of response and risk of adverse events leading to graft failure requires further investigation.

INTRODUCTION

Hepatocellular carcinoma (HCC), which arises from a background of chronic liver disease, is a highly lethal malignancy, with 42,810 new diagnoses and 30,160 cancer-related deaths estimated in the United States during 2020.[1] Worldwide, HCC is the fifth most common cancer and the third most common cause of cancer death.[2] Risk factors predisposing patients to HCC include hepatitis B virus (HBV), hepatitis C virus (HCV), hereditary hemochromatosis, and alcoholic as well as nonalcoholic cirrhosis.[3] Through research, we now have a better understanding of the molecular mechanisms of HCC, but there is still a paucity of therapeutic options, and local surgical resection still poses a significant risk of recurrence owing to underlying cirrhosis.[4] Liver transplantation has the lowest recurrence rates of 10% to 20%, but only in patients with early stage HCC.[5]

Sorafenib, an oral tyrosine kinase inhibitor (TKI), was the first systemic therapy for advanced HCC approved by the US Food and Drug Administration (FDA). Sorafenib was found to prolong median overall survival by approximately 3 months.[6,7] Sorafenib

Department of Medicine, Division of Hematology and Oncology, Lombardi Comprehensive Cancer Center, MedStar Georgetown University Hospital, 3800 Reservoir Road NW, Washington, DC, 20007, USA
* Corresponding author.
E-mail address: ARH29@GEORGETOWN.EDU

Clin Liver Dis 24 (2020) 739–753
https://doi.org/10.1016/j.cld.2020.07.007
1089-3261/20/© 2020 Elsevier Inc. All rights reserved.

remained the only FDA approved systemic therapy for 10 years until regorafenib and nivolumab were approved in 2017, closely followed by pembrolizumab in 2018 and cabozantinib and ramucirumab in 2019, for patients previously treated with sorafenib. In 2018, a sorafenib competitor, lenvatinib, was approved for first-line treatment of patients with HCC. By the end of 2019, 7 systemic therapeutic agents were available for the treatment of patients with HCC, but there are limited data on how to sequence these treatments for maximum survival benefit to patients. Five of the 7 approved treatments—namely, sorafenib, regorafenib, lenvatinib, cabozantinib, and ramucirumab—were shown to prolong patient survival by targeting tumor angiogenesis and signaling pathways for tumor proliferation. Nivolumab and pembrolizumab are immune checkpoint inhibitors that overcome tumor immune evasion. The novel mechanism of action of immune checkpoint inhibitors and their durable response has reshaped the treatment landscape for HCC.

IMMUNOTHERAPY RATIONALE

HCC is a potentially highly immune-responsive tumor, given its origins from an inflammatory background, making immunotherapy more likely to be effective. There have been cases of spontaneous remission of HCC after removal of patients from therapy, indicating a delayed antitumor immune response, occurring only after removal of immunosuppression.[8–10] A strong relationship between HCC and the patient's immune system is seen for cases that have a high tumor proinflammatory T-cell infiltrate, a high tumor CD4:CD8 ratio, a decreased risk of recurrence, and improved disease-free survival and overall survival.[11–14]

The liver has a natural immune tolerance—through upregulation of cytotoxic T-lymphocyte-associated protein-4 (CTLA-4) and programmed cell death protein-1 (PD-1)—to avoid unnecessary inflammation from antigens in the portal venous system. This may lead to impaired antitumor response in HCC. Superior disease-free survival and overall survival are seen in HCC tumors with lower levels of PD-1 and programmed death-ligand 1 and 2 (PD-L1 and PD-L2)[15,16]; hence, immune checkpoint blockade is hypothesized to overcome immune tolerance in the liver leading to a robust antitumor response where other treatments have failed.

Immune Checkpoint Inhibitor Monotherapy in Hepatocellular Carcinoma

Durable response to anti–programmed cell death protein-1 therapy

An early signal of the antitumor activity of immune checkpoint inhibitors in HCC was demonstrated in a phase II study of tremelimumab in patients with advanced disease.[17] Tremelimumab is a monoclonal antibody that binds to CTLA-4 expressed on the surface of activated T lymphocytes, resulting in inhibition of B7-CTLA-4–mediated downregulation of T-cell activation. Study investigators evaluated 21 patients treated with 15 mg/kg intravenous (IV) tremelimumab every 90 days for about 2 cycles. Tumor burden was decreased in 2 patients, and disease stabilization was observed in 11 patients, which lasted for more than 1 year. Concerns about liver toxicity and/or reactivation of viral hepatitis led to additional testing of immune checkpoint inhibitors in patients with HCC; however, the anti–PD-1 agent nivolumab was used for this testing owing to its better safety profile. The BMS-initiated dose escalation and expansion trial (CheckMate 040) tested nivolumab in adults (≥18 years) with histologically confirmed advanced HCC with or without HCV or HBV infection (NCT01658878). Patients received IV nivolumab at doses of 0.1 to 10 mg/kg every 2 weeks in the dose-escalation phase (3 + 3 design) of this trial. Then, in the dose expansion phase, 3 mg/kg nivolumab was administered every

2 weeks to 4 different patient cohorts: sorafenib untreated or intolerant without viral hepatitis, sorafenib progressors without viral hepatitis, HCV infected, and HBV infected. The primary end points were safety and tolerability and objective response rate (Response Evaluation Criteria In Solid Tumors version 1.1). The objective response rate was 20% (95% confidence interval [CI], 15–26) in patients treated with nivolumab in the dose expansion phase and 15% (95% CI 6–28) in the dose-escalation phase. The median duration of response was 17 months and the median overall survival was 15 months. The adverse events (AEs) were comparable with those experienced in patients with other types of cancer receiving nivolumab treatment.[18–20] Based on data from this trial, the FDA granted accelerated approval of nivolumab for patients with advanced HCC who have progressed or are intolerable to sorafenib treatment, pending confirmation of survival benefit in a randomized phase III study.

The CheckMate 040 study details are outlined in **Fig. 1**.

Negative phase III studies of nivolumab and pembrolizumab

In CheckMate 459, an international, multicenter, randomized phase III trial, 743 treatment-naïve patients with HCC were randomized to standard sorafenib (400 mg twice daily) or nivolumab (240 mg every 2 weeks).[21] Although study results did not meet statistical significance, the overall survival was improved with nivolumab over sorafenib (16.4 months vs 14.7 months; hazard ratio [HR], 0.85; 95% CI, 0.72–1.02; P = .0752).[21] The median progression-free survival was similar between the 2 groups, but the response rate for nivolumab was higher than sorafenib at (15% vs 7%).[21]

Investigators in the phase III KEYNOTE-240 trial randomized 408 patients at a 2:1 ratio to pembrolizumab (200 mg IV every 3 weeks) + best supportive care versus placebo (every 3 weeks) + best supportive care for up to 35 cycles or until disease progression or unacceptable toxicity. The objective response rate was 16.9% (95% CI, 12.7%–21.8%) for pembrolizumab versus 2.2% (95% CI, 0.5%–6.4%) for placebo (nominal one-sided P = .00001). Pembrolizumab responses were durable (median duration of response, 13.8 months [95% CI, 1.5–23.6+]), and although overall survival and progression-free survival were improved, prespecified statistical criteria were such that significance was not reached (overall survival, 13.6 vs 10.6 months [hazard ratio, 0.78; 1-sided P = .0238]; progression-free survival, 4.2 vs 3.8 months [hazard ratio, 0.78; 1-sided P = .0209]).[22]

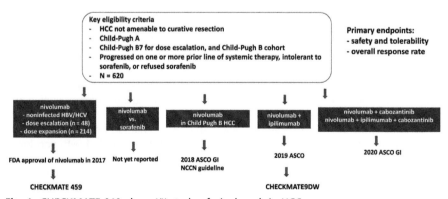

Fig. 1. CHECKMATE 040 phase I/II study of nivolumab in HCC.

Interestingly, the overall survival was higher in the control arms of both of these negative studies compared with the control arms from other earlier studies. Taking the CheckMate 459 study (2019), the median overall survival was 14.7 months in the sorafenib control arm, which is higher than the 10.2 months observed in the original SHARP study (2007).[6] Taking the KEYNOTE-240 trial, the median overall survival for patients receiving best supportive care after first-line sorafenib treatment was higher (10.6 months) than that in the RESOURCE study of second-line regorafenib (7.8 months)—the study that led to the approval of regorafenib in this setting.

Patient demographics (key prognostic parameters) were similar between the CheckMate 459 and SHARP trials. However, the quantity and quality of second-line therapies have changed from supportive care or continuation of sorafenib treatment to an additional TKI as well as immune therapy. In studies, it follows that these second-line treatments may significantly build on overall survival measures from first-line treatments.

Also, considering the KEYNOTE 240 study and its negative findings, the use of dual co-primary study end points of progression-free survival and overall survival, and 2 interim analyses resulted in stricter prespecified P values compared with a single primary study end point and fewer interim analyses. Hence, these phase III studies likely still demonstrate meaningful clinical benefit from experimental treatment, even though they do not statistically meet the primary study end points.

Immune Checkpoint Inhibitor Combination Therapy in Hepatocellular Carcinoma

Early promising results from anti–cytotoxic T-lymphocyte-associated protein-4 and anti–programmed cell death protein-1 combined therapy

After it was found that the anti–CTLA-4 and anti–PD-1 therapies acted synergistically and increased response rates in patients with metastatic melanoma, advanced renal cell carcinoma, and metastatic colorectal cancer with deficient mismatch repair/microsatellite instability—high, studies of this type of combination therapy ensued in patients with HCC,[23–25] with the hope of improving on monotherapy results. Two combinations, nivolumab plus ipilimumab and durvalumab plus tremelimumab, were evaluated in HCC with promising results. Ipilimumab is another anti–CTLA-4 antibody and durvalumab is an antibody raised against PD-L1. The safety and efficacy of the durvalumab plus tremelimumab combination compared with either drug alone was evaluated in a phase I/II study.[26] Forty patients with HCC were enrolled (11 HBV positive, 9 HCV positive, 20 uninfected); 30% had no prior systemic therapy and 93% were Child-Pugh class A. The confirmed response rate was 15%. The most common (≥15%) treatment-related AEs were fatigue (20%), increased alanine aminotransferase (18%), pruritus (18%), and increased aspartate aminotransferase (15%). The most common grade 3 or higher related AE was asymptomatic increased aspartate aminotransferase (10%). The combination is being investigated in the phase III HIMALAYA trial (NCT03298451), which is enrolling patients with unresectable, advanced HCC who have not previously received systemic treatment and are ineligible for locoregional therapy. The HIMALAYA trial is comparing sorafenib to durvalumab alone and in combination with tremelimumab (in 2 different combination regimens) with a primary end point of overall survival (NCT03298451).

The Checkmate 040 trial opened a nivolumab plus ipilimumab treatment cohort.[27] Patients with advanced stage HCC (n = 148) who had been treated with sorafenib were randomized to 3 nivolumab and ipilimumab dose and schedule variation arms. The objective response rate was found to be around 30%, with any ipilimumab plus nivolumab regimen—twice that of nivolumab monotherapy at comparable doses.[27] A median overall survival of 23 months was seen in patients who received nivolumab

(1mg/kg) plus ipilumumab (3mg/kg) every 3 weeks for 4 doses followed by nivolumab 240mg every 2 weeks (arm A), with a rate of 61% median overall survival at 12 months and 48% median overall survival at 24 months.[27] The reported treatment-related AEs were consistent with the known safety profiles of the individual components of the combination treatments and were reversible.

The doubled response rate and prolonged median overall survival in patients receiving second-line systemic therapy for advanced HCC supports the FDA approval of the combination of nivolumab and ipilimumab in patients with HCC who have been treated with sorafenib. Moreover, the ongoing, randomized, phase III CheckMate 9DW trial is treating patients with the combination of ipilimumab (1 mg/kg) plus nivolumab (3 mg/kg) every 3 weeks for 4 doses followed by maintenance nivolumab at a straight dose of 480 mg every 4 weeks and comparing the response of these patients with those receiving sorafenib or lenvatinib in the frontline setting. The primary end point is overall survival (NCT04039607) (**Table 1**).

Combinations of immunotherapy and antiangiogenesis inhibitors

Strong scientific rationale and emerging clinical data suggest that the combined vascular endothelial growth factor (VEGF)/PD-L1 blockade may be clinically beneficial in patients with HCC.

Bevacizumab and atezolizumab combination

It is known that HCC is a highly vascularized tumor and that several proangiogenic factors play a role in HCC pathogenesis. For example, in HCC, increased VEGF correlates with vascular density, tumor invasiveness, metastasis, and poor prognosis.[28–30] The VEGF pathway also plays a crucial role in exerting and maintaining an immunosuppressive tumor microenvironment through several mechanisms. The VEGF inhibitor bevacizumab can restore and/or maintain the antigen presentation capacity of dendritic cells, leading to enhanced T-cell infiltration in tumors.[31,32] In addition to increased trafficking of T cells into tumors,[33] several publications have illustrated that anti-VEGF therapies can also decrease the frequency of myeloid-derived suppressor cells, decrease production of suppressive cytokines, and lower expression of inhibitory checkpoints on $CD8^+$ T cells in tumors.[34,35] Therefore, the immunomodulatory effect of bevacizumab is expected to increase CD8-positive T-cell recruitment, and relieve intratumoral immunosuppression, thereby boosting the effects of immune checkpoint inhibitors.

The combination of bevacizumab and atezolizumab, an anti–PD-L1 antibody, was first tested in patients with HCC in a phase I multicenter study GO30140. In this study, systemic treatment-naïve patients with locally advanced or metastatic HCC received 1200 mg of atezolizumab plus 15 mg/kg of bevacizumab every 3 weeks. Investigators found that 23 of the 73 efficacy-evaluable patients (31.5%; 95% CI, 21.1–43.4) achieved confirmed objective responses, and 1 patient (1.4%) achieved a durable complete response. The median progression-free survival was 14.9 months (95% CI, 7.4–NE). No new safety signals related to the combination therapy were identified beyond the established safety profile for each individual agent.[36]

The follow-up phase III, open-label, randomized IMbrave 150 trial is comparing combination atezolizumab (1200 mg IV every 3 weeks) plus bevacizumab (15 mg/kg IV every 3 weeks) to oral sorafenib (400 mg twice a day) in patients with unresectable advanced HCC (NCT03434379). The primary end points include overall survival and progression-free survival, and the trial completed enrollment in December 2018. All primary end points were reportedly met at a median of 8.6 months of follow-up: the median overall survival was 13.2 months in the sorafenib arm but not yet met in the

Table 1
Clinical trials on HCC treatment approved by FDA or pending FDA approval

Trial	Phase	Therapy	Mechanism	Lines of Therapy	Outcome
SHARP NCT00105443	3	Sorafenib	Inhibitor of VEGFR, PDGFR, and RAF kinases	First	Overall survival of 10.7 mo vs overall survival of 7.9 mo for placebo
REFLECT NCT01761266	3	Lenvatinib	Inhibitor of VEGFR1, 2 and 3, fibroblast growth factor 1, 2, 3 and 4, PDGFR alpha, c-Kit, and the RET proto-oncogene	First	Overall survival of 13.6 mo vs overall survival of 12.3 mo for Sorafenib
RESORCE NCT01774344	3	Regorafenib	Inhibitor of VEGFR2-TIE2 tyrosine kinase	Second	Overall survival of 10.6 mo vs overall survival of 7.8 mo for placebo
CELESTIAL NCT01908426	3	Cabozantinib	Inhibitor of c-Met, VEGFR2, AXL, and RET	Second	Overall survival of 10.2 mo vs overall survival of 8.0 mo for placebo
REACH-2 NCT02435433	3	Ramucirumab	Inhibitor of VEGFR2	Second	Overall survival of 8.5 mo vs overall survival of 7.3 mo for placebo
CHECKMATE 040 NCT01658878	1/2	Nivolumab	Immune checkpoint inhibitor	Second	Response rate of 15%, 4% complete response
KEYNOTE 224 NCT02702414	2	Pembrolizumab	Immune checkpoint inhibitor	Second	Response rate of 17%, 1% complete response
CHECKMATE 040 NCT01658878	1/2	Nivolumab + ipilimumab	Immune checkpoint inhibitor	Second	Response rate of 32%, 8% complete response; median overall survival of 23 mo
IMBRAVE 150 NCT03434379	3	Bevacizumab + atezolizumab	Immune checkpoint inhibitor	First	Median overall survival not estimable (NE) compared with 13.2 mo with sorafenib (P = .0006). Median progression-free survival 6.8 mo vs 4.5 mo with sorafenib (P<.0001).

Abbreviations: PDGFR, platelet-derived growth factor receptor; VEGFR, vascular endothelial growth factor receptor.

experimental arm (HR, 0.58; 95% CI, 0.42–0.79; P = .0006); the median progression-free survival was 4.5 months versus 6.8 months (HR, 0.59; 95% CI, 0.47–0.76; P<.0001).[37] Response rates from the combination therapy were double that of sorafenib (objective response rate, 27% vs 12%; P<.0001). There were no new safety signals identified and overall this novel combination has the potential to be practice changing.

Tyrosine kinase inhibitors and immune checkpoint inhibitor combination

Multitargeted TKIs such as lenvatinib can inhibit cancer cell proliferation and modulate the tumor immune environment. There lies a rationale for the combination of lenvatinib with immune checkpoint inhibitors for the management of HCC.

Multi-TKI lenvatinib inhibits VEGF receptors 1, 2, and 3; fibroblast growth factors 1, 2, 3, and 4; platelet-derived growth factor-α; c-Kit; and RET. The REFLECT trial found that in patients with advanced HCC, lenvatinib provides a similar overall survival improvement to sorafenib, leading to FDA approval of lenvatinib in systemic treatment-naïve patients with advanced HCC. The phase I trial of lenvatinib plus pembrolizumab revealed grade 3 or higher treatment-related AEs in 60% of patients, with only 5% requiring discontinuation of therapy, and a preliminary response rate of 42%.[38] The combination of lenvatinib and pembrolizumab is being compared with first-line lenvatinib monotherapy in the double-blind, randomized LEAP002 study. The primary end points are progression-free survival and overall survival (NCT03713593).

Multi-TKI cabozantinib inhibits c-Met, VEGF receptor 2, AXL, and RET, showing prolongation of overall survival in patients with advanced HCC who had received sorafenib or additional systemic therapy in the Celestrial study. The phase III COSMIC-312 trial is now investigating the benefits of cabozantinib with and without atezolizumab compared with sorafenib in patients with advanced untreated HCC (NCT03755791).

The expanding landscape of immunotherapy use in HCC is reviewed in **Fig. 2.**

Triple combination

A CHECKMATE 040 study cohort enrolled 35 patients to receive nivolumab (3 mg/kg every 2 weeks), ipilimumab (1 mg/kg every 6 weeks), and cabozantinib (40 mg daily).[39] Early promising efficacy data are as follows: response rate, 29%; disease control rate, 80%; progression-free survival, 6.8 months; and median duration of response and median overall survival, not yet reached at 19 months follow-up. The rate of treatment-related grade 3 or 4 AEs was 71% and manageable (17% hypertension, 23% increase in aspartate aminotransferase, 17% increase in alanine aminotransferase, and 17% increase in lipase).

Management of adverse event of immune checkpoint inhibitors

Immune checkpoint inhibitors are well-tolerated by patients with HCC. When nivolumab was compared with sorafenib in the randomized phase III study (Keynote 459 study), grade 3 and 4 treatment-related AEs were reported in 81 patients (22%) in the nivolumab arm compared with 179 (49%) in the sorafenib arm.[21] Treatment discontinuation owing to an AE was reported for 16 patients (4%) receiving nivolumab versus 29 (8%) patients receiving sorafenib. Patient-reported findings suggest that those in the nivolumab arm experienced a better quality of life.

Immune-mediated AEs from pembrolizumab therapy were reported at a rate of 18.3%, and the most commonly observed toxicities were hypothyroidism, hyperthyroidism, and pneumonitis.[40] These events were grade 3 or higher in 7.2% of patients, and approximately 90% of these were resolved. Just over 8% of patients received steroids for possible immune-mediated AEs.

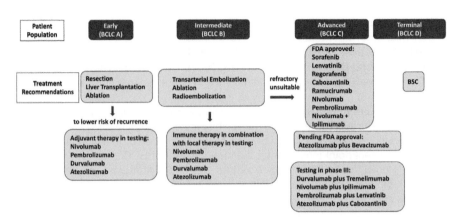

Fig. 2. The expanding landscape of immunotherapy use in patients with HCC.

The improved efficacy observed from the combination of nivolumab and ipilimumab is at the apparent cost of increased toxicity compared with single-agent immune checkpoint inhibitor therapy. As shown in Checkmate 040 study (Nivolumab package inset, Princeton NJ, Bristol Myers Squibb Company, 2020), 59% of patients receiving nivolumab and ipilimumab experienced grade 3 or higher AEs. Of these AEs, the following occurred at a rate of 4% or more: pyrexia, diarrhea, anemia, increased aspartate aminotransferase, adrenal insufficiency, ascites, esophageal variceal hemorrhage, hyponatremia, increased blood bilirubin, and pneumonitis. Adverse reactions led to treatment delay in 65% of patients and treatment discontinuation in 29%. A handful of patients (8.2%) received high-dose corticosteroids for a median of 1.6 weeks (range, 0.4–147.6 weeks). Most of the immune-mediated AEs could be resolved, including 80% of pneumonitis, 100% of colitis, 90% of hepatitis, and 82% of rashes. It was concluded that adverse reactions from the combination of nivolumab and ipilimumab are common but manageable. Physicians and other medical staff taking care of patients with HCC receiving immune checkpoint inhibitors need to be vigilant about monitoring for and managing patient AEs in an efficient and timely manner, especially if combination therapy is the chosen treatment.

Expanding on immune checkpoint treatment combinations

Local therapies including radiofrequency ablation, transarterial chemoembolization, transarterial radioembolization, and microwave embolization stimulate tumor destruction, the release of tumor antigens, and ultimately increase the production of tumor-specific T cells.[41,42] The combination of immune checkpoint blockade with these therapies activates CD4 and CD8 T cells and enhances antitumor activity.[43] Emerging clinical trials evaluating the combination of local therapy and immune checkpoint treatment are under way.

IMMUNOTHERAPY USE IN TRANSPLANT CANDIDATES

Adjuvant immunotherapy after resection or ablation is being explored in the Emerald-2 (NCT03847428), CheckMate 9Dx (NCT03383458), and KEYNOTE 937 (NCT03867084) trials, and results are pending.

One issue arising from the unique transplant-eligible population of patients with HCC is the role of immunotherapy before or after liver transplantation and potential complications that may arise. The HCC liver transplant population has been excluded

Table 2
Cases of immunotherapy use after liver transplant

Case	Reason for Liver Transplant	Immuno-Suppression	Immunotherapy	Reason for Immunotherapy	Response of Malignancy to Immunotherapy	Toxicity to Transplant
Morales et al,[45] 2015	Fulminant liver failure, HCV, HCC	Tacrolimus and mycophenolate mofetil	Ipilimumab	Cutaneous melanoma	Partial response	Mild liver enzyme elevation, no evidence of graft rejection
Ranganath et al,[48] 2015	Cirrhosis from alpha-1 antitrypsin deficiency	Tacrolimus	Ipilimumab	Cutaneous melanoma	No response	No AEs or graft rejection
Schvartsman et al,[49] 2017	Biliary atresia	Tacrolimus	Pembrolizumab	Cutaneous melanoma	Complete response	Hepatitis 10 d after second dose requiring steroids and mycophenolate
De Toni et al,[50] 2017	HCC	Tacrolimus	Nivolumab	Recurrent HCC	Partial response	No AEs or graft rejection
Friend et al,[51] 2017	HCC	Sirolimus	Nivolumab	Recurrent HCC	NA	Elevated liver enzymes, acute and chronic graft rejection leading to death
	HCC	Tacrolimus	Nivolumab	Recurrent HCC	NA	Elevated liver enzymes, acute graft rejection leading to death
Rai et al,[52] 2017	NA	NA	Pembrolizumab	Melanoma	NA	Acute graft rejection leading to death
Varkaris et al,[53] 2017	HCC	Tacrolimus	Pembrolizumab	Recurrent HCC	Disease Progression	No AEs or graft rejection
Kuo et al,[54–63] 2018	HCC	Sirolimus and mycophenolate mofetil	Ipilimumab followed by pembrolizumab at time of progression	Malignant peripheral nerve sheath tumor-like melanoma	Partial response to both agents	No AEs or graft rejection

(continued on next page)

Table 2
(continued)

Case	Reason for Liver Transplant	Immuno-Suppression	Immunotherapy	Reason for Immunotherapy	Response of Malignancy to Immunotherapy	Toxicity to Transplant
DeLeon et al,[47] 2018	HCC	Tacrolimus	Nivolumab	HCC	Disease progression	No AEs or graft regression
	HCC	Everolimus and mycophenolate mofetil	Pembrolizumab	Melanoma	Complete response	No AEs or graft regression
	HCC	Mycophenolate mofetil and sirolimus	Nivolumab	HCC	Disease Progression	No AEs or graft regression
	HCC	Tacrolimus	Nivolumab	HCC	Disease progression	No AEs or graft regression
	HCC	Tacrolimus	Nivolumab	HCC	NA	No AEs or graft regression
	HCC	Sirolimus	Nivolumab	HCC	NA	Acute graft rejection
	Cholangiocarcinoma	Mycophenolate Mofetil and prednisone	Pembrolizumab	Melanoma	NA	Acute graft rejection

from clinical trials testing the safety and efficacy of immunotherapy because of their need for chronic immunosuppression and concern surrounding the induction of acute organ rejection and ultimately organ failure. Although no large trial has been or is being conducted in this specific population, there have been conflicting published case reports. On the one hand, successful treatment with immunotherapy after organ transplant has been reported, with a trend toward reduced toxicity if the transplant was received several years before immunotherapy and the patient was able to tolerate a reduction in immunosuppressant (antirejection) medication,[44–46]; but on the other hand, rapid acute transplant rejection in the setting of single agent or combination immunotherapy has been seen within 5 days of treatment initiation.[44] One retrospective pilot evaluation of immunotherapy use after liver transplantation involved 7 patients, 2 of whom rejected their organ within approximately 24 days of initiation of immunotherapy.[47] **Table 2** highlights cases of immunotherapy use after liver transplantation and their specific outcomes.

POTENTIAL BIOMARKERS

Currently, there are no confirmed roles for molecular biomarkers in HCC to guide specific targeted therapies or identify specific subgroups likely to respond, or not respond to immunotherapy. Biomarkers of interest include tumor mutational burden and PD-L1. Tumors with the highest rates of mutations per megabase include melanoma, non-small cell lung cancer, and bladder cancer,[64,65] and all tend to respond to immunotherapy. However, the value of tumor mutational burden as a predictive biomarker for immunotherapy response in HCC has not yet been explored, and in one retrospective study of 1170 HCC samples, it was found that a higher tumor mutational burden was associated with significantly worse progression-free survival and overall survival ($P<.0072$ and $P<.0001$, respectively).[66] Further study is needed. In the CheckMate 459 trial, higher response rates were seen with nivolumab in tumors that expressed PD-L1.[21] Tumors with less than 1% PD-L1 expression had a 12% response versus a 28% response in those with greater than 1% PD-L1 expression.[21] The role of PD-L1 in predicting HCC response to checkpoint inhibitors needs to be further explored.

SUMMARY

HCC holds a high patient mortality rate despite multiple local and systemic treatments. Immunotherapy is currently changing the landscape of treatment for patients with advanced disease, but in patients who have undergone transplantation or are transplant candidates, the use of immune therapy remains controversial. In some cases, there is a reported absence of adverse reactions, whereas in other cases, life-threatening acute graft rejections are observed. Further research is needed in all HCC scenarios to help guide the sequencing of treatments and improve strategies for patient selection and prognosis.

ACKNOWLEDGMENTS

The authors would like to thank Marion L. Hartley, PhD, for her edits and suggestions during the writing of this review.

DISCLOSURE

A.R. He received a research grant from Merck and Genentech; serves on the speaker's bureau for Bayer, BMS, Eisai, and Exelixis; and served on the advisory board for Merck, Genentech, and AstraZeneca. S. Armstrong has nothing to disclose.

REFERENCES

1. Siegel RL, Miller KD, Jemal A. Cancer statistics, 2020. CA Cancer J Clin 2020; 70(1). https://doi.org/10.3322/caac.21590.
2. Ferlay J, Colombet M, Soerjomataram I, et al. Estimating the global cancer incidence and mortality in 2018: GLOBOCAN sources and methods. Int J Cancer 2018;144(8):1941–53.
3. Fattovich G, Stroffolini T, Zagni I, et al. Hepatocellular carcinoma in cirrhosis: incidence and risk factors. Gastroenterology 2004;127:S35–50.
4. Portolani N, Coniglio A, Ghidoni S, et al. Early and late recurrence after liver resection for hepatocellular carcinoma: prognostic and therapeutic implications. Ann Surg 2006;243:229–35.
5. Vivarelli M, Cucchetti A, La Barba G, et al. Liver transplantation for hepatocellular carcinoma under calcineurin inhibitors: reassessment of risk factors for tumor recurrence. Ann Surg 2008;248:857–62.
6. Llovet JM, Ricci S, Mazzaferro V, et al, SHARP Investigators Study Group. Sorafenib in advanced hepatocellular carcinoma. N Engl J Med 2008;359:378–90.
7. Cheng AL, Kang YK, Chen Z, et al. Efficacy and safety of sorafenib in patients in the Asia-Pacific region with advanced hepatocellular carcinoma: a phase III randomised, double-blind, placebo-controlled trial. Lancet Oncol 2009;10(1):25–34.
8. Parks AL, McWhirter RM, Evason K, et al. Cases of spontaneous tumor regression in hepatobiliary cancers: implications for immunotherapy? J Gastrointest Cancer 2015;46:161–5.
9. Iwanaga T. Studies on cases of spontaneous regression of cancer in Japan in 2011, and of hepatic carcinoma, lung cancer and pulmonary metastases in the world between 2006 and 2011. Gan To Kagaku Ryoho 2013;40:1475–87.
10. Kumar A, Le DT. Hepatocellular carcinoma regression after cessation of immunosuppressive therapy. J Clin Oncol 2016;34(10):e90–2.
11. Unitt E, Marshall A, Gelson W, et al. Tumour lymphocytic infiltrate and recurrence of hepatocellular carcinoma following liver transplantation. J Hepatol 2006;45:246–53.
12. Gao Q, Qiu SJ, Fan J, Zhou J, Wang XY, Xiao YS, Xu Y, Li YW, Tang ZY. Intratumoral balance of regulatory and cytotoxic T cells is associated with prognosis of hepatocellular carcinoma after resection. J Clin Oncol 2007;25(18):2586–93.
13. Flecken T, Schmidt N, Hild S, et al. Immunodominance and functional alterations of tumor-associated antigen-specific CD8+ T-cell responses in hepatocellular carcinoma. Hepatology 2014;59(4):1415–26.
14. Liang J, Ding T, Guo ZW, et al. Expression pattern of tumour-associated antigens in hepatocellular carcinoma: association with immune infiltration and disease progression. Br J Cancer 2013;109:1031–9.
15. Jung HI, Jeong D, Ji S, et al. Overexpression of PD-L1 and PD-L2 is associated with poor prognosis in patients with hepatocellular carcinoma. Cancer Res Treat 2017;49(1):246–54.
16. Liao H, Chen W, Dai Y, et al. Expression of programmed cell death-ligands in hepatocellular carcinoma: correlation with immune microenvironment and survival outcomes. Front Oncol 2019;9:883.
17. Melero I, Sangro B, Riezu-Boj JI, et al. Abstract 4387: antiviral and antitumoral effects of the anti-CTLA4 agent tremelimumab in patients with hepatocellular carcinoma (HCC) and chronic hepatitis C virus (HCV) infection: results from a phase II clinical trial. Immunology 2012. https://doi.org/10.1158/1538-7445.am2012-4387.

18. El-Khoueiry AB, Sangro B, Yau T, et al. Nivolumab in patients with advanced hepatocellular carcinoma (CheckMate 040): an open-label, non-comparative, phase 1/2 dose escalation and expansion trial. Lancet 2017;389(10088): 2492–502.

19. Kudo M, Matilla A, Santoro A, et al. Checkmate-040: nivolumab (NIVO) in patients (Pts) with advanced hepatocellular carcinoma (AHCC) and child-Pugh B (CPB) status. J Clin Oncol 2019;37(4_suppl):327.

20. Kambhampati S, Bauer KE, Bracci PM, et al. "Nivolumab in patients with advanced hepatocellular carcinoma and child-Pugh Class B cirrhosis: safety and clinical outcomes in a retrospective case series. Cancer 2019;125(18):3234–41.

21. Yau T, Park JW, Finn RS, et al. CheckMate 459: a randomized, multi-center phase III study of nivolumab (NIVO) vs sorafenib (SOR) as first-line (1L) treatment in patients (Pts) with advanced hepatocellular carcinoma (AHCC). Ann Oncol 2019;30: v874–5.

22. Finn RS, Ryoo B-Y, Merle P, et al. Results of KEYNOTE-240: phase 3 study of pembrolizumab (Pembro) vs best supportive care (BSC) for second line therapy in advanced hepatocellular carcinoma (HCC). J Clin Oncol 2019;37(15_suppl): 4004.

23. Wolchok JD, Chiarion-Sileni V, Gonzalez R, et al. Overall survival with combined Nivolumab and Ipilimumab in advanced melanoma. N Engl J Med 2017;377(14): 1345–56.

24. Motzer RJ, Tannir NM, McDermott DF, et al. Nivolumab plus ipilimumab versus sunitinib in advanced renal-cell carcinoma. N Engl J Med 2018;378(14):1277–90.

25. Overman MJ, Lonardi S, Wong KYM, et al. Nivolumab (NIVO) + low-dose ipilimumab (IPI) in previously treated patients (pts) with microsatellite instability-high/mismatch repair-deficient (MSI-H/dMMR) metastatic colorectal cancer (mCRC): long-term follow-up. J Clin Oncol 2019;37(4_suppl):635.

26. Kelley RK, Abou-Alfa GK, Bendell JC, et al. Phase I/II study of durvalumab and tremelimumab in patients with unresectable hepatocellular carcinoma (HCC): phase I safety and efficacy analyses. J Clin Oncol 2017;35(15_suppl):4073.

27. Yau T, Kang Y-K, Kim T-Y, et al. Nivolumab (NIVO) + ipilimumab (IPI) combination therapy in patients (pts) with advanced hepatocellular carcinoma (AHCC): results from CheckMate 040. J Clin Oncol 2019;37(15_suppl):4012.

28. Boige V, Malka D, Bourredjem A, et al. Efficacy, safety, and biomarkers of single-agent bevacizumab therapy in patients with advanced hepatocellular carcinoma. Oncologist 2012;17(8):1063–72.

29. Frenette C, Gish R. Targeted systemic therapies for hepatocellular carcinoma: clinical perspectives, challenges and implications. World J Gastroenterol 2012; 18(6):498–506.

30. Motz GT, Santoro SP, Wang LP, et al. Tumor endothelium FasL establishes a selective immune barrier promoting tolerance in tumors. Nat Med 2014;20(6): 607–15.

31. Oelkrug C, Ramage JM. Enhancement of T Cell recruitment and infiltration into tumours. Clin Exp Immunol 2014;178(1):1–8.

32. Wallin JJ, Bendell JC, Funke R, et al. Atezolizumab in combination with bevacizumab enhances antigen-specific T-cell migration in metastatic renal cell carcinoma. Nat Commun 2016;7:12624.

33. Manning EA, Ullman JG, Leatherman JM, et al. A vascular endothelial growth factor receptor-2 inhibitor enhances antitumor immunity through an immune-based mechanism. Clin Cancer Res 2007;13(13):3951–9.

34. Roland CL, Lynn KD, Toombs JE, et al. Cytokine levels correlate with immune cell infiltration after anti-VEGF therapy in preclinical mouse models of breast cancer. PLoS One 2009;4(11):e7669.

35. Voron T, Colussi O, Marcheteau E, et al. VEGF-A modulates expression of inhibitory checkpoints on CD8+ T cells in tumors. J Exp Med 2015;212(2):139–48.

36. Lee M, Ryoo B-Y, Hsu C-H, et al. Randomised efficacy and safety results for atezolizumab (Atezo) + bevacizumab (Bev) in patients (pts) with previously untreated, unresectable hepatocellular carcinoma (HCC). Presented at 2019 ESMO Congress. Barcelona, Spain, September 27 to October 1, 2019. Abstract LBA39.

37. Cheng AL, Qin S, Ikeda M, et al. LBA3 - IMbrave150: efficacy and safety results from a ph III study evaluating atezolizumab (atezo) + bevacizumab (bev) vs sorafenib (Sor) as first treatment (tx) for patients (pts) with unresectable hepatocellular carcinoma (HCC). ESMO Asia 2019. Singapore, November 22-24, 2019.

38. Ikeda M, Sung MW, Kudo M, et al. A phase 1b trial of lenvatinib (LEN) plus pembrolizumab (PEM) in patients (pts) with unresectable hepatocellular carcinoma (UHCC). J Clin Oncol 2018;36(15_suppl):4076.

39. Yau T, Zagonel V, Santoro A, et al. Nivolumab (NIVO) + ipilimumab (IPI) + cabozantinib (CABO) combination therapy in patients (pts) with advanced hepatocellular carcinoma (aHCC): results from CheckMate 040. J Clin Oncol 2020;38(suppl 4). abstr 478.

40. Zhu AX, Knox JJ, Kudo M, et al. KEYNOTE-224: phase II study of pembrolizumab in patients with previously treated advanced hepatocellular carcinoma. J Clin Oncol 2017;35(4_suppl):TPS504.

41. Ali MY, Grimm CF, Ritter M, et al. Activation of dendritic cells by local ablation of hepatocellular carcinoma. J Hepatol 2005;43(5):817–22.

42. Dromi SA, Walsh MP, Herby S, et al. Radiofrequency ablation induces antigen-presenting cell infiltration and amplification of weak tumor-induced immunity. Radiology 2009;251:58–66.

43. Aerts M, Benteyn D, Van Vlierberghe H, et al. Current status and perspectives of immune-based therapies for hepatocellular carcinoma. World J Gastroenterol 2016;22(1):253–61.

44. Chae YK, Galvez C, Anker JF, et al. Cancer immunotherapy in a neglected population: the current use and future of T-cell-mediated checkpoint inhibitors in organ transplant patients. Cancer Treat Rev 2018;63:116–21. Available at: https://www.ncbi.nlm.nih.gov/pubmed/29276997.

45. Morales RE, Shoushtari AN, Walsh MM, et al. Safety and efficacy of ipilimumab to treat advanced melanoma in the setting of liver transplantation. J Immunother Cancer 2015;3:22.

46. Lipson EJ, Bodell MA, Kraus ES, et al. Successful administration of ipilimumab to two kidney transplantation patients with metastatic melanoma. J Clin Oncol 2014; 32(19):e69–71.

47. DeLeon T, Salomao M, Bashar A. Pilot evaluation of PD-1 inhibition in metastatic cancer patients with liver transplantations: the Mayo Clinic experience. J Clin Oncol 2018;(suppl 4S). abstr 328.

48. Ranganath HA, Panella TJ. Administration of ipilimumab to a liver transplant recipient with unresectable metastatic melanoma. J Immunother 2015;38(5):211.

49. Schvartsman G, Perez K, Sood G, et al. Immune checkpoint inhibitor therapy in a liver transplant recipient with melanoma. Ann Intern Med 2017;167(5):361–2.

50. De Toni EN, Gerbes AL. Tapering of immunosuppression and sustained treatment with nivolumab in a liver transplant recipient. Gastroenterology 2017;152(6): 1631–3.

51. Friend BD, Venick RS, McDiarmid SV, et al. Fatal orthotopic liver transplant organ rejection induced by a checkpoint inhibitor in two patients with refractory, metastatic hepatocellular carcinoma. Pediatr Blood Cancer 2017;64(12). https://doi.org/10.1002/pbc.26682. Available at: https://www.ncbi.nlm.nih.gov/pubmed/28643391.
52. Rai R, Ezeoke OM, McQuade JL, et al. Immunotherapy in patients with concurrent solid organ transplant, HIV, and hepatitis B and C. Ann Oncol 2017;28:403–27.
53. Varkaris A, Lewis DW, Nugent FW. Preserved liver transplant after PD-1 pathway inhibitor for hepatocellular carcinoma. Am J Gastroenterol 2017;112(12):1895–6.
54. Kuo JC, Lilly LB, Hogg D. Immune checkpoint inhibitor therapy in a liver transplant recipient with a rare subtype of melanoma: a case report and literature review. Melanoma Res 2018;28(1):61–4.
55. Ungerechts G, Engeland CE, Buchholz CJ, et al. Virotherapy research in Germany: from engineering to translation. Hum Gene Ther 2017;28(10):800–19.
56. Li N, Zhou J, Weng D, et al. Adjuvant adenovirus-mediated delivery of herpes simplex virus thymidine kinase administration improves outcome of liver transplantation in patients with advanced hepatocellular carcinoma. Clin Cancer Res 2007;13(19):5847–54.
57. Abudoureyimu M, Lai Y, Tian C, et al. Oncolytic adenovirus-A Nova for gene-targeted oncolytic viral therapy in HCC. Front Oncol 2019;9:1182. Available at: https://www.ncbi.nlm.nih.gov/pubmed/31781493.
58. Sangro B, Mazzolini G, Ruiz M, et al. A phase I clinical trial of thymidine kinase-based gene therapy in advanced hepatocellular carcinoma. Cancer Gene Ther 2010;17(12):837–43.
59. Martinez M, Moon EK. CAR T cells for solid tumors: new strategies for finding, infiltrating, and surviving in the tumor microenvironment. Front Immunol 2019;10:128.
60. Liu C, Liu H, Wang Y, et al. ET140202 t-cells: a novel therapy targeting AFP/MHC complex, that is both safe and effective in treating metastatic hepatocellular carcinoma. J Clin Oncol 2019;37(15_suppl). https://doi.org/10.1200/jco.2019.37.15_suppl.e15614.
61. Zhai B, Shi D, Gao H, et al. A phase I study of anti-GPC3 chimeric antigen receptor modified T cells (GPC3 CAR-T) in Chinese patients with refractory or relapsed GPC3+ hepatocellular carcinoma (r/r GPC3+ HCC). J Clin Oncol 2017;35(15_suppl):3049.
62. Wang Y, Chen M, Wu Z, et al. CD133-directed CAR T cells for advanced metastasis malignancies: a phase I trial. Oncoimmunology 2018;7:e1440169.
63. Yao W, He JC, Yang Y, et al. The prognostic value of tumor-infiltrating lymphocytes in hepatocellular carcinoma: a systematic review and meta-analysis. Sci Rep 2017;7(1). https://doi.org/10.1038/s41598-017-08128-1.
64. Alexandrov LB, Nik-Zainal S, Wedge DC, et al. Signatures of mutational processes in human cancer. Nature 2013;500(7463):415–21.
65. Lawrence MS, Stojanov P, Polak P, et al. Mutational heterogeneity in cancer and the search for new cancer-associated genes. Nature 2013;499(7457):214–8.
66. Shrestha R, Prithviraj P, Anaka M, et al. Monitoring immune checkpoint regulators as predictive biomarkers in hepatocellular carcinoma. Front Oncol 2018;8:269.

Management of Side Effects of Systemic Therapies for Hepatocellular Carcinoma

Guide for the Hepatologist

Adam C. Winters, MD, Fatima Bedier, BS, Sammy Saab, MD, MPH*

KEYWORDS

- Hepatocellular carcinoma • Liver cancer • Liver cirrhosis • Chemotherapy
- Tyrosine kinase inhibitors • Checkpoint inhibitors • Immune-related adverse effects

KEY POINTS

- The number of agents approved in the United States for the treatment of advanced hepatocellular carcinoma has increased dramatically in the past few years.
- Although these discoveries provide patients additional opportunities for therapy, they also introduce adverse events that provide challenges for the treating physician.
- Common side effects of systemic therapies for HCC are predictable, manageable, and many improve with appropriate intervention.

INTRODUCTION

Liver cancer is the sixth most commonly diagnosed cancer and accounts for the fourth leading cause of cancer-related death worldwide.[1] Hepatocellular carcinoma (HCC) is by far the most common histologic cell type, accounting for 90% of all liver cancer in the United States.[2] The incidence of HCC in the United States has increased, with a 115% rise between the years 2000 and 2012, and is projected to continue to rise.[3] Because of its aggressive nature and that, typically, it is a sequela of advanced liver disease or cirrhosis, the mortality for patients with HCC is high: between 12% and 28% at 5 years.[4,5] Surgical therapy, either resection or orthotopic liver transplant, are options for patients diagnosed early in the disease course with small lesions. Unfortunately, most patients presenting with HCC are diagnosed with advanced disease that is not amenable to curative therapies.[6]

Until recently, sorafenib, a molecular targeting agent first introduced for HCC in 2007, was the only systemic therapy indicated for the treatment of unresectable

Pfleger Liver Institute, 200 Medical Plaza Driveway, Suite 214, Los Angeles, CA 90095, USA
* Corresponding author. Pfleger Liver Institute, UCLA Medical Center, 200 Medical Plaza, Suite 214, Los Angeles, CA 90095.
E-mail address: Ssaab@mednet.ucla.edu

Clin Liver Dis 24 (2020) 755–769
https://doi.org/10.1016/j.cld.2020.07.008
1089-3261/20/© 2020 Elsevier Inc. All rights reserved.

HCC in patients. The landscape has changed drastically with the introduction of new molecular targeting agents and agents with additional mechanisms of action, such as immune checkpoint inhibitors (CIs) **(Table 1)**. With the promise of new therapies for incurable HCC also comes the prospect of new and challenging side effects **(Table 2)**. Thus, it is incumbent on the hepatologist to recognize these adverse effects and manage them effectively to reduce overall symptom burden and maximize the efficacy of these drugs. The treatment of liver cancer often involves managing two conditions: the malignancy itself and the underlying environment from which it developed, specifically cirrhosis and, often, decompensated cirrhosis. As such, the gastroenterologist and hepatologist will undoubtedly be intimately involved in the treatment of these patients. This review uses existing evidence to show that the common side effects of systemic therapies for HCC are predictable, manageable, and improve with appropriate intervention.

MOLECULAR TARGETING AGENTS

The molecular targeting agents are made up of medications that target specific molecules necessary for increases in tumor growth and further tumor progression. In HCC, this encompasses the two agents currently approved as first-line therapy by the Food and Drug Administration (FDA): sorafenib and lenvatinib. The other molecular targeting agents (regorafenib, cabozantinib, and ramucirumab) are approved as second-line therapy for those who did not respond or have stopped responding to sorafenib or lenvatinib. The side effect profile for these agents is similar but includes important differences that require attention from the hepatologist.

The First Line

Sorafenib and lenvatinib
Sorafenib is a multikinase inhibitor, acting through inhibition of the serine–threonine kinases Raf-1 and B-Raf, the activity of vascular endothelial growth factor (VEGF)

Table 1
Food and Drug Administration–approved systemic therapies for hepatocellular carcinoma

	Name of Agents	Mechanism of Action
First-line therapy	Sorafenib	Multikinase inhibitor acting through inhibition of the serine–threonine kinases Raf-1 and B-Raf, VEGF receptors 1–3, and PDGF receptor.[7,8]
	Lenvatinib	Multikinase inhibitor, targeting VEGF receptors 1–3, FGF receptors 1–4, PDGF receptor α, RET, and KIT.[11]
Second-line therapy	Regorafenib	Multikinase inhibitor, targeting VEGFR 1–3, KIT, RET, BRAF, and PDGFR.[30]
	Cabozantinib	Multikinase inhibitor, targeting VEGFR 1–3, MET, AXL, RET, KIT, and FLT3.[32,33]
	Ramucirumab	Recombinant human monoclonal antibody that binds to VEGFR-2, blocking endothelial proliferation.[40,42]
	Nivolumab Pembrolizumab	Inhibitor of PD-1, a receptor expressed on the surface of T cells allowing for increased immune response against tumor cells.[48]

Abbreviations: FGF, fibroblast growth factor; FLT, fms like tyrosine kinase; PDGF, platelet-derived growth factor; Raf, rapidly accelerating fibrosarcoma; RET, rearranged during transfection; VEGF, vascular endothelial growth factor.

Table 2
Common terminology criteria for adverse events for common events of systemic therapy for hepatocellular carcinoma

Side Effects	Grade 1	Grade 2	Grade 3	Grade 4	Grade 5
AST/ALT elevation	>ULN -3.0 x ULN if baseline was normal; 1.5–3.0 x baseline if baseline was abnormal	>3.0–5.0 x ULN if baseline was normal; >3.0–5.0 x baseline if baseline was abnormal	>5.0–20.0 x ULN if baseline was normal; >5.0–20.0 x baseline if baseline was abnormal	>20.0 x ULN if baseline was normal; >20.0 x baseline if baseline was abnormal	—
Diarrhea	Having 4 more stools daily than patient's baseline	Having 4–6 more stools a day than a person's baseline	Having 7 or more stools a day than a person's baseline	10 or more than baseline, life-threatening condition	Death
Hand-foot skin reaction	Painless dermatitis, such as erythema and edema	Skin changes; painful blistering or peeling of the skin, which limits instrumental ADL	Skin changes, such as blisters, bleeding, peeling and edema; limits self-care ADLs	—	—
Fatigue	Fatigue relieved by rest	Fatigue not relieved by rest; limiting instrumental ADL	Fatigue not relieved by rest, limiting self-care ADL	—	—
Hyperbilirubinemia	>ULN -1.5 x ULN if baseline was normal; > 1.0–1.5 x baseline if baseline was abnormal	>1.5–3.0 x ULN if baseline was normal; >1.5–3.0 x baseline if baseline was abnormal	>3.0–10.0 x ULN if baseline was normal; >3.0–10.0 x baseline if baseline was abnormal	>10.0 x ULN if baseline was normal; >10.0 x baseline if baseline was abnormal	—
Hypertension	Systolic BP of 120–139 mm Hg; diastolic BP of 80–89 mm Hg	Systolic BP of 140–159 mm Hg; diastolic BP of 80–89 mm Hg; recurrent or persistent for 24 h	Systolic BP of ≥160 mm Hg; diastolic BP of ≥100 mm Hg	Life-threatening condition; immediate intensive care	Death
Peripheral edema	5%–10% interlimb discrepancy in volume or circumference at point of greatest visible difference; swelling or obscuration of anatomic architecture on close inspection	>10%–30% interlimb discrepancy in volume or circumference at point of greatest visible difference; readily apparent obscuration of anatomic architecture; obliteration of skin folds; readily apparent deviation from normal anatomic contour; limiting instrumental ADL	>30% interlimb discrepancy in volume; gross deviation from normal anatomic contour; limiting self-care ADL		

(continued on next page)

Table 2
(continued)

Side Effects	Grade 1	Grade 2	Grade 3	Grade 4	Grade 5
Rash	Papules and/or pustules covering <10% BSA	Papules and/or pustules covering 10%–30% BSA; limiting instrumental ADL	Papules and/or pustules covering >30% BSA with moderate or severe symptoms; limiting self-care ADL	—	—

Abbreviations: ADL, activity of daily living; ALT, alanine aminotransferase; AST, aspartate aminotransferase; BP, blood pressure; BSA, body surface area; ULN, upper limit of normal.
From Cancer.gov. https://ctep.cancer.gov/protocoldevelopment/electronic_applications/docs/CTCAE_v5_Quick_Reference_8.5x11.pdf Accessed 09/26, 2019.

receptors 1 to 3, and the platelet-derived growth factor (PDGF) receptor.[7,8] Sorafenib, 400 mg twice daily, was established as the standard of care for advanced HCC following the results of two large trials that demonstrated a survival benefit over placebo. The SHARP trial, a multinational phase 3, placebo-controlled trial encompassing nearly 600 patients, showed median survival and time to radiologic progression was nearly 3 months longer for the sorafenib group.[9] These results were corroborated shortly thereafter by the Asia-Pacific trial, another multinational placebo-controlled trial consisting of more than 200 patients, which similarly showed a significant yet modest survival benefit of 2.3 months.[10] Sorafenib was approved in 2007 as first-line therapy for unresectable HCC in the United States.

Unsurprisingly, both trials reported significantly higher adverse events for patients in the treatment group than those in the placebo group. In the SHARP trial, the incidence of treatment-related adverse events (TRAE) was 80% for the sorafenib group versus 52% for the placebo group. In the Asia-Pacific trial, nearly 82% of patients experienced TRAEs compared with about 39% for those receiving placebo. The incidence of TRAEs has important clinical ramifications, causing more than 50% of patients in both trials to either drop out or require dose reduction. The most common TRAEs identified in clinical trials include gastrointestinal symptoms, fatigue, hand-foot skin reaction (HFSR), rash, and hypertension (HTN).

Lenvatinib is a multikinase inhibitor that targets VEGF receptors 1 to 3, fibroblast growth factor receptors 1 to 4, PDGF receptor α, RET, and KIT.[11] Its noninferiority to sorafenib in patients with advanced HCC was demonstrated in a large randomized, phase 3, multicenter noninferiority trial. Median survival for lenvatinib dosed at 12 mg daily for patients greater than 60 kg and 8 mg daily for patients less than 60 kg was 13.6 months compared with 12.3 months for sorafenib (hazard ratio, 0.92; 95% confidence interval, 0.79–1.06), meeting criteria for noninferiority.[12] Lenvatinib also showed better progression-free survival and median time to progression than sorafenib. It was received approval by the FDA in August of 2018 for first-line therapy for advanced HCC in the United States.

Adverse events occurred in a similar proportion in the lenvatinib and sorafenib arms. Drug interruption in the lenvatinib arm occurred in 40% of patients, dose reduction in 37% of patients, and withdrawal in 9% of patients. Because of its similar mechanism of action, the adverse effects of lenvatinib and many of the other molecular targeting agents, specifically the second-line agents discussed separately later, are similar to those of sorafenib. For example, tyrosine kinase inhibitors as a class have been implicated in abnormal thyroid function tests and these levels should be monitored while on treatment.[13] Details regarding important adverse events that occur in more than 20% of patients treated with sorafenib and lenvatinib are outlined later.

Diarrhea Dose reduction caused by diarrhea occurs between 7.4% and 8% of patients receiving sorafenib for HCC, with an overall incidence of 38% to 39%. The incidence for patients receiving lenvatinib is similar. Most diarrhea symptoms are low-grade; however, grade 3 to 4 symptoms have occurred in up to 9% of HCC patients on sorafenib and 4% of patients on lenvatinib. Patients receiving sorafenib with sarcopenia may experience higher rates of dose-limiting diarrhea than those without.[14] Those patients who also suffer from hepatic encephalopathy should be counseled to adjust their lactulose doses if they experience diarrhea. In term of dietary modification, caffeine and dairy in particular can exacerbate diarrhea.[15] Patients should be encouraged to document and avoid other trigger foods. The mainstay of therapy refractory to supportive care is loperamide. Diphenoxylate/atropine may be used if loperamide is ineffective. For grade 3 or 4 symptoms, dose interruption may be required until symptoms become low grade or return to baseline.[15,16]

Proteinuria The use of lenvatinib for HCC has been associated with development of proteinuria in up to 25% of treated patients.[12] For those with grade 1 proteinuria (1+ protein or 0.15–1.0 g/24 hours) treatment may be continued with close monitoring.[17] For grade 2 (2–3+ urine protein or >1–3.5 g/24 hours) lenvatinib should be held and urinalysis should be repeated until protein levels are less than 2 g/24 hours before restarting. For patients with grade 3 proteinuria (>4+ proteinuria or 3.5 g/24 hours) lenvatinib should be held and the patient should be evaluated by a nephrologist.

Hand-foot skin reaction Along with diarrhea, HFSR is one of the most common causes of dose reduction in sorafenib therapy for HCC. HFSR is a toxic dermatologic reaction causing a painful hyperkeratotic, erythematous rash of the hands and feet. It typically presents within the first 6 weeks of sorafenib therapy.[15,18] Among patients being treated with sorafenib regardless of cancer cause, the incidence of all-grade HFSR of is around 34%.[19] Most patients with HCC present with Common Terminology Criteria for Adverse Events grade 1 or 2 disease, which typically does not require dose reduction. Grade 3 disease is the most severe and often requires at least temporary discontinuation of the drug.

Patients receiving sorafenib or lenvatinib should have a full skin examination before starting therapy, be monitored closely for development of symptoms, and instructed to use emollients on pressure-receptive areas of the hands.[20] Urea-based creams have been shown in one randomized trial to have a prophylactic effect on the development of HFSR.[21] Common Terminology Criteria for Adverse Events grade 1 disease encompasses painless skin changes/erythema and is treated with keratolytic emollients with topical urea 10% three times daily. Grade 2 disease is characterized by painful blistering or peeling of the skin that limits instrumental activities of daily living. Treatment of grade 1 is continued and augmented with potent steroid ointments, such as clobetasol 0.05%, twice daily and topical analgesia (ie, lidocaine 4% creams or patches).[20] Dose reduction of lenvatinib is considered for grade 2 symptoms.[16] For grade 3 disease, or that which limits self-care activities of daily living, the medication is held for at least 7 days or until there is sign of disease resolution.[22] Treatment dose is typically reduced. If the patient does not develop recurrence, dose escalation to full treatment is considered.[16,20,22] The incidence of grade 3 disease for lenvatinib seems to be lower than that of sorafenib.[12,16]

Fatigue Reports of fatigue are common in treatment with molecular targeting agents. Fortunately, fatigue typically does not require dose reduction and usually subsides by Month 6 of treatment.[15] It is incumbent on the treating physician to exclude alternative causes of fatigue, including comorbid conditions, other medication effects, and psychosocial effects. Counseling patients about the possibility of fatigue and identifying and treating other etiologies is essential to managing the fatigued patient on molecular targeting agents.

Rash An often self-limiting macular papular skin rash is a common adverse effect of both medications, occurring between 16% and 30% of patients treated with sorafenib and about 10% of patients treated with lenvatinib in clinical trials.[9,10,12] Care is largely symptomatic and includes a change to milder, perfume-free soaps; encouraging loose fitting clothing; and avoidance of hot water.[15]

Hypertension Treatment induced HTN is a well-established adverse effect of sorafenib and lenvatinib. Three separate meta-analyses have shown that the incidence of all-grade HTN in patients with any cancer treated with sorafenib is between 19.1% and 23.4%, with the incidence of high-grade HTN ranging between 4.3% and 5.7%.[23–25] The incidence seems to be higher in the treatment of renal cell carcinoma, because the incidence reported in the HCC trials are between 5% and 18.8%. Given sorafenib's inhibition of angiogenesis, an association has been found between the presence of HTN and favorable treatment effect.[26,27] The incidence of HTN and high-grade HTN seems to be higher with lenvatinib.[12,28] Patients with preexisting HTN should be identified and treated before starting therapy. Once therapy is initiated, all patients should have their blood pressure measured every 2 to 3 weeks to allow for prompt treatment.[29] Initiation of standard anti-HTN agents are recommended, including calcium channel blockers and angiotensin-converting enzyme inhibitors.

The Second Line

Regorafenib and cabozantinib
Regorafenib is an oral multikinase inhibitor affecting tumor angiogenesis (VEGFR 1–3), oncogenesis (KIT, RET, and BRAF), and metastasis (PDGFR).[30] Regorafenib, 160 mg daily, is currently FDA-approved as second-line therapy for patients with HCC previously treated with sorafenib. The efficacy of regorafenib as second-line therapy for HCC was suggested by a large double-blind, phase 3 multicenter trial of 567 patients with Child-Pugh A liver function and evidence of progression on sorafenib. Patients who received regorafenib had a median survival of 10.6 months versus 7.8 months for placebo.[31]

Similarly, cabozantinib is an inhibitor of multiple tyrosine kinases, including VEGF receptor 1, 2, and 3; the stem cell growth receptor KIT; MET; and AXL.[32,33] It is approved as second-line therapy at a dose of 60 mg daily for patients with HCC who have failed sorafenib, based on data published in 2018 from a phase 3 randomized, placebo-controlled trial. In a population of more than 700 patients who had previously progressed on sorafenib, those receiving cabozantinib displayed longer overall survival by more than 2 months.[34]

The incidence and nature of adverse effects for regorafenib and cabozantinib are similar to those seen in sorafenib and lenvatinib. For regorafenib, drug-related adverse events led to treatment interruption or dose reduction in 54% of patients and drug discontinuation in 10%. Adverse effects led to dose reduction in 62% of patients on cabozantinib and discontinuation in 16%. Similar to the previously mentioned first-line agents, the most common adverse effects seen with regorafenib/cabozantinib were HFSR (52%/46%; 13%/17% grade 3), diarrhea (33%/54%; 2%/10% grade 3), fatigue (29%/45%; 6%/10% grade 3), and HTN (23%/29%; 13%/16% grade 3 or 4). Because of their mechanistic similarity, the management of these conditions is similar to that described previously for sorafenib and lenvatinib. **Table 3** provides specifics regarding HFSR management. Liver dysfunction, described next, is an adverse effect commonly described with regorafenib.

Hepatic dysfunction Increased bilirubin and transaminase concentrations are a common adverse effect of regorafenib. The incidence of treatment-related hyperbilirubinemia in the treatment of HCC with regorafenib was found to be 19%, whereas an elevated aspartate aminotransferase (AST) was seen in 13% and increases in alanine aminotransferase (ALT) observed in 8%.[31] Severe (grade 3 or higher) events were rare. Although these abnormalities may be confounded by the presence of underlying advanced liver disease, increases in these markers were also seen in trials of patients with gastrointestinal stromal tumors and colon cancer.[35,36]

Grade 2 elevations are defined by 2.5 times the upper limit of normal (ULN) for AST and ALT, and 1.5 times ULN for bilirubin. These laboratory studies should be drawn

Table 3
Management of hand-foot skin reaction caused by molecular targeting agents

Before Initiation	Grade 1	Grade 2	Grade 3
Full skin examination	Continue prophylactic	Continue prophylactic	Continue measures
Pedicure to address	measures from	measures from before	from before
areas of	before initiation	initiation and for	initiation and
hyperkeratosis	Encourage use of	grade 1 symptoms	grade 1–2
Avoidance of hot	urea-based creams	Clobetasol 0.05%	symptoms
water	and topical	ointment	Stop agent for 7 d
Avoidance of bare	moisturizers	Analgesia using topical	until symptoms
feet or tight	Maintain current	lidocaine, pregabalin,	improve to at
shoes	dosing regimen	and opiates, as	least grade 1
		needed	If improved, restart
		Consider 50% dose	at 50% full dose
		reduction for at least	and re-escalate as
		7 d if symptoms do	tolerated
		not improve to at	If persistent
		least grade 1	recurrence with
		If no improvement to	reintroduction,
		reduced dose,	consider
		discontinue therapy	permanently
		for 7 d until symptoms	discontinuing
		improve to at least	offending agent
		grade 1; resume at	
		half-normal dose	

Data from Refs.[20–22]

twice per week and then each week for a month to ensure stability and/or a return to baseline. If these laboratory studies continue to rise to grade 2 elevations (>2.5–5.0 x ULN for AST/ALT; 1.5–3.0 x ULN for bilirubin), the drug is delayed until laboratory studies return to grade 1 levels. The drug can then be restarted at a lower dose. If the patient experiences a grade 2 elevation from laboratory values that were previously normal, the drug is continued with laboratory monitoring twice weekly for 2 weeks and then weekly for 1 month. For Grade 3 elevations (5–20 x ULN for AST/ALT; 3–10 x ULN for bilirubin), the drug should be held until laboratory studies return to baseline. If the drug is restarted, it should be done so at a lower dose with frequent laboratory monitoring. For any grade 4 elevation (>20 x ULN for AST/ALT; >10 x ULN for bilirubin), the drug should be discontinued.[37,38]

Ramucirumab
Ramucirumab is a monoclonal antibody that binds with high specificity to the extracellular domain to VEGFR-2, blocking endothelial proliferation.[39,40] It was initially studied as a therapy for HCC in a phase 2 study of 42 patients who received no prior therapy and showed a median overall survival of 12 months.[39] A subsequent placebo-controlled trial in patients who had previously been treated with sorafenib did not demonstrate a survival benefit, except for a subset analysis that suggested patients with elevated α-fetoprotein (AFP) greater than 400 ng/mL (median survival of 7.8 months vs 4.2 months for placebo).[41] Ramucirumab was further evaluated in a phase 3 trial of patients who previously demonstrated disease progression on sorafenib, had no worse than Child-Turcotte-Pugh class A cirrhosis, and a serum AFP greater than 400 ng/mL.[42] Patients receiving ramucirumab had a 1.2-month increased overall survival (8.5 months vs 7.3 months). In light of these results, ramucirumab was

FDA-approved in 2019 at a dose of 8 mg/kg every 2 weeks as second-line therapy for patients with advanced HCC who have previously failed sorafenib and have an AFP level of greater than 400 ng/mL.

From an adverse event standpoint, one of the major advantages of ramucirumab is that it does not seem to cause HFSR. This makes it an ideal agent for patients who failed first-line therapy because of significant HFSR, have less advanced cirrhosis, and an elevated AFP. The most common side effects encountered by patients with HCC receiving ramucirumab in the phase 3 trial were fatigue (36%; 5% grade 3), peripheral edema (25%; 2% grade 3), HTN (25%; 13% ≥grade 3), abdominal pain (25%; 2% ≥grade 3) decreased appetite (23%; 2% >grade 3), and the onset of ascites (18%; 4% ≥grade 3).[42] The most common laboratory abnormality was thrombocytopenia (46%; 8% ≥grade 3).

Checkpoint inhibitors: nivolumab and pembrolizumab

Tumor cells are able to avoid immunosurveillance through several methods, including activation of immune checkpoint pathways that suppress immune responses against tumor cells. CIs act to interrupt these signaling pathways and revive antitumor immune surveillance.[43] CIs have been shown to be effective either in combination or as monotherapy for treatment in several advanced malignancies, including melanoma,[44] renal cell carcinoma,[45] non–small cell lung cancer,[46] and urothelial cell carcinoma.[47] There are two CIs approved by the FDA for second-line treatment of HCC: nivolumab and pembrolizumab. These agents are both inhibitors of programmed cell death protein 1 (PD-1), a receptor expressed on the surface of T cells that, when bound to the programmed cell death protein 1 (PDL-1) on the surface the tumor cell, act to dampen the immune system and prevent attack on the tumor cell.[48]

The efficacy for nivolumab is derived from a phase 1/2 dose escalation and expansion trial of adults with advanced HCC. Of the 255 patients who were studied for response, about 19% experienced an objective tumor response, including three complete responses.[49] An 83% of patients experienced at least one TRAE, but only one patient stopped treatment. Similarly, the initial benefit for pembrolizumab was demonstrated in a phase 2 trial of patients with HCC who had failed sorafenib, which showed objective response in 17% of those studied.[50] A 73% of patients experienced at least 1 TRAE, with 5% requiring discontinuation of therapy. In a subsequent placebo-controlled, phase 3 trial of pembrolizumab for patients previously treated with sorafenib, pembrolizumab showed a survival benefit over placebo in median overall survival (13.9 months vs 10.6 months) and progression-free survival (3 months vs 2.6 months), although these failed to meet statistical significance.[51]

Although the novel CI mechanism has been shown to be effective in the treatment of malignancy, it has been associated with a unique class of adverse events, termed immune-related adverse events (irAEs).[52] These events are thought to arise from the increased immune response created by checkpoint inhibition. Intuitively, the treatment of these conditions is administration of glucocorticoids or other immunosuppressive agents, which opens the risk of opportunistic infections in patients who require treatment of irAEs.

Broadly, in patients who experience moderate irAEs (grade 2), CI therapy is held and not restarted until symptoms become mild (grade 1) or better. If moderate symptoms persist for more than a week, initiate corticosteroids (ie, 0.5–1 mg/kg/d oral prednisone or equivalent doses of intravenous methylprednisolone if unable to tolerate by mouth). Patients experiencing more severe irAEs (grade 3 and 4) require indefinite withdrawal of CIs and higher doses of corticosteroids (ie, 1–2 mg/kg/d of prednisone or methylprednisolone equivalent) until symptoms retreat to at least grade 1. At this point, steroids can begin to be tapered over at least a 4-week period.[53]

Specific irAEs often have nuanced management considerations, particularly in the setting of chronic liver disease. Immune related hepatitis (irH) is particularly common for patients receiving CIs for HCC and specifics related to this condition are outlined next. Notably, the reported mortality rates for pembrolizumab and nivolumab are 0.1% and 0.3%, respectively.[54]

Immune-related hepatitis The incidence of irH, mainly in the form of elevated transaminases, occurs in up to 21% of patients treated with nivolumab and 14% of those treated with pembrolizumab in data published from clinical trials.[49,50] The incidence has elsewhere been reported to be 30% and is the most common reason for CI treatment discontinuation in this patient population.[55] Notably, the reported incidence of irH in the treatment of melanoma with nivolumab and pembrolizumab is 1% to 3% because patients with HCC are likely more susceptible to irH.[56–58] Liver injury may occur at any time during treatment, but is typically seen between 6 and 14 weeks after initiation of therapy.[55,59] The differential diagnosis for patients on CIs with elevated liver tests is broad but requires careful consideration to ensure proper treatment and avoid unwarranted use of corticosteroids. Considerations include:

- Drug-related liver injury, particularly in patients who have recently started a new medication
- Herbal supplement use
- Alcohol use
- Opportunistic infection, such as Epstein-Barr virus or cytomegalovirus
- Thromboembolic disease, such as portal vein thrombosis or Budd-Chiari syndrome (hepatic vein thrombosis)
- Progression of underlying liver disease and/or cancer, particularly in the case of those with active hepatitis B or hepatitis C infection

Before initiation of CI therapy, viral hepatitis serologies should be sent and baseline liver tests should be established. Work-up for elevations in liver tests while on treatment should be targeted at ruling out the previously mentioned etiologies, including a careful history and physical examination, a thorough medication reconciliation, repeat viral hepatitis serologies, Epstein-Barr virus, and cytomegalovirus polymerase chain reaction. Autoantibodies may be positive in patients with irH, including anti–nuclear antibody, anti–smooth muscle antibody and anti–liver/kidney, although the impact of antibody positivity is unknown and therapy remains the same.[59] Imaging via ultrasonography or computerized tomography should be used to assess for disease progression, and to rule out the possibility of thromboembolic disease. Liver biopsy has been shown to accurately identify patients suffering from irH.[60] The pattern observed histologically with PD-1 irH is described as "heterogenous" but includes lesions of active hepatitis with areas of necrosis and mild to moderate periportal activity largely without granulomatous inflammation.[60] The lobular hepatitis seen on biopsy may be indistinguishable from autoimmune hepatitis.[61] There is no consensus about when to perform a liver biopsy in these patients; however, some advocate biopsy in patients with grade 3 and higher hepatoxicity (5–20 x ULN for AST/ALT; 3–10 x ULN for bilirubin).[59]

Treatment of CI-induced hepatitis is complex, although the mainstay of therapy is corticosteroids for grade 2 disease and higher.[61,62] There have been no clinical trials identifying the best agent or dosing regimen for irH. If there is no improvement in liver function tests after 1 week, addition mycophenolate mofetil is recommended.[63] **Fig. 1**

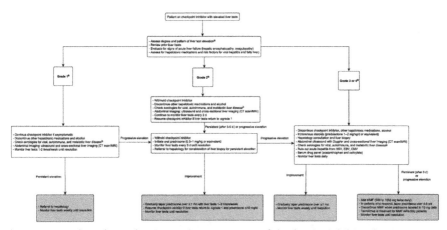

Fig. 1. Approach to the evaluation and management of checkpoint inhibitor hepatotoxicity. ANA, antinuclear antibody; ASMA, anti–smooth muscle antibody; CMV, cytomegalovirus; CT, computed tomography; CTCAE, Common Terminology Criteria for Adverse Events; EBV, Epstein-Barr virus; HBcAb, hepatitis B core antibody; HBsAb, hepatitis B surface antibody; HBsAg, hepatitis B surface antigen; HCV, hepatitis C; HCVAb, hepatitis C antibody; HSV, herpes simplex virus; LKM, liver kidney microsomal; MMF, mycophenolate mofetil. [a] Elevations in liver tests as per CTCAE version 5.0. Grade 1: AST or ALT >ULN - 3.0 x ULN if baseline was normal; 1.5 to 3.0 x baseline if baseline was abnormal and/or total bilirubin >ULN -15 x ULN if baseline was normal; >1.0 to 1.5 x baseline if baseline was abnormal. Grade 2: AST or ALT >3.0 to 5.0 x ULN and/or total bilirubin >1.5 to 3.0 x ULN. Grade 3: AST or ALT >5.0 to 20.0 x ULN if baseline was normal; >5.0 to 20.0 x baseline if baseline was abnormal and/or total bilirubin >3.0 to 10.0 x ULN if baseline was normal; >3.0 to 10.0 x baseline if baseline was abnormal. Grade 4: >20.0 x ULN if baseline was normal. >20.0 x baseline if baseline was abnormal and/or total bilirubin >10.0 x ULN if baseline was normal; >10.0 x baseline if baseline was abnormal. [b] Hepatitis serologies (HBsAg HBcAb, HBsAb, HCVAb, HCV RNA), iron panel, ANA, ASMA, anti-LKM, gamma globulin, ceruloplasmin, α-1 antitrypsin. (*From* Grover S et al., Gastrointestinal and Hepatic Toxicities of Checkpoint Inhibitors: Algorithms for Management, *American Society of Clinical Oncology Educational Book* 38 (May 23, 2018) 13-19. Reprinted with permission. © 2018 American Society of Clinical Oncology. All rights reserved.)

highlights the current expert consensus management guidelines from the American Society for Clinical Oncology. Resumption of CI is typically only considered for those who have suffered at most grade 2 hepatitis once liver tests have returned to the patient's baseline. Patients with more severe (grades 3 and 4) presentation should not be restarted on CIs.[62]

SUMMARY

The incidence of HCC in the United States is rising. For patients with advanced disease who are not candidates for curative therapies, treatment options have historically been limited. Recently, however, the approval of many new agents has increased the number of patients who can be treated for HCC. With the availability of new drugs, the hepatologist is faced with the specter of new and challenging adverse events that threaten to limit the ability to treat patients with advanced disease. Through prompt recognition and treatment, many of these adverse events can be managed, allowing patients to derive the maximum benefits of these therapies.

DISCLOSURE

The authors of this article have no conflicts of interest to disclose.

REFERENCES

1. Bray F, Ferlay J, Soerjomataram I, et al. Global cancer statistics 2018: GLOBO-CAN estimates of incidence and mortality worldwide for 36 cancers in 185 countries. CA Cancer J Clin 2018;68(6):394–424.
2. Altekruse SF, McGlynn KA, Reichman ME. Hepatocellular carcinoma incidence, mortality, and survival trends in the United States from 1975 to 2005. J Clin Oncol 2009;27(9):1485–91.
3. White DL, Thrift AP, Kanwal F, et al. Incidence of hepatocellular carcinoma in all 50 United States, from 2000 through 2012. Gastroenterology 2017;152(4):812–20.e5.
4. El-Serag HB. Hepatocellular carcinoma. N Engl J Med 2011;365(12):1118–27.
5. Thein HH, Khoo E, Campitelli MA, et al. Trends in relative survival in patients with a diagnosis of hepatocellular carcinoma in Ontario: a population-based retrospective cohort study. CMAJ Open 2015;3(2):E208–16.
6. Ronot M, Bouattour M, Wassermann J, et al. Alternative response criteria (Choi, European association for the study of the liver, and modified Response Evaluation Criteria in Solid Tumors [RECIST]) versus RECIST 1.1 in patients with advanced hepatocellular carcinoma treated with sorafenib. Oncologist 2014;19(4):394–402.
7. Wilhelm SM, Carter C, Tang L, et al. BAY 43-9006 exhibits broad spectrum oral antitumor activity and targets the RAF/MEK/ERK pathway and receptor tyrosine kinases involved in tumor progression and angiogenesis. Cancer Res 2004;64(19):7099–109.
8. Chang YS, Adnane J, Trail PA, et al. Sorafenib (BAY 43-9006) inhibits tumor growth and vascularization and induces tumor apoptosis and hypoxia in RCC xenograft models. Cancer Chemother Pharmacol 2007;59(5):561–74.
9. Llovet JM, Ricci S, Mazzaferro V, et al. Sorafenib in advanced hepatocellular carcinoma. N Engl J Med 2008;359(4):378–90.
10. Cheng AL, Kang YK, Chen Z, et al. Efficacy and safety of sorafenib in patients in the Asia-Pacific region with advanced hepatocellular carcinoma: a phase III randomised, double-blind, placebo-controlled trial. Lancet Oncol 2009;10(1):25–34.
11. Yamamoto Y, Matsui J, Matsushima T, et al. Lenvatinib, an angiogenesis inhibitor targeting VEGFR/FGFR, shows broad antitumor activity in human tumor xenograft models associated with microvessel density and pericyte coverage. Vasc Cell 2014;6:18.
12. Kudo M, Finn RS, Qin S, et al. Lenvatinib versus sorafenib in first-line treatment of patients with unresectable hepatocellular carcinoma: a randomised phase 3 non-inferiority trial. Lancet 2018;391(10126):1163–73.
13. Illouz F, Braun D, Briet C, et al. Endocrine side-effects of anti-cancer drugs: thyroid effects of tyrosine kinase inhibitors. Eur J Endocrinol 2014;171(3):R91–9.
14. Mir O, Coriat R, Blanchet B, et al. Sarcopenia predicts early dose-limiting toxicities and pharmacokinetics of sorafenib in patients with hepatocellular carcinoma. PLoS One 2012;7(5):e37563.
15. Brose MS, Frenette CT, Keefe SM, et al. Management of sorafenib-related adverse events: a clinician's perspective. Semin Oncol 2014;41(Suppl 2):S1–16.
16. Takahashi S, Kiyota N, Tahara M. Optimal use of lenvatinib in the treatment of advanced thyroid cancer. Cancers Head Neck 2017;2:7.

17. Cabanillas ME, Takahashi S. Managing the adverse events associated with lenvatinib therapy in radioiodine-refractory differentiated thyroid cancer. Semin Oncol 2019;46(1):57–64.

18. Porta C, Paglino C, Imarisio I, et al. Uncovering Pandora's vase: the growing problem of new toxicities from novel anticancer agents. The case of sorafenib and sunitinib. Clin Exp Med 2007;7(4):127–34.

19. Chu D, Lacouture ME, Fillos T, et al. Risk of hand-foot skin reaction with sorafenib: a systematic review and meta-analysis. Acta Oncol 2008;47(2):176–86.

20. Lacouture ME, Wu S, Robert C, et al. Evolving strategies for the management of hand-foot skin reaction associated with the multitargeted kinase inhibitors sorafenib and sunitinib. Oncologist 2008;13(9):1001–11.

21. Ren Z, Zhu K, Kang H, et al. Randomized controlled trial of the prophylactic effect of urea-based cream on sorafenib-associated hand-foot skin reactions in patients with advanced hepatocellular carcinoma. J Clin Oncol 2015;33(8):894–900.

22. Anderson R, Jatoi A, Robert C, et al. Search for evidence-based approaches for the prevention and palliation of hand-foot skin reaction (HFSR) caused by the multikinase inhibitors (MKIs). Oncologist 2009;14(3):291–302.

23. Wu S, Chen JJ, Kudelka A, et al. Incidence and risk of hypertension with sorafenib in patients with cancer: a systematic review and meta-analysis. Lancet Oncol 2008;9(2):117–23.

24. Funakoshi T, Latif A, Galsky MD. Risk of hypertension in cancer patients treated with sorafenib: an updated systematic review and meta-analysis. J Hum Hypertens 2013;27(10):601–11.

25. Li Y, Li S, Zhu Y, et al. Incidence and risk of sorafenib-induced hypertension: a systematic review and meta-analysis. J Clin Hypertens (Greenwich) 2014;16(3):177–85.

26. Estfan B, Byrne M, Kim R. Sorafenib in advanced hepatocellular carcinoma: hypertension as a potential surrogate marker for efficacy. Am J Clin Oncol 2013;36(4):319–24.

27. Ravaud A, Sire M. Arterial hypertension and clinical benefit of sunitinib, sorafenib and bevacizumab in first and second-line treatment of metastatic renal cell cancer. Ann Oncol 2009;20(5):966–7 [author reply: 967].

28. Ikeda K, Kudo M, Kawazoe S, et al. Phase 2 study of lenvatinib in patients with advanced hepatocellular carcinoma. J Gastroenterol 2017;52(4):512–9.

29. Maitland ML, Bakris GL, Black HR, et al. Initial assessment, surveillance, and management of blood pressure in patients receiving vascular endothelial growth factor signaling pathway inhibitors. J Natl Cancer Inst 2010;102(9):596–604.

30. Schmieder R, Hoffmann J, Becker M, et al. Regorafenib (BAY 73-4506): antitumor and antimetastatic activities in preclinical models of colorectal cancer. Int J Cancer 2014;135(6):1487–96.

31. Bruix J, Qin S, Merle P, et al. Regorafenib for patients with hepatocellular carcinoma who progressed on sorafenib treatment (RESORCE): a randomised, double-blind, placebo-controlled, phase 3 trial. Lancet 2017;389(10064):56–66.

32. Yakes FM, Chen J, Tan J, et al. Cabozantinib (XL184), a novel MET and VEGFR2 inhibitor, simultaneously suppresses metastasis, angiogenesis, and tumor growth. Mol Cancer Ther 2011;10(12):2298–308.

33. Kelley RK, Verslype C, Cohn AL, et al. Cabozantinib in hepatocellular carcinoma: results of a phase 2 placebo-controlled randomized discontinuation study. Ann Oncol 2017;28(3):528–34.

34. Abou-Alfa GK, Meyer T, Cheng AL, et al. Cabozantinib in patients with advanced and progressing hepatocellular carcinoma. N Engl J Med 2018;379(1):54–63.

35. Demetri GD, Reichardt P, Kang YK, et al. Efficacy and safety of regorafenib for advanced gastrointestinal stromal tumours after failure of imatinib and sunitinib (GRID): an international, multicentre, randomised, placebo-controlled, phase 3 trial. Lancet 2013;381(9863):295–302.

36. Grothey A, Van Cutsem E, Sobrero A, et al. Regorafenib monotherapy for previously treated metastatic colorectal cancer (CORRECT): an international, multicentre, randomised, placebo-controlled, phase 3 trial. Lancet 2013;381(9863): 303–12.

37. Pharmaceuticals PIB. Stivarga (regorafenib)[package insert].Whippany, NJ; Bayer Pharmaceutical Company; 2016.

38. Krishnamoorthy SK, Relias V, Sebastian S, et al. Management of regorafenib-related toxicities: a review. Therap Adv Gastroenterol 2015;8(5):285–97.

39. Zhu AX, Finn RS, Mulcahy M, et al. A phase II and biomarker study of ramucirumab, a human monoclonal antibody targeting the VEGF receptor-2, as first-line monotherapy in patients with advanced hepatocellular cancer. Clin Cancer Res 2013;19(23):6614–23.

40. Franklin MC, Navarro EC, Wang Y, et al. The structural basis for the function of two anti-VEGF receptor 2 antibodies. Structure 2011;19(8):1097–107.

41. Zhu AX, Park JO, Ryoo BY, et al. Ramucirumab versus placebo as second-line treatment in patients with advanced hepatocellular carcinoma following first-line therapy with sorafenib (REACH): a randomised, double-blind, multicentre, phase 3 trial. Lancet Oncol 2015;16(7):859–70.

42. Zhu AX, Kang YK, Yen CJ, et al. Ramucirumab after sorafenib in patients with advanced hepatocellular carcinoma and increased alpha-fetoprotein concentrations (REACH-2): a randomised, double-blind, placebo-controlled, phase 3 trial. Lancet Oncol 2019;20(2):282–96.

43. Darvin P, Toor SM, Sasidharan Nair V, et al. Immune checkpoint inhibitors: recent progress and potential biomarkers. Exp Mol Med 2018;50(12):165.

44. Hodi FS, O'Day SJ, McDermott DF, et al. Improved survival with ipilimumab in patients with metastatic melanoma. N Engl J Med 2010;363(8):711–23.

45. Motzer RJ, Tannir NM, McDermott DF, et al. Nivolumab plus ipilimumab versus sunitinib in advanced renal-cell carcinoma. N Engl J Med 2018;378(14):1277–90.

46. Reck M, Bondarenko I, Luft A, et al. Ipilimumab in combination with paclitaxel and carboplatin as first-line therapy in extensive-disease-small-cell lung cancer: results from a randomized, double-blind, multicenter phase 2 trial. Ann Oncol 2013;24(1):75–83.

47. Balar AV, Galsky MD, Rosenberg JE, et al. Atezolizumab as first-line treatment in cisplatin-ineligible patients with locally advanced and metastatic urothelial carcinoma: a single-arm, multicentre, phase 2 trial. Lancet 2017;389(10064):67–76.

48. Prasad V, Kaestner V. Nivolumab and pembrolizumab: monoclonal antibodies against programmed cell death-1 (PD-1) that are interchangeable. Semin Oncol 2017;44(2):132–5.

49. El-Khoueiry AB, Sangro B, Yau T, et al. Nivolumab in patients with advanced hepatocellular carcinoma (CheckMate 040): an open-label, non-comparative, phase 1/2 dose escalation and expansion trial. Lancet 2017;389(10088): 2492–502.

50. Zhu AX, Finn RS, Edeline J, et al. Pembrolizumab in patients with advanced hepatocellular carcinoma previously treated with sorafenib (KEYNOTE-224): a non-randomised, open-label phase 2 trial. Lancet Oncol 2018;19(7):940–52.

51. Finn RS, Ryoo B-Y, Merle P, et al. Results of KEYNOTE-240: phase 3 study of pembrolizumab (Pembro) vs best supportive care (BSC) for second line therapy

in advanced hepatocellular carcinoma (HCC). J Clin Oncol 2019;37(15_suppl): 4004.

52. Naidoo J, Page DB, Li BT, et al. Toxicities of the anti-PD-1 and anti-PD-L1 immune checkpoint antibodies. Ann Oncol 2015;26(12):2375–91.

53. Puzanov I, Diab A, Abdallah K, et al. Managing toxicities associated with immune checkpoint inhibitors: consensus recommendations from the Society for Immunotherapy of Cancer (SITC) Toxicity Management Working Group. J Immunother Cancer 2017;5(1):95.

54. Khoja L, Day D, Wei-Wu Chen T, et al. Tumour- and class-specific patterns of immune-related adverse events of immune checkpoint inhibitors: a systematic review. Ann Oncol 2017;28(10):2377–85.

55. Personeni N, Pressiani T, Capogreco A, et al. Liver injury by immune checkpoint inhibitors in patients with hepatocellular carcinoma. J Clin Oncol 2019; 37(4_suppl):341.

56. Robert C, Ribas A, Wolchok JD, et al. Anti-programmed-death-receptor-1 treatment with pembrolizumab in ipilimumab-refractory advanced melanoma: a randomised dose-comparison cohort of a phase 1 trial. Lancet 2014;384(9948): 1109–17.

57. Robert C, Long GV, Brady B, et al. Nivolumab in previously untreated melanoma without BRAF mutation. N Engl J Med 2015;372(4):320–30.

58. Brown ZJ, Heinrich B, Steinberg SM, et al. Safety in treatment of hepatocellular carcinoma with immune checkpoint inhibitors as compared to melanoma and non-small cell lung cancer. J Immunother Cancer 2017;5(1):93.

59. Reynolds K, Thomas M, Dougan M. Diagnosis and management of hepatitis in patients on checkpoint blockade. Oncologist 2018;23(9):991–7.

60. De Martin E, Michot JM, Papouin B, et al. Characterization of liver injury induced by cancer immunotherapy using immune checkpoint inhibitors. J Hepatol 2018; 68(6):1181–90.

61. Haanen J, Carbonnel F, Robert C, et al. Management of toxicities from immunotherapy: ESMO Clinical Practice Guidelines for diagnosis, treatment and follow-up. Ann Oncol 2017;28(suppl_4):iv119–42.

62. Brahmer JR, Lacchetti C, Schneider BJ, et al. Management of immune-related adverse events in patients treated with immune checkpoint inhibitor therapy: American Society of Clinical Oncology Clinical Practice Guideline. J Clin Oncol 2018;36(17):1714–68.

63. Reddy HG, Schneider BJ, Tai AW. Immune checkpoint inhibitor-associated colitis and hepatitis. Clin Transl Gastroenterol 2018;9(9):180.

Multidisciplinary Team Management of Hepatocellular Carcinoma Is Standard of Care

Dekey Lhewa, MD[a], Ellen W. Green, MD, PhD[b],
Willscott E. Naugler, MD[a],*

KEYWORDS

- Multidisciplinary team • Hepatocellular carcinoma (HCC) • Bioinformatics

KEY POINTS

- Burden of HCC management is rising.
- HCC is unique amongst cancers in that it usually arises in a diseased liver, which competes with HCC to drive mortality.
- Multidisciplinary team (MDT) management of HCC should be considered standard of care.
- Liver cancer MDT has challenges regarding documentation and research, which may be facilitated with real-time bioinformatics tools.

Multidisciplinary teams (MDT) for the management of cancers probably had their origins in the tumor boards created in the 1970s, although the primary function of boards at that time was educational.[1] A shift in this paradigm arose in part due to the realization that wide variations in cancer outcomes existed in different countries. For example, a 1995 UK report showed lower survival for colorectal cancer compared with other European countries.[2] This realization led to development of national guidelines to standardize care based on available evidence, often with recommendations for cancer management through an MDT, although the recommendations vary by cancer type. Significant hope has been pinned on technological advances using artificial

All authors contributed substantially to the conception, analysis, writing, and critical revision of this article.

This article was not supported financially or otherwise by any commercial interests, and no author has any financial conflicts of interest concerning material in this work.

[a] Department of Medicine, Division of GI & Hepatology, Oregon Health & Science University, 3181 Southwest Sam Jackson Park Road, MC L461, Portland, OR 97212, USA; [b] Department of Medicine, Internal Medicine Residency, Oregon Health & Science University, 3181 Southwest Sam Jackson Park Road, Portland, OR 97212, USA

* Corresponding author.

E-mail address: nauglers@ohsu.edu

intelligence (AI) to understand the relevant aspects of patients with cancer and deliver evidence-based treatment recommendations. The most notable such example is IBM's Watson for Oncology, a computing system using AI algorithms to generate treatment recommendations, but which has run into multiple challenges since its inception in 2012. Although such technology may one day significantly minimize the necessity for MDTs (and their work), it seems clear that this day is not in the near future. For hepatocellular carcinoma (HCC), that day may be even more removed given the added level of complexity in its management, a notion affirmed in IBM's choice of cancers for which Watson for Oncology works (lung, breast, colorectal, along with 8 others not including HCC).

HCC is the fifth leading cause of cancer-related death in the United States, but although the top 4 cancers have realized long-term declines in mortality, the annual death rate for HCC has been increasing.[3] The vast majority (~90% in Western countries)[4] of HCC arises in livers with underlying cirrhosis (or significant fibrosis), making it relatively unique among malignancies: a deadly cancer that occurs coincident with a second comorbidity that is often fatal in its own right. This combination of liver cancer and liver dysfunction has led to difficulties in accurately staging HCC. Traditional cancer staging systems take into account primary tumor size, lymph node involvement, and degrees of malignant spread. These systems work well when the cancer is the driver of mortality. In the case of HCC, however, cirrhosis competes with the tumor to drive mortality, thus making staging systems solely focused on the cancer characteristics perform poorly.[5] Several different staging systems from around the world do take into account the degree of liver dysfunction, and the one favored by most Western countries including the United States is the Barcelona Clinic Liver Cancer (BCLC)[6] system. In the United States, the National Cancer Institute sponsors the "Physician Data Query" (PDQ), a frequently updated evidence-based resource that offers guidance for treatment of HCC based on current literature and relying on the BCLC staging system.[7] The American Association for the Study of Liver Diseases (AASLD) also bases treatment recommendations on BCLC staging.[8] However, the US National Comprehensive Cancer Network (NCCN) guidelines do not use a particular staging system in outlining treatment recommendations for HCC, instead focusing on operability.[9]

MULTIDISCIPLINARY TEAM FOR HEPATOCELLULAR CARCINOMA MANAGEMENT

The troublesome reality for HCC is that matching patients at various stages with increasing numbers of treatment modalities has become so complex that no trial or set of trials is able to inform a robust evidence-based treatment algorithm. How then to make clinical decisions for patients in the absence of clear guiding evidence? In asking ourselves (and our patients) what the best treatment might be, it seems clear that all available, potentially beneficial treatment modalities should be considered. And given the complex interactions between treatment decisions, it follows that input from providers of all treatment modalities should be brought to bear where the available evidence does not provide straightforward answers. The logical conclusion from the preceding is that (in the case of HCC) multiple providers from different disciplines must interact on many or most treatment decisions, and the vehicle for accomplishing this has become the liver cancer MDT. Although this logic is sound and nearly all of US centers providing comprehensive liver cancer care us a liver cancer MDT (thus making it standard of care), none of the aforementioned evidence-based treatment guidelines include use of an MDT in their treatment algorithms. In the 2010 version of AASLD's practice guidelines for the management of

HCC, the investigators do recommend that all patients with HCC should be managed with MDTs,[10] but in the 2018 update the MDT recommendation is absent.[8] Why is this? The likely answer is that no clear published data show that use of liver cancer MDTs reliably improves patient outcomes. In the absence of evidence, it is impossible for evidence-based guidelines to recommend MDT use, despite its widespread adoption in clinical practice. It thus behooves us to ask if liver cancer MDTs help patients and providers, and if so how? First we can define the liver cancer MDT, then examine why we should be using it.

DEFINING THE LIVER CANCER MULTIDISCIPLINARY TEAM

The simplest definition of an MDT suggests at least 2 health care providers working collaboratively with patients to achieve coordinated care. Such a basic definition needs expansion for the liver cancer MDT, especially given need to measure defined outcomes and advocate for institutional policy changes that support the team. A good definition was suggested in 2015,[11] and included the following elements:

1. Representation on the MDT by at least 1 provider from each specialty involved in HCC care at the institution
2. Regular face-to-face (or virtual) meetings, weekly to monthly depending on volume
3. Use of an institutional algorithm, for example, based on one of the national guidelines, for treatment of HCC, taking advantage of local expertise
4. If all available treatment modalities are not offered at the institution, like liver transplant, some connection to an institution that does proved all available treatments

WHY USE A LIVER CANCER MULTIDISCIPLINARY TEAM TO MANAGE PATIENTS WITH HEPATOCELLULAR CARCINOMA?

Clinical Case 1: 60-year-old man presents with compensated cirrhosis (no ascites, no encephalopathy) but clear signs of portal hypertension (nonbleeding esophageal varices and thrombocytopenia) and a 1.5-cm liver lesion radiographically diagnostic for HCC.

A simple question might occur when examining the preceding case: what medical provider would be best suited to give the best, most evidence-based treatment recommendation for the patient? Using the BCLC-based AASLD practice guidelines, the suggested treatment is surgical resection if possible, and thus if there were one provider for the patient to see, a hepatobiliary surgeon would make sense. Unfortunately, many patients similar to that described in Case 1 are not surgical candidates because of tumor location, degree of portal hypertension, or comorbid medical conditions. If primary resection cannot be offered, then what is the next best treatment? Now the options broaden, and here data exist that would support use of local ablation (eg, with radiofrequency ablation (RFA), external beam radiation), chemo-embolization (with either drug-eluting beads or Ethiodol-based treatment), radioembolization (Yttrium-90), various systemic chemotherapies, or liver transplantation. The patient could be sequentially sent to each of the providers responsible for the noted treatments, but at the end who would make the decision? The easy answer is that the patient would make the decision, but in reality the possibilities are so complex that patients rely on providers for guidance. One may imagine one-to-one phone calls between all the providers, but sequential clinic visits and multiple phone calls become complicated and time-consuming! Wouldn't a face-to-face (or virtual) meeting between providers make more sense? Of course it does, thus the practical evolution of the liver cancer MDT, which as illustrated by this case would significantly decrease the time it would take to have all relevant treatment modalities examined and a consensus recommendation reached. *It is clear that decreasing time to initial recommendation and treatment is a goal in cancer treatment, and liver cancer MDTs support this goal.*[12,13]

Clinical Case 2: 60-year-old man with decompensated cirrhosis (refractory ascites, Model for End-Stage Liver Disease score = 15) listed for liver transplant is discovered on routine screening to have a 1.5-cm liver lesion radiographically diagnostic for HCC.

Although primary resection is clearly off the table for this patient, many other treatment modalities are available for Case 2. Guidelines suggest[8] that this patient should not receive treatment until the HCC grows to a point (2 cm) in which prioritization on the transplant list is possible. Such waiting to treat exposes the patient to a small risk that the cancer will grow out of control, even precluding transplant or other therapies. Such a decision to abstain from immediately treating newly found cancer cannot be taken lightly, and needs to involve the patient as well as the treating providers. Criteria for liver transplantation for HCC are complex and evolving, and addressed elsewhere in this issue. Transplantation is available for patients beyond Milan criteria but within so-called "down-staging" criteria,[14] and it is imperative that a provider expert in these principles be part of the management discussion. *A consensus recommendation from a liver cancer MDT (1) gives the patient confidence that the team of providers has examined all the possibilities and (2) provides medicolegal protection to involved providers in rare cases where the HCC progresses significantly during the observation ("not treating") period.*

Clinical Case 3: 60-year-old woman with compensated cirrhosis and clinically significant portal hypertension presents with a 6-cm infiltrative liver lesion that on biopsy revealed poorly differentiated HCC along with an alfa-fetoprotein = 900.

Here, the 2 treatment modalities that could be considered based on available evidence are radioembolization or systemic therapy. The patient is not within transplantable criteria, so this is not a consideration—or is it? Recent policy changes in the allocation of livers for transplantation now allow for so-called "down-staging" into Milan (transplantable) criteria, and this patient fits within down-staging criteria. Thus, to give this patient the best chance of cure, liver transplantation must be considered, even though it cannot be the initial treatment. This determination will likely influence the choice between the preceding 2 therapies, but given the complex and evolving transplant policies neither the interventional radiologist or medical oncologist alone are best suited to guide treatment to a point in which transplantation might be possible. *Solving this complex problem is clearly facilitated by all parties involved making a consensus "roadmap" treatment plan considering parallel or sequential treatments by multiple disciplines, a job well-addressed by the liver cancer MDT. In addition, the liver cancer MDT serves as an educational forum where expert providers from different disciplines are able to share the latest evidence in their respective fields with the group.* Only a superhuman could synthesize all new data regarding HCC management from the different disciplines—AI may one day help us in this regard, but until that day the liver cancer MDT best serves this function.

Clinical Case 4: 74-year-old woman with compensated cirrhosis and significant cardiovascular disease is found to have a 3-cm liver lesion radiographically diagnostic for HCC.

Liver transplantation and primary resection may be considered in this patient, but she is likely not a candidate for either. From here, guidelines suggest aggressive locoregional treatment, such as RFA or external beam radiation. But what treatment is the patient likely to receive? One study compared patients getting liver cancer MDT review with those who did not, with the finding that patients managed through a liver cancer MDT were more likely to receive transplantation, resection, or ablation.[15] Case 4 should be considered for these curative treatments, but in absence of liver cancer MDT management could easily receive systemic therapy or chemoembolization if only seen by one provider. One can see how treatment decisions in this case can and do affect patient survival, and of course the liver cancer MDT facilitates management that improves survival, one of the gold standards of cancer care but difficult to study in today's multimodal treatment landscape. Several studies of varying quality have attempted to show a survival benefit linked to liver cancer MDT use. **Table 1** details a comprehensive list of published studies looking at liver cancer MDTs and outcomes.

Clinical Case 5: 54-year-old man with previously compensated hepatitis C virus (HCV) cirrhosis developed multifocal HCC 4 years prior, at which time he was deemed ineligible for liver transplantation because of ongoing polysubstance use and homelessness. Since that time, the patient has been treated with chemoembolization 5 times, RFA twice, and most recently radioembolization. His latest scan shows a 1.5-cm HCC recurrence, but he has also developed refractory ascites. He is now 2 years abstinent from drugs and alcohol, has stable housing, and the HCV infection has been cured.

Where to start? Management of patients with HCC is often an iterative exercise, and detailed information about the treatment course is needed to make new decisions. A comprehensive data collection for such patients as Case 5 is necessary at each possible decision point. Gathering of data is time-consuming (and fraught with errors of omission), and it would be optimal if each involved provider did not have to gather the data again when management decisions must be addressed. *Liver cancer MDTs provide a practical forum for patient data to be gathered and retained for purposes of continuity of care so that individual providers do not have to repeat this work.* Similarly, providers in the liver cancer MDT may update the group on relevant details missed in the data collection so that one provider does not miss a key element observed by another provider. This facet of the liver cancer MDT streamlines the clinical workflow and minimizes overall work of the group.

Clinical Case 6: a 36-year-old woman with fatty liver disease is found to have 4 liver lesions, biopsy of which reveals hepatic adenomas.

Not everything seen in the liver cancer MDT is malignant! There is a significant need for some provider or entity to manage the ubiquitous liver lesion(s) so often turned up incidentally on fishing expeditions. Some may be malignant, and the liver cancer MDT certainly brings the expertise and tools to investigate these lesions and point the patient to appropriate care (if not the liver cancer MDT). Once confirmed, benign lesions (eg, hepatic hemangiomas, biliary hamartomas, focal nodular dysplasias) may be authoritatively noted as such with the recommendation that no further follow-up is necessary, often preventing years of fruitless imaging with attendant worries for the patient. There are a few lesions that are benign but have malignant potential, such as hepatic adenomas, as seen in this case, or biliary cystadenomas, varieties of choledochal cysts, and so on. *The liver cancer MDT best makes comprehensive plans for long-term management of benign lesions with malignant potential, especially because these rare entities have the least evidence-based data on which to rely for guidance.* **Table 2** notes all patients who presented over a 3-year period from November 2016 to December 2019 to the Oregon Health & Science University (OHSU) liver cancer MDT. Sixty-two percent of cases were HCC, but 21% had indeterminate lesions on initial presentation. Many of these later turned out to be malignancies of various kinds, but a significant number were benign, a distinction the liver cancer MDT is uniquely qualified to make.

Table 1
Summary of studies on multidisciplinary care for HCC

Study	Study Design	Key Findings	Limitations
Chang et al,[16] 2008 *Outcome studied:* Survival	• Survival of HCC patients pre- and post-establishment of MDT at SF VAMC • N = 121 • Median follow-up 4.5 mo for pre and 9.5 mo post MDT establishment	• Overall survival improved after MDT (21% survival pre vs 65% post, *P*<.0001) • Earlier stage of HCC in post MDT and greater no. of treatments (pre 37% vs 64% post MDT)	• Single center • Veterans only population
Gaba et al,[15] 2013 *Outcome studied:* Survival	• Retrospective • Impact of imaging surveillance and MDT review • N = 167 patients with HCC • Mean length of follow-up 451 ± 348 d	• 58% HCC patients underwent imaging surveillance and MDT review For MDT vs non-MDT patients: • More ablations/resection (16% vs 3%) and transplant (23% vs 4%), *P*>.006 • Less tumor progression less in MDT (45% vs 68%); *P* = .005	• Retrospective, non-RCT study • Single US center • Lead-time bias with surveillance and early diagnosis
Gashin et al,[17] 2014 *Outcome studied:* Survival	• Retrospective study • Impact of nonadherence to MDT recommendations on clinical outcomes • N = 137 patients, 419 MDT discussions • Mean follow-up 16.7 mo	• After first MDT, 62.0% received recommended treatment • Patients who received at least 1 treatment after their first MDT were more likely to be alive at 1 y than those w/o treatment (58.7% vs 39.5%; *P* = .043)	• Retrospective study • Single center • Self-selection bias in those who follow MDT recommendations
Ramanathan et al,[18] 2014 *Outcome studied:* Survival	• Prospective study • ITT study of transplantation vs palliative multimodality treatment vs no treatment • N = 715	• 1 and 5 y survival: • Post LT, 97.1% and 72.5% • Palliative multimodal, 73.1% and 46.5% • No treatment arm, 24.5% and 6.4%	• Newer treatments not included in this study due to timing of study • Potential biases from retrospective definition of cohorts

Yopp et al,[13] 2014 *Outcome studied:* Survival	• Survival in patients with HCC diagnosed pre and post MDT • N = 355 • Median follow-up 4.2 mo pre and 7.9 mo post MDT	• Longer median survival in post MDT vs pre MDT (13.2 mo vs 4.8 mo, P = .005) • MDT patients diagnosed at earlier stage • More curative treatments in MDT patients	• Retrospective collection of data before MDT • Most patients lacked insurance that covered LT
Chirikov et al,[19] 2014 *Outcome studied:* Survival	• Association between MDT care and mortality in HCC • Study of SEER Database: 2000–2007 • N = 3588 treated HCC patients • Multispecialist care as surrogate for MDT	• Patients w/ ≥3 specialist types were associated with 10% reduced mortality compared with 1 specialty (P = .04)	• Retrospective • Multispecialist care as surrogate for MDT
Agarwal et al,[20] 2017 *Outcome studied:* Survival	• Comparison of utilization of therapies and outcomes in patients with HCC with or w/o management through MDT • N = 349	• Earlier stage HCC in MDT vs non-MDT (48% vs 26%, P<.0001) • Treatments for HCC greater in MDT vs non-MDT (OR 2.80; 95% CI 1.71–4.59; P<.0001) • MDT: independent predictor of improved survival on multivariate analysis (HR 0.722; 95% CI 0.551–0.946; P = .018)	• Advancement in treatments with MDLT cohort (2007–2011) vs historical control group (2002–2011) • Retrospective data
Charriere et al,[21] 2017 *Outcome studied:* Survival	• Prospective data but retrospective cohort • MDT patients from 2006 to 2013 with proven untreated HCC with plan of curative treatment made in MDT • N = 387 • Median follow-up 27.5 mo	• Compliance with MDT recommendations associated with longer OS (HR 0.39; 95% CI 0.27–0.54; P<.0001)	• Retrospective cohort

(continued on next page)

Table 1
(continued)

Study	Study Design	Key Findings	Limitations
Serper et al,[22] 2017 *Outcome studied:* Survival	• Observational cohort study • Review of VA clinical data repository • N = 3988	• Care by >1 specialist was significantly associated with greater likelihood of receiving treatment (OR 1.60) • MDT associated with longer OS (HR 0.83; 95% CI 0.77–0.9)	• Observational study so probability of unmeasured confounders • Only veteran population
Kaplan et al,[23] 2018 *Outcome studied:* Survival, cost	• Cost of HCC in integrated health system • Review of HCC patients cost data in the Veterans Outcome and Cost Associated with Liver disease cohort from 2008 through 2010 • N = 3188 HCC and 12,722 controls	• Mean 3-y total cost of care in HCC patient = $154,688 vs $69,010 for controls • In LT patients 3 y incremental cost of $422,007 vs $396,735 in non-LT patients with HCC	• Observational cohort study • Veteran only population and health care system
Mokdad et al,[24] 2018 *Outcome studied:* Treatment recommendations, survival	• Treatment and survival in patients with HCC in low vs high proportion safety net hospitals (SNH) • Inference high SNH have less specialty services and difficulty accessing off-site specialty care • N = 17,489	• Significantly fewer treatments in high SNHs (32% vs 45%) • Fewer curative treatments for localized HCC in high SNH (OR 0.51) • Significantly lower survival in high SNHs (HR 0.93 vs 1.3)	• Retrospective data from registry: confounders and missing treatment information in 8%
Sinn et al,[25] 2019 *Outcome studied:* Survival	• Retrospective cohort study, prospective HCC registry • New HCC at single center in South Korea, 2005–2013 • Survival in MDT vs non-MDT HCC patients • N = 6619 • Median follow-up = 3.5 y	• 5-y survival were higher in MDT patients vs non-MDT patients (71.2% vs 49.5%, *P*<.001) • On multivariate analysis: MDT independent factor HR 0.47;95% CI, 0.41–0.53; *P*<.001)	• Retrospective study • Single center • Application outside South Korea (HBV predominant etiology of HCC)

Duininck et al,[26] 2019 *Outcome studied:* Survival	• Retrospective review of patients diagnosed with HCC from 2009–2016 at Grady Hospital in Atlanta • Pre and post MDT comparison of treatment and survival • N = 204	• MDT vs non-MDT: Increased referral to surgery (49% vs 30%; *P* = .019), LDT (58% vs 31%; *P* = .001) and XRT (13% vs 3%; *P* = .019) • Improved median OS (30.7 in MDT vs 4.9 mo in non-MDT; *P*<.001)	• Retrospective • Single center • Comparison of different time periods- improved treatments availability in MDT group • Lack of insurance affecting LT eligibility
Wiggans et al,[27] 2013 *Outcome studied:* How MDT aids in accurate HCC diagnosis	• Retrospective study of Peninsula regional HPB unit serving Devon and Cornwall regions in the United Kingdom • Hepatic tumor patients undergoing resection 2006-12 • Assessment of MDT accuracy diagnosis and final histologic path	• Histopathology confirmation of MDT diagnosis in 90.4% of patients (those with HCC: 70%) • N = 438 patients total, HCC patients n = 44	• Retrospective study • Application outside United Kingdom • Small no. of patients with HCC
Oxenberg et al,[28] 2015 *Outcome studied:* How MDT assessment affects best HCC treatment	• Assessment in change of treatment plan pre and post GI MDT discussion • N = 149, liver cancer: 32%	• Change in treatment plan occurred in >1/3rd of patients	• Single center • Small HCC N#

Abbreviations: CI, confidence interval; GI, gastrointestinal; HCC, hepatocellular carcinoma; HPB, Hepatobiliary; HR, hazard ratio; ITT, intention to treat; LDT, Liver Directed Therapy; LT, liver transplantation; MDLT, Multidisciplinary Liver Tumor; MDT, multidisciplinary team; OS, overall survival; RCT, randomized controlled trial; SEER, Surveillance Epidemiology and End Results; SF, San Francisco; VA, Veteran's Administration; VAMC, veterans affairs medical center; w/o, without; XRT, Radiation Therapy.

Table 2
Oregon Health & Science University liver cancer multidisciplinary team 2016 to 2019

Variable	N = 1077 (%)
Gender	
Female	389 (36.1)
Male	688 (63.9)
Age at diagnosis, y	
Median	63
Race	
White	965 (89.6)
Asian	49 (4.5)
Black	9 (0.8)
Ethnicity	
Not Hispanic	951 (88.3)
Hispanic	99 (9.2)
Primary lesion	
Hepatocellular carcinoma (HCC)	657 (61.9)
Cholangiocarcinoma	74 (7.0)
Hepatic adenoma	22 (2.1)
Hepatic hemangiomatosis	18 (1.7)
Focal nodular hyperplasia	22 (2.1)
Gallbladder cancer	6 (0.6)
Indeterminate/unknown lesion	223 (21.1)
No lesion	13 (1.2)
Etiology of liver disease	
Viral hepatitis (HBV, HCV)	508 (48.1)
No underlying liver disease	246 (23.3)
Fatty liver	129 (12.2)
Alcohol	113 (10.7)
Primary sclerosing cholangitis	19 (1.8)
Primary biliary cirrhosis	6 (0.6)

Abbreviations: HBV, hepatitis B virus; HCV, hepatitis C virus.

The preceding cases demonstrate the many reasons why the liver cancer MDT is the standard of care for managing patients with HCC, including arguments other than improving patient survival. An addition to the list is that the liver cancer MDT provides a local forum to enroll patients in various clinical trials available at the institution. The following list summarizes justifications for use of a liver cancer MDT for the management of patients with HCC or indeterminate liver masses.

Clinics Care Points: Justifications for use of the liver cancer MDT in HCC management.

- Decreases time to initial recommendation and treatment
- Maximizes patient confidence with liver cancer MDT consensus recommendations
- Limits medico-legal liability to providers
- Produces "roadmap" treatment plan involving multiple providers

Table 3
Patients with hepatocellular carcinoma treated at Oregon Health & Science University, no liver transplant

Variable	MDT to +365 d
Unique patients	316
Gross revenue per patient	$104,365
Total gross revenue	$32,979,367
Time period assessed: November 2016 to February 2019	

Abbreviation: MDT, multidisciplinary team.

- Educational forum to keep members of different disciplines updated on latest evidence
- Improves patient survival by providing the most evidence-based treatments
- Provides continuity of care between multiple providers executing diverse treatments
- Minimizes redundant collection of data between events necessitating decisions
- Makes comprehensive plans handling benign liver lesions with malignant potential
- Facilitates patient enrollment in clinical trials

CHALLENGES FACING THE LIVER CANCER MULTIDISCIPLINARY TEAM
Support

It takes significant time, effort, and commitment to sustain a liver cancer MDT. Busy providers cannot bill for time attending weekly meetings, and the team needs at least one support staff (usually more) to coordinate care, make agendas, and guide patients through the workflow. These "non-billable" needs must be supported by the institution for the liver cancer MDT to exist. How can such support be defended to hospital administrators looking to cut costs in uncertain times? In addition to educating administrators on benefits (preceding summary list), a look at what the patients bring financially to the institution can be helpful. For example, at OHSU from 2010 to 2012 the gross hospital revenue for 1 year starting at date of presentation at the liver cancer MDT was $89,763 per patient, a number that did not include patients receiving liver transplantation.[11] **Table 3** is an updated look at the same numbers in patients with HCC not receiving transplantation, and **Table 4** shows gross revenue from patients receiving liver transplantation for the primary indication of HCC. In the transplanted patients, the time period assessed was 12 months before transplantation to 6 months after transplantation. These timeframes obviously do not catch all revenue

Table 4
Patients with HCC treated at Oregon Health & Science University who received LT for HCC

Variable	LT −365 d to LT +180 d
Unique patients	59
Gross revenue per patient	$351,838
Total gross revenue	$20,758,471
Time period assessed: January 2016 to December 2018	

Abbreviations: HCC, hepatocellular carcinoma; LT, liver transplantation.

brought in by the patients, nor can the revenue be solely attributed to the liver cancer MDT. However, it makes a strong argument that this revenue depends on an active, cohesive, and well-supported liver cancer MDT.

Documentation

Although "multidisciplinary" seems to be the new buzz word in patient care, the form it takes varies by disease targeted, local resources, and complexity of care. A surprising problem has arisen in medicine as multidisciplinary teams evolve: how to document this care. The standard "SOAP" note is not appropriate, and though there is an intuitive knowledge from MDT members of what is relevant about MDT meetings/discussions, there is no standardized way to document this "outcome" of MDT summaries and recommendations. The result is that the rich MDT discussions and recommendations may be poorly documented in the electronic medical record (EMR) or perhaps not documented at all. This in turn leads to (1) poor communication to providers not present at the MDT, (2) poor communication to referring providers, (3) difficulty for MDT members to remember exactly the rationale behind prior presentation recommendations, (4) an implication that nothing was done based on the adage "if it wasn't documented, it didn't happen," and (5) difficulty in doing retrospective research about MDT efficacy.

Inadequate Provider Resources for a Liver Cancer Multidisciplinary Team

By definition, centers that provide comprehensive care for the patient with HCC must have liver transplantation, and the same goes for a liver cancer MDT. Unfortunately, there are simply too many patients with HCC for liver transplant centers and their liver cancer MDTs to manage. How can centers without liver transplant but with most/all of other required disciplines treat patients with HCC in a way that offers all options? And how can providers working in more rural areas provide HCC care with few/no other team members? Such are the real problems facing us, and they are problems that are only going to worsen given several converging factors (**Fig. 1**). Transplant and other large centers clearly need help in caring for so many patients, so what are ways we can give every patient all treatment options, yet allow for significant care to arise from centers or providers who do not have comprehensive treatment capabilities? The most organic solutions involve outreach clinics of larger institutions and collaborative virtual liver cancer MDTs. Also, there can be agreements of providers/smaller institutions with transplant centers that, for example, suggest all patients diagnosed with HCC go first to the transplant center for a liver cancer MDT discussion and

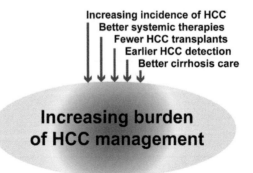

Fig. 1. Factors contributing to the increasing burden of HCC management.

development of a "roadmap" plan, pieces of which may be performed locally depending on available expertise. Finally, we are in the early stages of developing powerful bioinformatics tools that may aid in the decision-making process for management of complex diseases like HCC. At first, such tools will likely be used where expert liver cancer MDTs are not available, and could significantly change care for patients with more limited health care access.

RESEARCH

Although we have many studies comparing one treatment versus another, we do not have good studies to help us with how HCC is actually managed in the real world. Real world HCC management often involves sequential treatments with multiple modalities. Just retrospectively studying this kind of management is a tangle of confusion, even for single-center studies. Factor into this the fact that institutional algorithms radically differ in their approach to HCC treatment and we are left with a situation in which the kinds of randomized controlled studies we would like to do are simply not possible. Take for example, the patient with compensated cirrhosis with a 1.5-cm HCC. Some centers would primarily use transarterial chemoembolization (TACE) followed by ablation, others ablation alone, others radioembolization, and still others would preferentially await tumor growth in hopes of liver transplantation. A prospective study to answer this question is unlikely, so how can we study such a question? One solution is to study questions such as these through the liver cancer MDT. This has of course occurred to many a clinician researcher, but the hurdles are high. *First*, although there is a lot of HCC and the burden is growing, given the many treatment pathways available there are often very few patients going down a specific pathway at any one institution. *Second*, given such small numbers of patients going down a particular pathway one would like to have multicenter data to improve power and decrease biases inherent to single-institution treatment preferences. *Third*, there is so much work often without good institutional support that just maintaining a database is a herculean effort for the team. Having outlined the difficulties for research in the liver cancer MDT, it is also clear that this is where we need to be focusing research energy to better serve the increasing numbers of patients with HCC.

One solution to the preceding problems of documentation and research is the development of a bioinformatics tool that streamlines the clinical work of the liver cancer MDT, makes agendas and reports for MDT meetings, and compiles all data into a base for later clinical outcomes research. Several commercial and academic groups around the world are working on such tools. We developed such a Web-based tool at OHSU called "MD Capture—Liver" (MD = multidisciplinary), and have been using it clinically since November 2016 in the liver cancer MDT. Patient demographic and laboratory information is entered before MDT conferences, and the tool is used in real time to record what the group observes on latest scans, then documents summaries and recommendations along with automated liver function and cancer staging. The tool then produces a summary document that is put into the EMR and sent to the referring provider. When a new decision needs to be made concerning care, updated laboratory tests and scans are put into the tool; all prior data, rationales, and recommendations are immediately available for the group to see. We have found that the tool markedly streamlines the complex clinical workflow, and the reports have been very useful for both patient and provider communication. Because data collected by the Web-based tool are entered for clinical purposes, extra time and energy for data capture are minimized. We can easily pull out demographic, cancer stage, treatment recommendations for our own quality control or institutional research (**Table 5**). In

Table 5
Demographics and treatment recommendations for patients with HCC managed through the Oregon Health & Science University liver cancer MDT

Variable	n (%)
Gender	
Female	185 (27)
Male	500 (73)
Age at diagnosis, y	
Median	64
Race	
White	618 (90.2)
Asian	28 (4.1)
Black	6 (0.9)
Diagnosis method	
Determined radiographically	584 (85.3)
Determined by biopsy	101 (14.7)
Model for End-Stage Liver Disease	
Average	10
Median	9
Characteristics	
Cirrhosis	628 (91.7)
Ascites present	211 (30.8)
Encephalopathy present	125 (18.2)
Portal vein invasion	105 (15.3)
Extrahepatic disease	43 (6.3)
Barcelona Clinic Liver Cancer stage	
0	19 (10.1)
A	291 (42.5)
B	153 (22.3)
C	126 (18.4)
D	27 (3.9)
First treatment recommendation for new HCC	
Chemoembolization (TACE)	173 (25.3)
Radioembolization (Y90)	146 (21.3)
Systemic therapy (usually palliative)	115 (16.8)
RFA or MWA[a]	102 (14.9)
Palliative referral	44 (6.4)
External beam radiation	37 (5.4)
Surgical resection	21 (3.1)
Transplant referral[b]	92 (13.4)

Time period: Nov 2016 through Dec 2019.
Abbreviations: HCC, hepatocellular carcinoma; MDT, multidisciplinary team; MWA, microwave ablation; RFA, radiofrequency ablation; TACE, transarterial chemoembolization.
[a] Usually preceded by TACE, but both treatments recommended simultaneously.
[b] Usually in conjunction with other locoregional therapy.

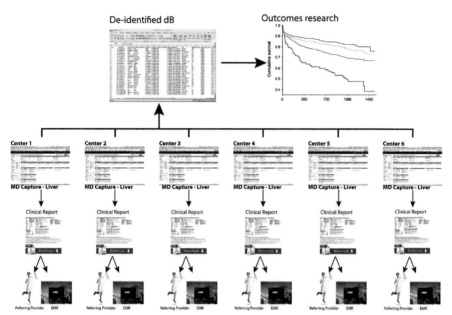

Fig. 2. Use of bioinformatics tool (MD Capture—Liver) for MDT documentation and multi-center outcomes research. MD Capture—Liver is a Web-based bioinformatics tool that records relevant patient data in the MDT conference as well as cancer staging, summaries, and recommendations of the group. The data are stored on a secure server at the local institution, and periodically the data are de-identified and sent to a central server from which research questions may be queried. The tool also automatically generates a documentation report for the EMR and referring providers.

addition, we are sending the tool to other institutions who will benefit from improving workflow and documentation, all while building a database of HCC patient management for use in outcomes research. Protected Health Information is stored on local secure servers, and de-identified data are automatically uploaded to a central secure server. Multicenter data can then be accessed by participating centers to answer research questions regarding patients that have come through the liver cancer MDT (**Fig. 2**).

Over time, tools like MD Capture—Liver will accrue thousands of patients, allowing real-time queries that will help us understand outcomes for various treatment pathways for a given patient. Such real-time use of big data will assist clinicians with decision making where no clear evidence otherwise exists, as is often the case for patients with HCC.

SUMMARY

MDTs in general are becoming more common in medical practice. The need for MDTs varies depending on disease complexity, and nowhere is an MDT more useful than in the management of HCC. Although robust data supporting the use of liver cancer MDTs is weak for management of patients with HCC, nearly all centers that provide comprehensive HCC care use a liver cancer MDT, and we argue here that its use should be considered standard of care for patients with HCC. Several challenges face the evolving liver cancer MDT, including frequent lack of institutional support, shortages of expert personnel, and difficulties documenting outcomes toward conducting clinical research on patients managed through the MDT. Some of these challenges can be met with use of bioinformatics tools now being built or tested and will certainly be in widespread use in the near future.

REFERENCES

1. Berman HL. The tumor board: is it worth saving? Mil Med 1975;140(8):529–31.
2. The Expert Advisory Group on Cancer to the Chief Medical Officers of England and Wales. A policy framework for commissioning cancer services (The Calman-Hine Report). Wales: Department of Health; 1995.
3. Siegel RL, Miller KD, Jemal A. Cancer statistics, 2020. CA Cancer J Clin 2020; 70(1):7–30.
4. Fattovich G, Stroffolini T, Zagni I, et al. Hepatocellular carcinoma in cirrhosis: incidence and risk factors. Gastroenterology 2004;127(5 Suppl 1):S35–50.
5. Liu PH, Hsu CY, Hsia CY, et al. Prognosis of hepatocellular carcinoma: assessment of eleven staging systems. J Hepatol 2016;64(3):601–8.
6. Llovet JM, Bru C, Bruix J. Prognosis of hepatocellular carcinoma: the BCLC staging classification. Semin Liver Dis 1999;19(3):329–38.
7. PDQ Adult primary liver cancer treatment. Available at: https://www.cancer.gov/types/liver/hp/adult-liver-treatment-pdq. Accessed March 30, 2020.
8. Heimbach JK, Kulik LM, Finn RS, et al. AASLD guidelines for the treatment of hepatocellular carcinoma. Hepatology 2018;67(1):358–80.
9. NCCN clinical practice guidelines in oncology: hepatobiliary cancers. 2020. Available at: http://www.nccn.org/professionals/physician_gls/pdf/hepatobiliary.pdf. Accessed March 30, 2020.
10. Bruix J, Sherman M. Management of hepatocellular carcinoma: an update. Hepatology 2011;53(3):1020–2.
11. Naugler WE, Alsina AE, Frenette CT, et al. Building the multidisciplinary team for management of patients with hepatocellular carcinoma. Clin Gastroenterol Hepatol 2015;13(5):827–35.
12. Gardner TB, Barth RJ, Zaki BI, et al. Effect of initiating a multidisciplinary care clinic on access and time to treatment in patients with pancreatic adenocarcinoma. J Oncol Pract 2010;6(6):288–92.
13. Yopp AC, Mansour JC, Beg MS, et al. Establishment of a multidisciplinary hepatocellular carcinoma clinic is associated with improved clinical outcome. Ann Surg Oncol 2014;21(4):1287–95.
14. OPTN/UNOS. US liver allocation policy. Available at: https://optn.transplant.hrsa.gov/media/1200/optn_policies.pdf. Accessed April 12, 2020.
15. Gaba RC, Kallwitz ER, Parvinian A, et al. Imaging surveillance and multidisciplinary review improves curative therapy access and survival in HCC patients. Ann Hepatol 2013;12(5):766–73.
16. Chang TT, Sawhney R, Monto A, et al. Implementation of a multidisciplinary treatment team for hepatocellular cancer at a Veterans Affairs Medical Center improves survival. HPB (Oxford) 2008;10(6):405–11.
17. Gashin L, Tapper E, Babalola A, et al. Determinants and outcomes of adherence to recommendations from a multidisciplinary tumour conference for hepatocellular carcinoma. HPB (Oxford) 2014;16(11):1009–15.
18. Ramanathan R, Sharma A, Lee DD, et al. Multimodality therapy and liver transplantation for hepatocellular carcinoma: a 14-year prospective analysis of outcomes. Transplantation 2014;98(1):100–6.

19. Chirikov VV, Mullins CD, Hanna N, et al. Multispecialist care and mortality in hepatocellular carcinoma. Am J Clin Oncol 2013;38(6):557–63.
20. Agarwal PD, Phillips P, Hillman L, et al. Multidisciplinary management of hepatocellular carcinoma improves access to therapy and patient survival. J Clin Gastroenterol 2017;51(9):845–9.
21. Charriere B, Muscari F, Maulat C, et al. Outcomes of patients with hepatocellular carcinoma are determined in multidisciplinary team meetings. J Surg Oncol 2017;115(3):330–6.
22. Serper M, Taddei TH, Mehta R, et al. Association of provider specialty and multidisciplinary care with hepatocellular carcinoma treatment and mortality. Gastroenterology 2017;152(8):1954–64.
23. Kaplan DE, Chapko MK, Mehta R, et al. Healthcare costs related to treatment of hepatocellular carcinoma among veterans with cirrhosis in the United States. Clin Gastroenterol Hepatol 2018;16(1):106–14.e5.
24. Mokdad AA, Murphy CC, Pruitt SL, et al. Effect of hospital safety net designation on treatment use and survival in hepatocellular carcinoma. Cancer 2018;124(4): 743–51.
25. Sinn DH, Choi GS, Park HC, et al. Multidisciplinary approach is associated with improved survival of hepatocellular carcinoma patients. PLoS One 2019;14(1): e0210730.
26. Duininck G, Lopez-Aguiar AG, Lee RM, et al. Optimizing cancer care for hepatocellular carcinoma at a safety-net hospital: the value of a multidisciplinary disease management team. J Surg Oncol 2019;120(8):1365–70.
27. Wiggans MG, Jackson SA, Fox BM, et al. The preoperative assessment of hepatic tumours: evaluation of UK regional multidisciplinary team performance. HPB Surg 2013;2013:861681.
28. Oxenberg J, Papenfuss W, Esemuede I, et al. Multidisciplinary cancer conferences for gastrointestinal malignancies result in measureable treatment changes: a prospective study of 149 consecutive patients. Ann Surg Oncol 2015;22(5): 1533–9.

1. Publication Title	2. Publication Number	3. Filing Date
CLINICS IN LIVER DISEASE	016 – 754	9/18/2020

4. Issue Frequency	5. Number of Issues Published Annually	6. Annual Subscription Price
FEB, MAY, AUG, NOV	4	$313.00

7. Complete Mailing Address of Known Office of Publication (Not printer) (Street, city, county, state, and ZIP+4®)

ELSEVIER INC.
230 Park Avenue, Suite 800
New York, NY 10169

Contact Person
Malathi Samayan

Telephone (Include area code)
91-44-4299-4507

8. Complete Mailing Address of Headquarters or General Business Office of Publisher (Not printer)

ELSEVIER INC.
230 Park Avenue, Suite 800
New York, NY 10169

9. Full Names and Complete Mailing Addresses of Publisher, Editor, and Managing Editor (Do not leave blank)

Publisher (Name and complete mailing address)

DOLORES MELONI, ELSEVIER INC.
1600 JOHN F KENNEDY BLVD. SUITE 1800
PHILADELPHIA, PA 19103-2899

Editor (Name and complete mailing address)

KERRY HOLLAND, ELSEVIER INC.
1600 JOHN F KENNEDY BLVD. SUITE 1800
PHILADELPHIA, PA 19103-2899

Managing Editor (Name and complete mailing address)

PATRICK MANLEY, ELSEVIER INC.
1600 JOHN F KENNEDY BLVD. SUITE 1800
PHILADELPHIA, PA 19103-2899

10. Owner (Do not leave blank. If the publication is owned by a corporation, give the name and address of the corporation immediately followed by the names and addresses of all stockholders owning or holding 1 percent or more of the total amount of stock. If not owned by a corporation, give the names and addresses of the individual owners. If owned by a partnership or other unincorporated firm, give its name and address as well as those of each individual owner. If the publication is published by a nonprofit organization, give its name and address.)

Full Name	Complete Mailing Address
WHOLLY OWNED SUBSIDIARY OF REED/ELSEVIER, US HOLDINGS	1600 JOHN F KENNEDY BLVD. SUITE 1800 PHILADELPHIA, PA 19103-2899

11. Known Bondholders, Mortgagees, and Other Security Holders Owning or Holding 1 Percent or More of Total Amount of Bonds, Mortgages, or Other Securities. If none, check box ▶ ☐ None

Full Name	Complete Mailing Address
N/A	

12. Tax Status (For completion by nonprofit organizations authorized to mail at nonprofit rates) (Check one)
The purpose, function, and nonprofit status of this organization and the exempt status for federal income tax purposes:
☒ Has Not Changed During Preceding 12 Months
☐ Has Changed During Preceding 12 Months (Publisher must submit explanation of change with this statement)

PS Form **3526**, July 2014 [Page 1 of 4 (see instructions page 4)] PSN: 7530-01-000-9931 PRIVACY NOTICE: See our privacy policy on www.usps.com.

---

13. Publication Title	14. Issue Date for Circulation Data Below
CLINICS IN LIVER DISEASE	MAY 2020

15. Extent and Nature of Circulation		Average No. Copies Each Issue During Preceding 12 Months	No. Copies of Single Issue Published Nearest to Filing Date
a. Total Number of Copies (Net press run)		108	101
b. Paid Circulation (By Mail and Outside the Mail)	(1) Mailed Outside-County Paid Subscriptions Stated on PS Form 3541 (Include paid distribution above nominal rate, advertiser's proof copies, and exchange copies)	41	37
	(2) Mailed In-County Paid Subscriptions Stated on PS Form 3541 (Include paid distribution above nominal rate, advertiser's proof copies, and exchange copies)	0	0
	(3) Paid Distribution Outside the Mails Including Sales Through Dealers and Carriers, Street Vendors, Counter Sales, and Other Paid Distribution Outside USPS®	37	35
	(4) Paid Distribution by Other Classes of Mail Through the USPS (e.g. First-Class Mail®)	0	0
c. Total Paid Distribution [Sum of 15b (1), (2), (3), and (4)]	▶	78	72
d. Free or Nominal Rate Distribution (By Mail and Outside the Mail)	(1) Free or Nominal Rate Outside-County Copies included on PS Form 3541	15	14
	(2) Free or Nominal Rate In-County Copies Included on PS Form 3541	0	0
	(3) Free or Nominal Rate Copies Mailed at Other Classes Through the USPS (e.g. First-Class Mail)	0	0
	(4) Free or Nominal Rate Distribution Outside the Mail (Carriers or other means)	0	0
e. Total Free or Nominal Rate Distribution (Sum of 15d (1), (2), (3) and (4))	▶	15	14
f. Total Distribution (Sum of 15c and 15e)	▶	93	86
g. Copies not Distributed (See Instructions to Publishers #4 (page 83))	▶	15	15
h. Total (Sum of 15f and g)	▶	108	101
i. Percent Paid (15c divided by 15f times 100)	▶	83.87%	83.72%

* If you are claiming electronic copies, go to line 16 on page 3. If you are not claiming electronic copies, skip to line 17 on page 3.

16. Electronic Copy Circulation		Average No. Copies Each Issue During Preceding 12 Months	No. Copies of Single Issue Published Nearest to Filing Date
a. Paid Electronic Copies	▶		
b. Total Paid Print Copies (Line 15c) + Paid Electronic Copies (Line 16a)	▶		
c. Total Print Distribution (Line 15f) + Paid Electronic Copies (Line 16a)	▶		
d. Percent Paid (Both Print & Electronic Copies) (16b divided by 16c × 100)	▶		

☒ I certify that 50% of all my distributed copies (electronic and print) are paid above a nominal price.

17. Publication of Statement of Ownership

☒ If the publication is a general publication, publication of this statement is required. Will be printed in the NOVEMBER 2020 issue of this publication.   ☐ Publication not required.

18. Signature and Title of Editor, Publisher, Business Manager, or Owner

Malathi Samayan - Distribution Controller   *Malathi Samayan*   Date 9/18/2020

I certify that all information furnished on this form is true and complete. I understand that anyone who furnishes false or misleading information on this form or who omits material or information requested on the form may be subject to criminal sanctions (including fines and imprisonment) and/or civil sanctions (including civil penalties).

PS Form **3526**, July 2014 (Page 3 of 4)   PRIVACY NOTICE: See our privacy policy on www.usps.com

Moving?

Make sure your subscription moves with you!

To notify us of your new address, find your **Clinics Account Number** (located on your mailing label above your name), and contact customer service at:

Email: journalscustomerservice-usa@elsevier.com

800-654-2452 (subscribers in the U.S. & Canada)
314-447-8871 (subscribers outside of the U.S. & Canada)

Fax number: 314-447-8029

Elsevier Health Sciences Division
Subscription Customer Service
3251 Riverport Lane
Maryland Heights, MO 63043

*To ensure uninterrupted delivery of your subscription, please notify us at least 4 weeks in advance of move.

Printed and bound by CPI Group (UK) Ltd, Croydon, CR0 4YY

03/10/2024

01040402-0009